**The Future Role of the
State Hospital**

The Future Role of the State Hospital

Edited by

Jack Zusman
Elmer F. Bertsch
Department of Psychiatry
School of Medicine
State University of New York at Buffalo

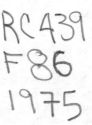

Lexington Books

D.C. Heath and Company
Lexington, Massachusetts
Toronto   London

Grateful acknowledgment is made for permission to use material reprinted herein: from *The Theory and Practice of Psychiatry*, by Fredrick C. Redlich and Daniel X. Freedman, © 1966 by Fredrick C. Redlich and Daniel X. Freedman, Basic Books, Inc. Publishers, New York; from J. Gilboy and J. Schmidt, " 'Voluntary' Hospitalization of the Mentally Ill," reprinted by special permission of the *Northwestern University Law Review*, copyright © 1971 by Northwestern University School of Law, vol. 66, no. 4; from L.Z. Freedman, "Forensic Psychiatry," in A.M. Freedman and H.T. Kaplan, eds., *Comprehensive Textbook of Psychiatry*, © 1967 The Williams & Wilkins Co., Baltimore; from A.L. McGarry and M. Greenblatt, "Conditional Voluntary Mental Hospital Admission," reprinted, by permission, from A.L. McGarry and the *New England Journal of Medicine*, vol. 287 (1972).

Library of Congress Cataloging in Publication Data

Main entry under title:

The Future role of the state hospital.

    Includes papers presented at a conference organized by the Division of Community Psychiatry of the State University of New York at Buffalo and held in November 1973.
    Includes index.

    1. Psychiatric hospitals—Congresses. I. Zusman, Jack, 1934-   ed. II. Bertsch, Elmer F., ed. [DNLM: 1. Community mental health services— United States. 2. Hospitals, Psychiatric—United States. WM27 AA1 Z9f]
RC439.F85   362.2'1   74-16940
ISBN 0-669-95612-0

Published simultaneously in Canada

Printed in the United States of America

International Standard Book Number: 0-669-95612-0

Library of Congress Catalog Card Number: 74-16940

Contents

List of Figures

List of Tables

Foreword

The state mental hospital is not dead, nor is it necessarily dying—but it most certainly is headed for a radical change. In many states throughout the country the decision has already been made to transform the mental hospital system substantially; in many other states the decision is about to be made. And these decisions have been made, or are being made, because over the past decades two experiences occurred that literally compelled a shift in orientation of the state mental hospital system as we have traditionally known it.

First was the increasing widespread use of psychotropic drugs that facilitated the treatment and rehabilitation of the mental patient, and thereby sharply diminished the need for institutional care.

Second—and really the most compelling—was the flowering of *first* the concept and *then* the realization of treatment in the community setting, a happening that was crystallized by the community mental health center's program.

By 1966 or 1967 when the center's program was fully underway—underway in the sense that a number of facilities were then operating and delivering services pursuant to the comprehensive model—it was rapidly becoming clear that the community setting had dramatic advantages over the state mental hospital for the treatment of the mentally ill, advantages in terms of dollar savings to both the patient and to the state, as well as savings in terms of human suffering—separations from family, job, and friends. With the comprehensive community program the patient can get treatment sooner and complete the therapy sooner so that his "time out of circulation"—if there is any—is drastically reduced.

With these experiences—the psychotropic drugs and community mental health centers—the public state mental hospital experienced a dramatic decline in the number of resident patients from 540,604 in 1963 to 275,995 in 1972; and the population continues to decline.

Where, then, goes the state mental health facility—the sometimes old, rural facility that too often has been used to warehouse the mentally ill?

Several states, we know, have made the decision to get out of the business of operating state hospitals. In some cases, the ownership has simply been transferred to another level of government, usually the county, but in most cases the change has been a sincere one designed to alter the mode of treatment—to really capitalize on the advantages of the community model.

The text of Dr. Roy's remarks, first presented at the 1973 conference, "The Future Role of the State Hospital," at the State University of Buffalo, was entered into the *Congressional Record* of October 18, 1973.

The most typical reassignment scheme for a state mental hospital is for it to take on the role of a community service facility, most likely with broader responsibilities than it formerly had. In such cases, as the facility takes on a new role, it also takes on a new image. The walls and fences come down; the spacious campuses are opened up to general public use; and the inhibitions of the community towards use of the facility tend to drop.

This is essentially the change that is taking place at St. Elizabeth's Hospital in Washington, D.C. One unit was turned into a community mental health center to serve one of the city's four catchment areas. Other parts of the hospital have changed their style of service or orientation—and the public has begun to think of St. Elizabeth's as a resource for them, rather than as just a huge but isolated facility that divided the community.

In Wisconsin another technique was used for its two state mental hospitals—they were turned into specialized treatment and research facilities. Each of the hospitals has several such specialized facilities, and the purpose is to develop new insights, new skills, new techniques in the treatment of particular mental illness problems, as well as to treat those who are residents of the facilities and therefore part of the research effort. Such a scheme is patterned after the National Institutes of Health, which, although consisting primarily of research facilities, treat people with specialized problems as part of their research.

In some instances, conversion to community treatment may not be so simple. Where there is no viable use for the state mental hospital for the treatment of the mentally ill, and the facility is still a good one, then it should be turned over to other pursuits that are in the public interest—schools, general health care facilities, recreational units, and the like. And some state mental hospitals, indeed, will simply need to be abandoned, such as old facilities that are sufficiently dilapidated that they will require near-total rebuilding to be useful. Perhaps these buildings should be torn down and the land used for a totally different purpose.

There are, of course, many problems connected with the transfer of a state mental hospital to new functions. Where these facilities are the main—perhaps the only significant—employer in a community, the community understandably views such a shift as a serious threat to its economic well-being.

But there is no need for serious concern here. The employees of a state mental hospital can be retrained to provide similar types of services within the community-oriented program, or even retrained to serve in the new program to be operated out of the facility.

In those instances where the residents of the facilities continue to need residential care and the hospital is abandoning that role, often the solution has been to find an alternative residential facility, but one that is—it often turns out—more appropriate. The elderly constitute a large segment of this population, and often the change to smaller residential facilities that are more a part of the community and particularly adapted to the needs of the elderly has proven beneficial.

So I foresee no problem in continuing the transition away from the traditional mental hospital. It is happening; it will continue to happen. The real question is how swift the transition will be. One of the important questions remaining relative to this transition is what the appropriate role is for federal government.

Although the federally sponsored community mental health center's program has played a key role in developing the community programs and demonstrating their viability—and thus creating the countervailing force to the state hospital system—much of the impetus for redesigning the use of state hospitals, or for closing them down, has come from leaders within the states themselves.

This leadership has come mainly from two directions: those responsible for the fiscal stability of the state—the money managers who see the savings in terms of dollars primarily, and only secondarily in terms of benefits to human beings; and those responsible for the delivery of an effective mental health service program, who do see the savings primarily in terms of improved well-being for those receiving care.

The momentum is there. The thrust is there at the state level, but what the Congress and the administration does in Washington will also have a significant impact on the rapidity with which the transition is made. For example, one of the proposals for national health insurance—S 11, the Kennedy-Griffiths bill—has in it a provision relating to coverage of treatment for mental illness that says, in effect, that there should be unlimited coverage for services provided within the setting of a community mental health center, but that the coverage should be restricted for those services provided in a hospital setting. Obviously, enactment of such a provision tomorrow would intensely accelerate the rate at which states move from delivering services through a system of hospitals to delivery through a system of community programs.

National health insurance is still some distance off. But enactment of legislation that will have an impact on the kind of change I am talking about is probably not so far off. One very real possibility has to do with a change in the medicaid law. Under the program as presently designed, the provision of clinic—or outpatient—mental health services is optional within the state plan. The administration all along has opposed the inclusion of required outpatient mental health services because of a fear that the cost would be too great, although it has accepted—and this is part of the Medicaid law—that inpatient hospital services for the mentally ill shall be covered; and Congress has gone along with this distinction.

But now that the administration is proposing that federal support for the community mental health centers program be eliminated, it is under pressure—as well as a moral obligation—to help develop alternative sources of funding for community mental health programs. Since the federal community mental health center staffing grant—once the center is fully operational—essentially goes toward paying the cost of delivering services to the poor, an obvious device for supplying some relief is by broadening the medicaid law to require the inclusion of outpatient mental health services in a state medicaid plan. And if the change were accomplished in such a way as to make the delivery of such services in the clinic or community program setting more attractive financially than for those provided in the state mental hospital, then there would be another impetus for states to accelerate the conversion process.

But I think the administration and Congress can do more to speed the shift. Every time we in Congress consider and pass a piece of legislation that relates in some way to the delivery of mental health services, then we ought to make it clear—through the establishment of incentives—that the way of the future is service delivery within the community program setting. Similarly, every time the administration deals with such issues through the implementation of rules and regulations or other devices, then it, too, should make sure that the emphasis is on community service programs. For the momentum is underway. It is now only a question of how swiftly the transition shall take place.

Congressman William Roy
Second District, Kansas

**Part I
General Overview**

Introduction to Part I

Rapidly changing public attitudes toward state hospital care of the mentally ill and governmental responses to these changes have produced a crisis in state hospital systems all over the country. The number of patients in state hospitals had been systematically reduced throughout the 1960s. Piecemeal efforts to decrease the number of hospital facilities had been superseded in the 1970s by plans for dismantling entire systems of state hospitals in California, New York, Pennsylvania, and Massachusetts. State central office staffs, once devoted to supporting and monitoring state hospitals, are now being given other functions. Organizations and facilities built up at great cost over many years are being abandoned. Although professional consensus and much public sentiment appears to be that these changes are all to the good, should they prove to be a mistake, reversing them, unfortunately, is likely to be extremely expensive if not impossible.

Regrettably, the dismantling process so far has taken place with relatively little critical examination of the theories underlying the change and with little experimentation to verify planners' predictions. As this dismantling process continues, and its impact is more strongly felt, evidence mounts that there was only limited understanding of what was being dismantled. Easy acceptance of the characterization of state hospitals as human warehouses has blunted careful examination of the full range of functions served by state hospitals. Their intricate involvement in providing convenient, if sometimes inappropriate, resolutions for social problems such as control of borderline criminal behavior and care for those judged incapable of caring for themselves is now becoming clear.

Mental health professionals now often declare that it is inappropriate to use state hospitals or other parts of the mental health system to resolve these social problems. Professionals in many instances have effectively closed off use of facilities under their control for the care of the large class of social misfits for whom they formerly accepted responsibility. Most mental health professionals, however, do not see it as their job to suggest alternative solutions to the problems created by the sudden redefinition of their responsibilities. Yet, the general public does expect these problems to be handled by the mental health establishment in part, as a result of many years of campaigning by professionals to have the public believe that every social problem had a major mental health component. The implicit and at times stated promise to the public had been that most if not all social problems could be resolved if only

3

the public were to provide the necessary support to the mental health professionals who were supposedly trained to handle them.

Absent also has been the discussion of how best to use the considerable resources that will potentially be available if state hospital operations significantly decrease or cease. As anyone experienced with governmental agencies is aware, such agencies rarely die quietly when their function has been completed. They live on, sometimes as empty shells, wasting public resources. At other times they find new sources of clients who will be processed through the system regardless of need.

State hospitals should not—cannot—be left to wither on the vine or fend for themselves. Their potential value is too great. The state governments, which over the years have invested millions of dollars in land, buildings, and manpower, must preserve and make appropriate use of these facilities. Because of neglect of considerations such as these, mental health professionals stand in great danger of losing their leadership position and credibility with the public.

The state mental hospital grew out of a nineteenth century concern that local communities were neither interested in nor able to take adequate care of their mentally ill. Apparently it was assumed that by centralizing care in large hospitals that would be operated by state governments, many of the difficulties of the locally operated units would be solved. For example, state operated units have a large funding base, and in theory need not be jeopardized fiscally in case of a sudden downturn in local economic conditions. The gathering in one place of a large number of patients makes it economical and efficient to employ highly competent, specialized, and expensive personnel and to construct expensive specialized facilities. With the accumulation of large numbers of mental patients in one institution, it would neither be necessary nor efficient to mix the mentally ill, chronically physically ill individuals, indigents, and petty offenders in one institution as local governments had done.

Needless to say, the state hospitals were hailed as a major advance in their day (is anything ever started in the United States without being hailed as a major advance?) and for many years the state hospitals worked very well. They worked in the sense that they did their jobs quietly and effectively without much public attention and at minimal expense. For many years the task consisted primarily of custody. Treatment ran a poor second, and understandably so; there were no effective treatments known for the serious mental illnesses.

That eventually the whole service system seemed to erupt and break down in chaos in the early twentieth century must be attributed to a number of factors, most of which were outside rather than inside the system. Increasing population growth and urbanization produced many more admissions of seriously ill patients than the hospitals were prepared to handle. Where moral (individualized psychological) treatment could work very well in the mid nineteenth century and patients and staff could seem like one happy family, this became impossible by the beginning of the twentieth century when the happy family outgrew its limits.

Over the years, as the quality of life and treatment in state hospitals decayed, the population of the United States began to raise its level of expectation both of psychiatric treatment and of general living conditions. Rather primitive conditions in a state hospital were no burden for a patient who came himself from an urban slum or a rural home with few comforts. A prosperous worker, however, was not content to make the best of the stringent living conditions produced by limited budgets in the hospitals, nor was his family likely to be content.

Finally, most recently there has been both an increasing tolerance of social deviance in society and a decreasing tolerance for large institutions and their problems. It was natural in such a situation that state hospitals would become a prime target.

Out of the "young Turk" movement in psychiatry, and the optimism about the future of public services in this country, both of which seem to be a part of the aftermath of World War II, grew the idea of the community mental health center and the related dismantling of the state hospitals. If a community mental health center were available to every area of the United States, as was hoped, it would be quite logical that state hospitals would shrink in size and eventually disappear.

Increasing interest in community mental health centers helped to produce the new subspecialty, community psychiatry, whose proponents at one point seemed to see the world as their patient. No human difficulty seemed to be beyond therapeutic reach. Even those individuals with a narrower view seemed unquestioningly to accept the value of the new community mental health approach in spite of lack of evidence of its effectiveness or even of its being workable. In the literature reflecting the early discussions about community mental health centers, one looks in vain for serious consideration of questions such as the use of the state hospitals that were to be abandoned and concern about the possible loss to mental health services of the many thousands of highly trained staff members and millions of dollars in real estate and equipment that were then being used to serve the psychiatric needs of the American people. Even if somehow all state hospital assets were to be converted to use of the community mental health centers, how was this to come about? What about staff retraining programs? Land sale and purchase? Building destruction and construction? Through all the discussion and turmoil, one looks in vain for a voice of leadership offering questions, if not answers. This would have been leadership in the sense of independent judgement, not in the sense of racing to stay ahead of the crowd.

In all of the anticipation and excitement about community health centers, there seems to have been little concern with quality of program and the measures necessary to see to it that the centers worked properly. It was almost as if it was assumed that simply by obtaining funds, putting up a building, and opening the doors, magical things were going to happen.

It is not surprising that now we see the signs of the professional and public backlash. A few studies and many newspaper stories suggest that patients moved precipitously out of state hospitals are living in "back wards" in the community. There has been little or no provision made for after-discharge follow-up and little or no effort expended to prepare patients for release. Hospitals (and mental health centers) spend little effort on rehabilitation—teaching patients how to get and keep a job, how to maintain a household, how to take care of themselves—but prefer to concentrate on "therapy." While therapy (whether pharmacologic, psychologic, or social) seems to produce in-hospital improvement and usually at the least does no harm, its lack of long-term effectiveness in keeping patients out of hospitals is becoming clear. Combine lack of practical preparation for hospital discharge with lack of special support facilities in the community for use after discharge and the scene is set for wide-scale failure. The backlash is beginning. One California study shows that discharged mental patients are convicted of violent crimes several times more frequently than are the general population. Long Beach, New York, has taken legal steps to prevent discharged patients from residing there, offering the perfectly reasonable justification that most of the patients sent to live there never came from there in the first place.

Out of concern for the unanswered questions about state hospitals and mental health centers and in the hope of stimulating useful discussion, the Division of Community Psychiatry of the State University of Buffalo arranged a conference in November 1973 on "The Future Role of the State Hospital."[a] The papers presented at this conference, plus others solicited to cover additional subjects, are collected here in the hope of providing a broad look at an issue of crucial importance to the mental health field.

The book is divided into four sections, with each section devoted to examination of a major aspect of the future of the state hospital. The foreword by Congressman William Roy examines the relationship between state hospitals and recent developments in general health care from a national perspective. An issue of major concern to mental health service planners and administrators is the likely impact of any form of national health insurance on the funding of mental health agencies. Should mental health services be excluded completely from insurance coverage most individuals requiring service will become responsibilities of state or local government. Even the significant number of individuals who presently are able to pay for psychiatric treatment through health insurance may lose this coverage as health insurance plans move to conform to the federal model.

[a]This conference was supported in part by funds made available by the New York State Department of Mental Hygiene; CIBA-GEIGY Corporation; Continuing Medical Education, SUNYAB; McNeil Laboratories, Inc.; Merck, Sharpe & Dohme; Roche Laboratories; Sandoz Pharmaceuticals; Smith, Kline & French Laboratories; and The Lilly Research Laboratories.

It is to be expected that exclusion of mental health services from any national health insurance plan would have a major effect in influencing definition and diagnosis of mental health problems in the future. State and local governments as well as individual physicians may reasonably be expected to respond to the public demand for increasing all types of services in ways likely to generate the greatest federal reimbursement. Symptoms that can be seen as indications of physical illness and thereby produce insurance coverage will certainly be diagnosed in that way. On the other hand, if mental health services are liberally supported in a national insurance plan, private psychiatric practice is likely to burgeon with a possible increase in the per case as well as total cost of mental health services and a diminution in the number of psychiatrists available for public agency service.

Congressman Roy, who is also a physician, offers a view of community mental health services quite likely held by many individuals outside of the mental health field. He shows concern for the problems, respect for the professionals, and a desire to deal positively with issues that fortunately have been so typical of national political leaders for a number of years, and that account in no small part for the rapid growth of community mental health centers. It is this willingness to follow the leadership of mental health professionals and to place public resources on the line in response to the professionals' requests that is currently in danger of being tragically dissipated.

Chapter 1, by Dr. Harold W. Demone, Jr. and Dr. Herbert C. Schulberg, provides an extensive review of the human services problems that state hospitals were designed to meet, and of the history of attempts to deal with these problems. One of the conclusions to be drawn from this chapter, that mental hospitals are not likely to survive because they are hardly needed or wanted, must be taken quite seriously. Dr. Demone has just completed an assignment as director of a statewide planning effort in Massachusetts to consider the future of the state hospital system there. One can hardly find, therefore, an individual more familiar with the complexities of state hospital operation but who is not, at the same time, part of the administration of the system and therefore committed to its continuance. Dr. Schulberg, who has been Dr. Demone's collaborator on many projects and publications, also has extensive experience as a planner of mental health services and as a consultant in this field.

In Chapter 2 Dr. Earl Pollack and Mr. Carl Taube review statistical trends in the service loads of state hospitals throughout the United States. Their projections suggest a continuing decrease in state hospital populations and suggest this question: At what point is it rational to eliminate state hospital services and either provide alternative facilities for those currently being admitted or provide no service at all? When the total state hospital population in the United States goes below some figure—perhaps 100,000, perhaps 50,000—then must we not consider the small size of this group and the magnitude of their needs in comparison with, for example, the millions of children not receiving adequate education or the hundreds of thousands who are undernourished? Should not funds going for expensive services in state hospitals be diverted to other more pressing needs?

Dr. Pollack and Mr. Taube are representatives of the group we consider to be among the unsung heroes of mental health services—Biometry Division of the National Institute of Mental Health. Year after year, through financial feast and famine, this group, headed by Dr. Morton Kramer, has continued to collect and analyze data of all sorts from mental health facilities across the United States. Sad to say, all too often their findings were ignored or forgotten by planners and administrators in the passionate drive for larger facilities and more funds. Yet, for those who were concerned with what was really happening, and not just with what theory said should be happening, the Biometry group was always available, always helpful, and always sensible.

No doubt, whatever direction state hospital and community mental health services take in the future, Biometry will be there describing what is happening.

1

Has the State Mental Hospital a Future as a Human Service Resource?

Harold W. Demone, Jr. and
Herbert C. Schulberg

The chronically impaired and the offender have long made up our institutionalized populations. Out-of-sight and out-of-mind institutional programs for the tuberculous, chronically ill and disabled, mentally ill, retarded, and juvenile and adult offenders reflected the spirit of the nineteenth century—and nursing homes for the aged the spirit of the twentieth century. All of these program developments, if seen in their time and context, legitimately reflect a desire to improve the plight of the less fortunate who often languished in town and county lock-ups and jails. These alternative physical sites were often magnificant; surely rustic countrysides had curative powers. Thus, by the middle of the twentieth century state governments were usually spending between five and ten percent of their annual operating budgets to sustain—but barely so— these nineteenth century solutions in spite of overwhelming evidence of their inadequacies as therapeutic measures. It is true that they did keep the streets reasonably free from certain low income, unpleasant people. Ironically, the coming of hippies, groupies, drop-outs, freaks, long-haired suburban youth, drug experimenters, political and social revolutionaries, and civil rights and antiwar militants in various combinations and permutations filled and over-filled the vacuum in the 1960s and 1970s.

Thus, as our physical institutions failed to keep our cities and towns free from antisocial people, failed to be humanitarian, and failed to be cost-effective (another attribute of the 1960s), a dismantling process that began in the 1950s accelerated. The turberculosis field moved earliest and fastest. Fresh air had not worked but medication was successful and all those lovely antebellum wooden fire traps (and occasional modern brick structures) situated in hilly, wooded locations were unneeded. Many of the people who made a living in this industry, and many of the politicians who saw patronage and contracts disappear, began to protest. Failing to stem the tide, they sought alternative populations to refill their wooden fire traps. Medicare, Medicaid, social security, and public welfare then combined to create a new and larger industry. In Massachusetts, in 1973 approximately one-tenth of the state budget went for geriatric care.

As with the tuberculosis field, the mid 1950s saw the beginning of deinstitutionalizing the American state mental hospital. By 1972 the national state hospital population had decreased 50 percent from its former peak in 1955 in spite of a considerable increase in the general population during the same time period. Deinstitutionalization was substantially hastened by the report of the

Joint Commission on Mental Illness and Health, the NIMH-supported state
mental health planning activities (1963-65), medication, and community mental
health programs. And the trend continues. By mid 1973 Massachusetts was
down 76 percent in its average daily mental hospital census from its prior high
in the mid 1950s.

Dealing with these planned and unplanned developments has required increasing energy and time from the mental health system's participants. Among the
many factors affecting the future are increased citizen participation; modified
professional staff roles and relations; active paraprofessional program involvement; and budget specialists at both the executive and legislative levels who see
the empty buildings as reflecting unneeded appropriations. Thus, mental health,
as all of the human services, is no longer the exclusive property of a small group
of self-appointed professionals.

The Human Services Movement

On balance many positive changes have occurred in the last decade, in both
the conceptual rationales underlying program development as well as the organizations offering services.[1] Psychoanalytic concepts, while still well-regarded,
no longer serve as the principal cornerstone for design of mental health programs.
Social psychiatric precepts are becoming equally relevant for structuring clinical
services and guiding personnel utilization. Community-based outpatient care
rather than inpatient hospitalization is now the treatment of choice for both
acutely as well as chronically disturbed individuals. Clinicians increasingly
acknowledge the complexity of behavioral problems and the significant role of
other community caregivers. The provision of indirect services such as consultation is now a legitimate function of mental health agencies, and many professionals quite comfortably assume this role. As a result of the clinician's
increased community orientation, local citizens are more involved in policy,
program, and budget planning.

Although the pace of these developments has varied, it is increasingly
acknowledged that a client's problems are often rooted in his community's
tumultuous social structure and fragmented caregiving system as in his personal
psyche. Personal distress can be as profound when it results from unstable
economic conditions, inadequate housing, and unresponsive human services as
the anxiety stemming from neurotic concerns and unresolved developmental
crises. If the mental health system is to contribute maximally, it must link much
more closely and effectively with the larger human service network.

In the past decade the mental health subsystem has expanded from the
single-purpose clinic or hospital to the more encompassing five essential services
of community mental health. During the 1970s it will be challenged to modify
even further by designing, or linking to caregiving, systems that provide clients

with comprehensive and coordinated assistance of a nonpsychiatric as well as a psychiatric nature. Human services' systems will be concerned programmatically with health care, vocational training, rehabilitation, and education. From an administrative perspective, March[2] and Demone[3] have described these new human services' systems as incorporating the following features: comprehensiveness; decentralized facilities located in areas of high population density; and integrated or linked program administration. Programs will be tested against a matrix that examines availability, accessibility, continuity, quality, and cost-effectiveness.

These changes are played against an evolving series of concepts and wide-ranging experimentation. Often practice precedes conceptual efforts to rationalize their validity, but it also is true that modified beliefs serve as an important precursor to action. Baker[4] has suggested that the community mental health ideology of the 1960s may well be supplanted by a human services ideology incorporating several new major attitude dimensions. Although still developing, the following five themes already characterize this system: systemic integration of services; comprehensiveness and accessibility; a problem-in-living definition of client troubles; helping activities containing generic qualities; and provider accountability to clients. A human services' orientation is not incompatible with community mental health concepts; rather, it is an extension of these ideas through evolutionary processes. Just as those subscribing to sociotherapeutic beliefs could comfortably adapt to community mental health beliefs,[5] so could these individuals also support a human services' ideology even though each of these successive belief systems is based upon ever broader parameters of meaningful professional practice.

The tendency to designate a community's health, recreation, and social welfare agencies as human services' organizations reflects not only the desire to provide services more efficiently and effectively but also a growing awareness of the common fundamentals inherent in the varied problems presented by clients. It also indicates a recognition of the generic quality of professional and nonprofessional caregivers. Traditional distinctions between the problems germane to a psychiatric clinic and an alcoholism clinic, for example, or the functions of different mental health professionals have become increasingly artificial, and many agencies have drastically revised their intake policies and clinical practices accordingly. Neighboring child guidance clinics and adult psychiatric clinics are being reorganized as family-oriented facilities, and family agencies that previously excluded alcoholics, drug addicts, and other special problem cases now routinely accept such individuals. Mental hospitals, which limited their services to psychiatrically defined problems, are undertaking such functions as after-care programs to parolees from correctional institutions and residential care for runaway youths.

As mental health and other public and private human service agencies extend their range of services, it will become all the more urgent that they forge systemic linkages to provide the complex array of resources, technologies, and skills required for optimal client care. Defenders of the status quo need only follow a few clients through the present system in order to realize that it is poorly designed for resolving their multiple problems. The alcoholic client of a community mental health center may be offered outpatient psychotherapy, but little effort is made to arrange employment counseling or to involve his wife and children in the resolution of related familial problems. The parents of an emotionally disturbed child might well have to negotiate with the local psychiatric facility, the school system, and the public welfare agency to insure that the youngster receives necessary educational and mental health services. Program coordination must also grapple with problems stemming from the fact that federal reimbursement for the identical service will vary according to whether it is provided by a health or social service agency.

In spite of the erratic pace of progress, concerted meaningful efforts that reorganize program components more effectively for the benefit of the client are apparent. At the heart of these efforts is the conception that human services' programs operate as a system of organizations whose participants are interdependent and must be appropriately linked.[6] Systems concepts are increasingly being applied to the design and operation of human services' programs, particularly relevant in defining the problems of management, of changing human services' organizational goals, of interorganizational relations, and of organizational-environmental interaction.

The application of systems concepts to the design and operation of human services' programs represents a rational, planned approach to the development of future caregiving arrangements. During the past decade, planning has been sanctioned within given categorical fields such as health or social welfare, but with change occurring at an exponential rate, the trend of the 1970s must be to broaden the planning base. Systems concepts are of singular value to illuminate a person's functioning and problems beyond the limited scope of a single, categorical field. They also highlight the fact that shifting program emphases from one categorical sector to another upsets delicate fiscal and personnel balances that must be reestablished.

Effective planning for human services, from an ecosystem's perspective, depends upon the involvement and cooperation of the target community, the participation of established professional groups affected by potential program change, and the sagacity of the planners themselves when faced with attractive alternatives in a turbulent environment. The temptation to move simultaneously in all directions must be resisted. The human service planner must understand that fundamental conflicts can be created if overly diverse philosophies, services, and human inputs are incorporated within a single enterprise. He must determine whether administrative controls are to be vested in professional or community representatives, whether clinical-type services or social action are to be emphasized, and whether cooperative or conflictual strategies are to be utilized. Furthermore, the planner must distinguish between his short- and long-term objectives since they may be antithetical, for example, providing "new career" training only to some of the poor can be of immediate benefit to the trainees, but it may reduce poor people's support for the more fundamental and long-range changes needed to alter the poverty cycle. Choice selection is also becoming more complex as legislative actions compel human services to develop within the scope of broader urban undertakings, for example, funds for corrections programs and preventive mental health activities are provided in the Safe Streets Act, and many social services are funded through Housing and Urban Development programs.

Impact on the Mental Hospital

The mental hospital, as a major component of the mental health subsystem, is now challenged by an unparalleled crisis as it is subjected to policy, fiscal, and programmatic pressures. Many of the hospital's functions (some would say all) are either anachronistic or performed better in other settings. Diminishing inpatient censuses, the development of effective alternatives, and the need to redeploy existing resources into higher priority community-based services, are leading many legislators and program administrators to challenge the current substantial fiscal investment in psychiatric institutions. As new funding sources for expanding human services become increasingly difficult to obtain, the billions of dollars required to support mental hospitals become highly visible targets.

Many planners and administrators are suggesting that the institutions be closed and a number of states already are implementing this policy. Protests have emanated from those who argue that some patients are being dumped in communities, that adequate alternative community facilities are lacking, that personnel rights are being abrogated, and that local economies are being disrupted. Nevertheless, the dye has been cast and the future role of mental hospitals already is the subject of intense scrutiny. When this change is seen (as suggested in the introduction), not as a phenomenon unique to mental health, but as one segment of a larger social movement in which the use of large, isolated institutions for all problems is being successfully challenged, then it can be assumed that the trend is irreversible.

Notwithstanding the strength of the deinstitutionalization movement, it should be remembered that current successes over time often become historical failures. This is not lamentable for this is how we learn. For example, for a while in the nineteenth century, the mental hospital movement embodied the same societal goals envisioned for community mental health programs in the 1960s. However, mental hospitals experienced many difficulties and failures over the decades in sustaining a therapeutic role and their plight became increasingly worse during the first half of the twentieth century. Public and professional concern for the welfare of persons treated in these nonthera-peutic institutions found expression in the late 1950s in the report of the Joint Commission on Mental Illness and Health.

The resulting 1963 Community Mental Health Centers Act is deemed by many to have specifically intended that all mental hospitals be replaced by newly funded and operated local facilities. In fact, the recent Nader critique of the act's accomplishments[7] is predicated upon this interpretation of its original intent. However, it is clear that the presumed federal goal of closing mental hospital was neither subscribed to nor did it even gain sympathy in many parts of the country. Certainly, it was not an unequivocal federal goal. In reality, financial and manpower needs and political pressures dictated that existing resources, including the mental hospital, be included in many of the local attempts to establish comprehensive community mental health pro-grams. Furthermore, federal funds for community mental health centers were severely limited and required maximum utilization of existing local resources. (In addition, in 1973 even these minimal federal efforts were revealed as demon-strations only.) Population growth and shifts and growing highway networks had reduced the physical, if not psychological, distance between many mental hospitals and their communities. The combination of these and other factors convinced many states by 1965 of the financial wisdom of using some or all mental hospitals as the core or major component of selected comprehensive programs, to provide the five essential services to their own local areas as well as additional services for which they were uniquely staffed and/or equipped.

Eight years later some assessment of results of a public policy designed to utilize the mental hospital as a contemporary, therapeutic facility seems rea-sonable. Such an evaluation is difficult under the best of circumstances, as noted by Baker and Schulberg,[8] and it has been made even more complex by the fact that assessment criteria now extend beyond the mental hospital's function as a community mental health center to include its potential as a human services' resource. Present parameters for defining a community mental health center's clients and services are clearly in flux because of chang-ing societal assumptions about client need, shifting funding patterns, swelling demands for services, and broadened role requirements for caregivers.

Given this evolving analytic framework for assessing the mental hospital's future as a viable human services' resource, the resulting picture is at best a mixed one.[9] There are many who contend that existing psychiatric institu-tions remain as outmoded today as they were in the past. Others, increasingly less, fervently profess that these facilities continue to warrant societal and legislative support. The facts and rationales behind these contradictory asser-tions and how they will influence the mental hospital's future as a contemporary human services' agency are explored below.

Clients

Any analysis of the mental hospital's fate must reflect on its input consti-tuency. For which individuals will society seek care and treatment in such facilities? How will this policy decision be made? Who will make it? With what frequency will such persons be admitted to these institutions? How are these epidemiologic projections affected by developments within a mental hospital and the broader human services' network of which it is a component? Schulberg and Baker's (in press) study of Boston State Hospital's transition to a community health center found that changing clinical programs within the institutions were related to altered client input patterns from the geographic catchment area and to modified clientele selection priorities. Do these findings from one urban community and its mental hospital reflect a unique situation in a large New England city, or can they be considered indicative of wider trends?

The literature suggests that the nature of mental hospital clientele and the services provided them are indeed changing around the country. A review by Ozarin and Feldman[10] found a drastic 50 percent reduction in state hospital populations between 1955 and 1970, as well as a shift in the focus of care from inpatient to outpatient service. In 1955, 71 percent of patient care episodes occurred in hospitals and 22 percent in outpatient clinics. In 1968 the figures were 43 percent for hospitals and 45 percent for clinics. Additionally, the number of admissions to mental hospitals represented only one-third of total admissions to psychiatric inpatient care in 1968 since admissions to general hospitals more than doubled since 1955.

The decreased need to utilize the residential facilities of mental hospitals generally is associated with the advent of tranquilizers in the mid 1950s, but the growth of community mental health centers and psychiatric programs in general hospitals in the late 1960s has lent further impetus to this trend. Stubblebine and Decker[11] and Wolford et al.[12] describe how state hospital-ization rates were reduced in San Francisco and Pittsburgh, respectively, as expanding community mental health programs assumed greater responsibilities. In the former city, for example, involuntary patients were treated locally because of a superior court ruling. In Pittsburgh the decision was made to substitute local care for mental hospital commitment. In both cities, and there are many other examples, the result was the virtual disappearance of institutional commitments.

An example of how shifting definitions of human problems and their causative factors affect input projections to human service networks in general, and mental hospitals in particular, is the movement by many states (thirteen by mid 1973) to define alcoholism as a medical rather than criminal problem, thus shifting the locus or responsibility to health and social welfare services away from correctional ones. One result could be a temporary increase in the demand on the mental hospital system with a substantial reduction in admissions over time as additional federal and state funds become available to other community caregivers such as general hospitals, detoxification centers, outpatient clinics, halfway houses, and sheltered workshops. Here, again, the increased use of the mental hospital is seen as either an interim or desperate resort but never as a first or permanent choice. The Holder and Stratas[13] description of a systems approach to alcoholism programming indicates the alternatives in designing comprehensive alcoholism networks, which may or may not include the mental hospital's resources. Thus, although alcoholics already comprise approximately one-third of mental hospital admissions and their number may temporarily rise, it is likely that as community alternatives evolve over a period of years, the number of alcoholics served by mental hospitals will dwindle.

Although more and more planners project the diminished use, even the abandonment, of mental hospitals in treating a community's emotionally disturbed citizens, some of those associated with these hospitals emphasize the continued need for these facilities in caring for the chronically ill. Few dispute that chronically ill persons will always represent a sector of the community's psychiatric caseload. Whether their needs can be met through community mental health centers and other resources, or whether mental hospitals are needed is a key ambiguity in forecasting future program trends. Reports such as those by Kraft, et al.[14] about the Ft. Logan Mental Health Center and Myerson[15] about Worcester State Hospital assert that chronic, unresponsive schizophrenics accumulate and constitute a substantial portion of a facility's treatment population in spite of efforts to avoid this "silting." All would agree that specialized input and treatment procedures are needed for these individuals, but there is less concensus as to whether these procedures are best organized and administered within the framework of mental hospitals or in alternative smaller, newer, and less costly arrangements.

Along with this specific uncertainty about the ability to dispense totally with mental hospital services in treating traditionally defined psychiatric clients, countertrends at some psychiatric institutions raise additional questions about the universality and inevitability of the declining volume of client admissions to mental hospitals. It is evident that given proper statutory and administrative sanctions, institutions located in urban centers and capable of establishing links to the local human services' system can generate major changes in the clients for whom they accept responsibility. At a number of Massachusetts institutions such as Boston and Worcester State Hospitals, the range of community-oriented services was expanded as the psychiatric custodial censuses dwindled. Buildings and staff were converted to other programs. Previously ignored populations like drug dependents and runaway youth are now being served.

Here, again, as other community alternatives are developed, these newly designed hospital-operated programs have begun to diminish in admissions. Nevertheless, it is likely that urban-based, maximally flexible psychiatric institutions can continue to provide selected and needed high priority programs on an interim basis as the community readies itself to meet new challenges. Their clientele will include individuals with a variety of social and physical problems, and the category of individuals now defined as psychiatrically ill will be but one of those served by these emerging centers. Whether these institutions will continue to bear the mental hospital label, be operated by mental health authorities, and be staffed by people skilled in psychological intervention tools is moot, however. If a TB sanatorium now specializes in runaway youth or the chronically ill, is it still a TB sanatorium? Should physicians specializing in diseases of the chest continue to administer it? And finally, how do its cost benefits compare to alternatives?

This expanded view of the mental hospital's potential future inputs clearly stems from the premise discussed earlier in this paper, that is, that there are sufficient common denominators in the personal needs of the psychiatrically disturbed, the parolee, the physically handicapped, and the alcoholic to warrant provision of a variety of general as well as unique services within a single, comprehensive, caregiving facility staffed by generalists. As such, all or part of its physical site, buildings, or staff may be involved. Conversely, if these client populations are viewed as having specific needs that can best, or only, be met in a categorical service center staffed by trained and experienced professionals, it is unlikely that they will be perceived as appropriate inputs for changing mental hospitals.

The experience of the tuberculosis field in the 1960s, the juvenile correction program in Massachusetts in 1972-73, and some recent state mental hospital closures are instructive. As suggested earlier in this paper, the changes implied by the elimination of physical institutions were and are politically very powerful. That the buildings are usually ancient, ill-fitted for any use, often fire hazards, and their location customarily in sites distant from population centers, mass transportation, and professional staff, makes little difference to their defenders. The employees are voters. They and their institutions expend funds and contribute to the local economy. The superordinate goal sometimes becomes the continuation of the institution for any purpose. The degree to which the program site or facility is an accurate reflection of client and consumer needs is seldom a significant issue.

As a consequence, paradoxes abound. In a new fiscal year in Massachusetts, staff are still assigned to youth correctional institutions empty of clients. A state hospital eliminated as a patient-serving institution still costs a million dollars to maintain. Obviously, the strength of the political, employment, and economic issues should never be underestimated even in the face of rational, client-focused program considerations.

Program Alternatives

This complex vision of a community's options and intentions for meeting diverse citizen needs produces differing forecasts of whether mental hospitals are to be incorporated within future human service networks. At the one extreme is the contention by many observers that most mental hospitals in both urban and rural settings have failed over a lengthy period to modify significantly their program philosophy and operating practices. These observers assert that although these institutions may have eliminated the worst characteristics of the snake pit era, they have undertaken few of the programmatic changes essential to contemporary functioning. The generally inadequate status of the physical plant and its replacement cost are also noted. The 1971 decision of a federal court in the case of *Wyatt* v. *Stickney*, requiring Alabama's mental hospitals to upgrade services and facilities, reveals the desperate situation that still exists in at least some of our psychiatric institutions.

In some cases the mental hospital's current failure to meet contemporary standards has resulted from a state's decision to expand community-based services and to phase out institutions. In other instances the hospital's own personnel have lacked the leadership required to develop and administer progressive programs even when given the mandate to do so. An even more fundamental issue about the mental hospital's viability is that raised by Mendel[16] and Polak and Jones,[17] who contend that existing mental hospitals by definition are antitherapeutic, since by admitting troubled persons they permit communities to avoid mobilizing the social and psychological support systems that these persons require. They also question the assumption that deviant behavior can better be assessed and diagnosed in the hospital than in the person's natural environment. From this perspective it is clear that regardless of whether the hospitals' limited progress is societally determined or organizationally induced, many existing institutions are not meeting people's needs. They should be phased out, and alternative provisions sought for the clientele whom they traditionally have served.

More optimistic prognoses of the mental hospital's future stem from the viewpoint that many of these facilities already are, or still are, capable of making constructive contributions to a community's need for the full spectrum of human services. Overviews by Ozarin and Levenson[18] and Greenblatt[19] point to several contemporary roles within the psychiatric institution's grasp, for example, serving as the core of a health system or undertaking community mental health functions within a larger caregiving network. Fisher, Mehr, and Truckenbrud[20] model a future mental hospital as follows: (1) a medical-freudian section for persons with physical disorders that clearly are causing behavioral reactions; (2) a voluntary human services' section for persons who cannot function in traditional community settings; and (3) an involuntary security section for people who do not seek admission but whose behavior violates the right of others.

A more circumscribed but nevertheless significant contribution to meeting a community's human services' needs through mental hospital facilities is suggested by Bartz, Loy, and Cook.[21] They view psychiatric institutions as caring only for those special populations that cannot be accommodated within community mental health centers, for example, alcoholics, acting-out adolescents, chronic no-family persons, and those dangerous to others. Bartz et al. view existing mental hospitals as appropriate residential settings for these populations since their treatment requires total-control environments in which intensive behavioral training and change can occur. Of course, none of these proposed models resembles current state mental hospitals.

Even these optimistic forecasts must be tempered, however, by the recognition that in spite of positive societal mandates and creative leadership efforts, even the best intended mental hospitals may be unable to overcome the legacies of deteriorating physical plants and staffing patterns inappropriate to contemporary programs. This problem is poignantly exemplified at Boston State Hospital. Over the past decade, this organization has given top priority to improved patient care and treatment environments and has moved in progressive program directions in spite of the profoundly constraining influence of poor plant conditions. In February 1973, however, the superintendent was forced to acknowledge publicly that "Boston State Hospital is physically dying." Capital improvement funds were again sought from the State Legislature after the Joint Commission on Hospital Accreditation rescinded the hospital's accreditation because its toilets and lighting were so bad. The superintendent warned that if these physical conditions were not quickly remedied, staff would be lost and programs and patient care surely would deteriorate in spite of the hard-won gains of the previous decade.

An equally frustrating dilemma in insuring the mental hospital's program growth is that of establishing personnel patterns appropriate to contemporary purposes. An analysis of staff employed at the Massachusetts mental hospitals in 1973, for example, revealed that although staff/patient ratios generally exceeded the long-standing goal of 1:1 (9,000 staff for 7,000 patients), few of the personnel were engaged in treatment. More than four times as many employees were maintaining Massachusetts hospital buildings and grounds as there were psychiatrists, psychologists, and social workers combined to treat the patients residing within them. Similarly, even in the face of the 1972 *Wyatt* v. *Stickney* court order to upgrade personnel patterns, the director of an Alabama mental hospital has acknowledged that "the volume of skills is not available and not likely to be available until Alabama establishes competitive pay grades and appropriates the necessary funds."[22]

The mental hospital's program options for the 1970s, thus, include the choice of (a) abandoning the ghost of relevance and closing down; (b) temporarily assuming highly specialized functions that cannot be currently performed elsewhere; and (c) undertaking full-scale human services' activities as a major caregiving organization. However, even when new mandates are

achieved and contemporary directions pursued, the constraints of antiquated
physical facilities, distant locations, low status, anachronistic state personnel,
civil service and administrative practices, and inappropriate staffing patterns
stand ready to thwart progress.

Mental Hospital Planning

A decision about the future of mental hospitals, given the cited options,
must include consideration of community alternatives, client need, staff
capability, geographic location, nature of physical plant, hospital status,
fiscal support, and political and economic realities. Careful planning is required
before action is undertaken. The Nader Report concluded similarly in emphasizing that "planning should immediately be initiated for the long-range demise
of state hospitals."[23] Statewide planning efforts comparable to the early 1960s
projects have recently been conducted in such states as Massachusetts[24] and
California.[25] It is meaningful to consider the approaches they have taken
and the reactions they are meeting in seeking to implement program and
facility recommendations. (Special attention will be given to the 1973 Massachusetts report, which the authors chaired and directed, respectively).[a]

An organization's future can be assessed along a variety of dimensions. In
considering the future of the mental hospital, planners can focus upon either
(a) the hospital's clients or (b) its organizational capacities. The first approach
identifies those currently being served by public psychiatric institutions and
examines and compares the range of treatment alternatives. This planning
strategy relies heavily upon data of the types described earlier in this paper
regarding the community's projected input patterns, and it is particularly
concerned with the use of public policy in altering utilization patterns of
diverse human services' facilities. It is entirely conceivable from this perspective to recommend the phased closing of all mental hospitals, as community-
based alternatives to large-scale institutions are established.

The second planning approach primarily focuses upon organizational
strengths and weaknesses, and places relatively less emphasis upon alternative
options to the mental hospital. It is fundamentally a survival strategy, seeking
ways and means to retain an organization rather than seeking optimal client
benefits and improved systemic caregiving patterns.

The 1972-73 Massachusetts effort to plan for the future of its public
mental hospitals focused initially upon the principal subpopulations then

---

[a]The Massachusetts Mental Hospital Planning Project was an eighteen-month joint
planning project of United Community Services of Metropolitan Boston (a nonprofit, voluntary, human services' planning agency) and the Massachusetts Department of Mental
Health. It was financed principally by the Committee of the Permanent Charity Fund, Inc.,
a Massachusetts-based community foundation.

being served by these institutions. By evaluating their clinical needs and assessing the optimal public voluntary service systems required to provide appropriate care, it was possible to compare the state hospital with the alternatives and then judge whether it had any long-term role vis-à-vis each subpopulation. Therefore, client characteristics, treatment technologies, and facility requirements were reviewed for the following populations: adult mentally ill, geriatrics, adult psychiatric offenders, children and youth, and substance abusers. This planning approach can be illustrated by a brief description of the issues raised, the recommendations made about each of these populations, and the implementation procedures that then would ensue. The danger of this approach is that by examining separately each of the populations at risk, the alternative interventions may be limited by the views and experiences of the involved professionals and specialists and a larger systemic intervention overlooked. To compensate for this potential shortcoming, each categorical report was then reviewed by an overall advisory council charged with considering broader systemic issues.

Adult Mentally Ill

The adult mentally ill have long been the major population served by mental hospitals, and it is around their gross needs and abilities that most institutional programs were designed. This organizational emphasis over the last century resulted in the construction of major inpatient psychiatric services, and it is only in the past decade or two that we have come to recognize the finer and subtler clinical needs of those persons who traditionally occupied these beds. Consequently, a planning approach to the needs of the adult mentally ill must consider the distinctions between those individuals requiring (1) acute intensive treatment, (2) longer term community-based care, and (3) continued residential care.

Although the mental hospital has long been used for and occupied by all three of these groups, the current thinking is that the first two groups of adults can better be treated in facilities other than the mental hospital and that the third group is rapidly diminishing in size. This position is based upon the rationale that community-based care is preferable to that in mental hospitals because it fosters the integration of emotionally disturbed individuals into the mainstream of normal life and diminishes disability and dependency. This position maintains that institutional settings tend to be depersonalizing and lacking in accountability regardless of how superior the leadership efforts may be. Therefore, communities must be encouraged to accept total responsibility for their mentally ill and this will occur only if extrusion to distant mental hospitals is no longer possible. By assuming that (1) the clinical needs of acutely ill adults can be met through such community facilities as the general hospital, and that (2) long-term chronically hospitalized individuals can be

supported in various community residencies, it is possible to project a caregiving network for the adult mentally ill that no longer utilizes the mental
hospital.

There are many professionals and citizens, to be sure, who view such a
program policy for the adult mentally ill as premature, if not naive. Acknowledging the competence of the community to cope with the acute phase of
illness, they contend that it still is not possible to maintain the chronically
ill in communities and that to preclude the availability of mental hospital
facilities is deleterious to the welfare of such individuals. This position is
based upon evidence of high readmission rates for those discharged from
mental hospitals (although it is going down); unwillingness by many cities
and towns to permit the establishment of community homes for the mentally
ill in residential neighborhoods (although this is improving); and growing
concern about neurological disorders stemming from prolonged use by chronic
schizophrenics of neuroleptic drugs.[26] Nevertheless, these negative voices have
not impeded public policy recommendations opposing continued use of
institutional facilities, and steps are being initiated in Massachusetts and other
parts of the country to minimize and eliminate mental hospitals for the adult
mentally ill.

Elderly

In May of 1969 about 40 percent of the patients in Massachusetts state
mental hospitals were aged, although as with all major groupings this census
has declined rapidly in recent years (from 4,500 in 1967 to 2,500 in 1972).

As state hospital residents, the elderly can be described as two major
groupings requiring different treatment orientation. They are (1) patients
who have become aged while in the hospital—usually the chronic schizophrenic,
the paranoid, and those with affective disorders; usually in good medical condition, they have become institutionalized over time,[27] and (2) patients admitted
as elderly. Three-quarters of these patients are said to suffer from organic brain
syndromes—usually with senile dementia. (The reliability of these diagnoses,
however, has been challenged.)[28] Many other problems are also evident in
this group—arthritis, sensory impairment, digestive diseases, cardio-vascular
and/or neoplastic diseases, and these patients have higher morbidity and
mortality rates.[29]

After reviewing experiences in Massachusetts and elsewhere, Massachusetts
planners have concluded that the majority of geriatric mental patients do not
need long-term *psychiatric* hospitalization, although alternative support
programs may be necessary for many. Appropriate programming in both the
hospitals and in the community can (1) prevent long-term psychiatric hospitalization; (2) return to the community many of those already in psychiatric

hospitals; and (3) prevent excessive unhappiness, deterioration, and withdrawal in those who do need long-term care in some facility.

Alcoholism

The many national programmatic changes in alcoholism have already been noted. About 30 percent of current admissions to state mental hospitals in Massachusetts are alcoholic and there is substantial reason to believe that although this rate may rise briefly, it will drop sharply in subsequent years and such trends are already evident. Planners saw the state hospital principally as an organization possessing a bundle of resources that should be reallocated from the institution to the community, some of which should go to alcoholic programs. If the hospital were to be used for alcoholics in any way as presently constituted or in some redesigned form, such a decision should be made at the local level. The possibility of alternative roles for state mental hospitals, however, would not include outreach, consultation, education, intermediate care, outpatient services, inpatient care, or emergency services. The limited possible role of the state hospitals in serving alcoholics was viewed as being in the provision of back-up services for those alcoholics who require intensive inpatient or other psychiatric care and/or those chronic alcoholics requiring long-term care.

The Drug Dependent

Although four of the eleven Massachusetts state hospitals currently provide direct services to drug-dependent persons, planners recommended that all future programs be community-based. The personnel and financial resources of the hospitals should be reallocated to local contractually operated services. The development of a comprehensive community-based program additionally would eliminate the need to detain drug-dependent persons within correctional facilities for the crime of drug dependency. The need is recognized for possibly using a separate section of a state hospital on an interim basis while appropriate community facilities are created.

Adult Psychiatric Offender

This highly diffuse population has two main characteristics: It is considered dangerous, and, therefore, usually dealt with in the criminal justice system; and it is mentally disturbed. Four explicit operational assumptions underlined the program analysis: (1) community-based care is preferred; (2) security may be necessary; (3) humane and competent treatment is required; and (4) the possible severity of illness combined with the possible disruption to communities and institutions created by the psychiatric offender makes the need for serving them greater than the absolute numbers of the population would otherwise indicate.

While this complex analysis will not be reviewed here, questions arise as to the responsibility of the mental health authority for those psychiatric offenders within its jurisdiction, customarily dealt with as the state mental hospital. Does the hospital still have a legitimate and useful role? What are the alternatives?

Court evaluations are one responsibility; in 1972 in Massachusetts referrals totalled 6,000 outpatients, and 1,000 inpatients. The other major state hospital responsibility is the care of those hospitalized mentally ill persons who are violent. The planners recommended regional centers for the diagnosis and treatment of violent mentally ill men and women serving both civilly committed mental patients and mentally ill offenders. Each of the centers would serve between fifteen and twenty inpatients at a time.

The major offender population now served by the state mental hospital—court referrals for evaluation—will probably be further reduced from 1,000 in 1972 to 500 in 1974 as court clinics are expanded and a new mental health code is fully implemented. As the regional centers for psychiatric offenders are developed, the number being sent for such evaluations to Bridgewater State Hospital would be minimal and drop to zero at other state hospitals. Thus, the evaluation function of the state mental hospital with one minor exception would be eliminated.

Children and Youth

The present use of Massachusetts state mental hospitals for children and youth is minimal. Excluding a single specialized facility, no inpatients aged twelve and under are reported in other hospitals; less than 500 children are treated in various outpatient programs. About 500 adolescents, some as outpatients, are also seen by state hospital programs. Thus, increased residential programs are required for children. Ideally, seven small (thirty to fifty) residential units for children are indicated. These and other services would be purchased, not operated by the State Department of Mental Health.

None of the planners consider the present state mental hospital facilities ideal locations for children's services. Nevertheless, they recognized that financial realities might require some use of selected hospital buildings until alternatives are more fully available. Residential facilities for children in Massachusetts have always been in short supply and at this point in time many advocates for services to children will use any resource made available to them. Except for the possible temporary use of state mental hospital buildings, recommendations regarding children would not affect the curtailed need for physical plants. Once again, the redistribution of the present budget allocations from the various hospitals to community services would, of course, have significant impact on these institutions.

Implementation Procedures

It already is evident that similar recommendations are or will be made about utilizing alternatives to the mental hospital in caring for the few remaining clinical populations now being served in these institutions. Though sympathetically inclined, no one interest group contacted by the project saw the state mental hospital as a primary intervention mechanism for their particular subpopulation. The financial resources—yes; the staff—yes, although retraining, it is suggested, may be necessary for many; and an occasional building—as a last and temporary resort, if convenient and in good condition. Thus, in less than a decade even the hospital's back-up role has lost most of its advocates. Some would suggest that the transition be cautious in order that the community alternatives be ready. Others are willing to be more precipitous. But even the more conservative are not defending the status quo; rather they are change incrementalists. It, therefore, is necessary to consider selected implementation issues and decisions that will confront program administrators undertaking transitions of this scope and complexity.

The fiscal dilemma is of central importance. The noninstitutional human services' network will require significant expansion as it assumes previous mental hospital responsibilities. However, funding austerities in fiscal 1974 and probably through 1977-78 make it unlikely that substantial additional revenue will be forthcoming from state or federal governments to augment these community-based services. Therefore, resources being spent for mental hospital support inevitably will have to be redeployed into alternative care-giving organizations if they are to flourish.

As with the nation, the mental health establishment over the last decade had assumed a "guns and butter" economic philosophy. As community mental health budgets were expanded, so were those for state hospitals and at a substantially greater absolute amount. But new choices have to be made. They will not be easy for they require taking away from one subsystem to allocate to another. The life of the public mental health administrator is complicated even further by another threat. His superiors in the executive and legislative branches are viewing with growing interest the large institutional budgets for possible use in other high priority, nonmental health areas. The simplicity or complexity of fiscal redeployment will vary among states, depending upon local budget-setting procedures and degree of legislative control over allocations and political implications.

In states where fiscal flexibility exists, Schulberg[30] has suggested that as a possible first step public funds not be appropriated directly to mental hospitals but rather to designated citizen groups, territorially based, and charged with the responsibility for purchasing those comprehensive services pertinent to the needs of local residents. Assuming that appropriately high standards can be imposed and maintained,[31] the citizen area board would have the prerogative of purchasing human services from whatever public or private resources it deems most effective, thus placing client need before provider interests. If the consumer has a choice in purchasing psychiatric and other services, the budget of a mental hospital would then have to be supported through the services that it sells in an open market to those mental health and nonmental health, public and private programs that choose to utilize its facilities and services. If the mental hospital can offer an appropriate product and can attract clients, it will survive; if it cannot compete in the marketplace, then it should not be maintained.

A strict purchase of service approach to human services programming admittedly produces problems, for example, local human services' administrators may decide to purchase clinical care solely upon the basis of cost rather than quality. This fiscal marketplace strategy could also jeopardize the minimal level of organizational stability needed to insure program continuity. Statewide standards would be critical. Nevertheless, it represents an attractive initial alternative to present budgetary mechanisms that often maintain programs out of traditional rather than functional concerns. Thus, this strategy deserves further consideration, particularly if it can be combined with a plan for adjustable base subsidies along the lines suggested by Boggs.[32]

Another key issue affecting the redesign of mental health and human services' efforts is the need to help local citizens and program administrators accept responsibility for not only the clients whom they traditionally viewed as coming within their purview, for example, neurotics and depressives, but also for those persons formerly perceived as falling within the mental hospital's jurisdiction, for example, chronic schizophrenics and the aged. Furthermore, the individual needs and job security of mental hospital employees must be viewed with respect rather than disdain if organized labor's support is to be enlisted in the task of implementing contemporary caregiving systems. We cannot be humane to patients and inhumane to employees.

Although each of these policy and program issues is formidable and not easily resolved, the evidence is growing that a public and steadfast commitment to new service delivery mechanisms can achieve success by better meeting client's needs. New programs can be established for those previously served by psychiatric institutions,[33] and organizational problems associated with the closing of a mental hospital can be overcome.[34] The human services' administrator's willingness to battle societal and professional resistance to deinstitutionalization is, of course, a sine qua non in these efforts and upon his fortitude rests the nature of future community programs for the mentally ill and emotionally disturbed.

These models, which in part move state mental health authorities out of the operation and management of direct services, are also part of a national trend similar to that of deinstitutionalization. They permit more adaptive and responsive administrative and structural arrangements for the public administrator. They require, however, new management and planning roles, one major feature of which is the more sophisticated use of standards and regulations that simultaneously promote more effective service delivery, stimulate experimentation and innovation, require evaluation and review, and constrain abuses.[35]

Summary

The caregiving network within which clients' problems are resolved has expanded in recent years to include nonpsychiatric as well as psychiatric concerns. New human services' systems are developing with an emphasis upon comprehensiveness, centralized facilities, and integrated program administration or network models insuring continuity of care. The implications for the mental hospital are profound and challenge its continued viability and very existence. It already is evident that given proper statutory and administrative sanctions, those mental hospitals capable of establishing links to the local human services' system can undergo major change in clients and functions so that within a period of years, some could function as multipurpose human services' centers. A second group of hospitals could provide a variety of residual functions changing over time as alternatives evolve. If they can develop the competence to continually modify and adapt, they may prove to be a very valuable community resource. But in neither case could they reasonably be considered state mental hospitals. They would be whatever they became: halfway house, detoxification center, sheltered residence, workshop, or a combination of these and similar functions. Finally, those mental hospitals that for societally determined or organizationally induced reasons are not functioning within a contemporary framework of systemically related human services should be phased down and closed. These choices and decisions are complex ones dependent upon projected client-utilization patterns, alternative community-based resources, cost benefits, options for fiscal redeployment, and personnel prerogatives. Nevertheless, a commitment to providing clients with optimal services must remain the basic motivation for pursuing change and the mental hospital's future should be resolved only within this framework.

Notes

1. Schulberg, H.C.; Baker, F.; and Roen, S. (eds.), *Developments in Human Services*, vol. I (New York, N.Y.: Behavioral Publications, 1973).

2. March, M., "The Neighborhood Center Concept," *Public Welfare* 26 (1968): 97-111.
3. Demone, H.W., "Human Services at State and Local Levels and the Integration of Mental Health," in G. Caplan (ed.), *American Handbook of Psychiatry*, vol. II (N.Y.: Basic Books, 1974).
4. Baker, F., "From Community Mental Health to Human Service Ideology," *Amer. J. Pub. Hlth.* 64 (1974):576-81.
5. Rabkin, J., "Opinions about Mental Illness: A Review of the Literature," *Psychol. Bull.* 77(1972):153-71.
6. Baker, F. and Schulberg, H.C., "Community Health Caregiving Systems: Integration of Inter-organizational Networks," in A. Sheldon, F. Baker, and C. McLaughlin (eds.), *Systems and Medical Care* (Cambridge, Mass.: M.I.T. Press, 1970), pp. 182-206; Boggs, E., "The Mad Tea Party: An Ecological Approach to Changing Human Service Systems" (Paper presented at Institute on Hospital and Community Psychiatry, St. Louis. Mo., September 26, 1972); Morris, R., "Welfare Reform 1973: The Social Services Dimension," *Science* (1973): 515-22.
7. Chu, F. and Trotter, S., "The Mental Health Complex, Part I," *Community Mental Health Centers* (Washington, D.C.: Center for Study of Responsive Law, 1972).
8. Baker, F. and Schulberg, H.C., "A System Model for Evaluating the Changing Mental Hospital," in F. Baker (ed.), *Organizational Systems* (Homewood, Ill.: Richard D. Irwin, 1973), pp. 476-88.
9. Schulberg, H.C., "The Mental Hospital in the Era of Human Services," *Hosp. & Comm. Psychiat.* 27 (1972): 566-73.
10. Ozarin, L. and Feldman, S., "Implications for Health Service Delivery: The Community Mental Health Centers Amendments of 1970," *Amer. J. Pub. Hlth.* 61 (1971): 1780-84.
11. Subblebine, J. and Decker, J., "Are Urban Mental Health Centers Worth It?" *Amer. J. Psychiat.* 127 (1971): 908-12.
12. Wolford, J.; Hitchcock, J.; Ellison, D.; Sonis, A.; and Smith, F., "The Effect on State Hospitalization of a Community Mental Health/Mental Retardation Center," *Amer. J. Psychiat.* 129 (1972): 202-206.
13. Holder, H. and Stratas, N., "A Systems Approach to Alcoholism Programming," *Amer. J. Psychiat.* 129 (1972): 32-37.
14. Kraft, A.; Binner, P.; and Dickey, B., "The Community Mental Health Program and the Longer-Stay Patient," *Arch. Gen. Psychiat.* 16 (1967): 64-70.
15. Myerson, D., "Can Institutionalization be Prevented?" *Mass. J. Ment. Hlth.* 2 (1972): 17-26.
16. Mendel, W., "On the Abolition of the Psychiatric Hospital," in L. Roberts, N. Greenfield, and M. Miller (Eds.), *Comprehensive Mental Health: The Challenge of Evaluation* (Madison, Wisconsin: University of Wisconsin Press, 1968), pp. 237-47.

17. Polak, P. and Jones, M., "The Psychiatric Nonhospital: A Model for Change," *Comm. Ment. Hlth. J.* 9 (1973): 123-32.
18. Ozarin, L. and Levenson, A., "The Future of the Public Mental Hospital," *Amer. J. Psychiat.* 125 (1969): 1647-52.
19. Greenblatt, M., "The Public Psychiatric Hospital: Room for Optimism," *Amer. J. Psychiat.* 127 (1971): 1397-98.
20. Fisher, M.; Mehr, J.; and Truckenbrud, P., *Power, Greed, and Stupidity in the Mental Health Racket* (Philadelphia, Pa.: Westminister Press, 1973).
21. Bartz, W.; Loy, D.; and Cook, W., "Mental Hospitals and the Winds of Change," *Ment. Hyg.* 55 (1971): 266-69.
22. Psychiatric News, "Alabama Struggles to Meet Court-Imposed Mental Hospital Standards," *Psychiat. News,*vol. VIII, no. 10, May 16, 1973.
23. Chu and Trotter, "The Mental Health Complex."
24. Schulberg, H.C., "The Mental Hospital in the Era of Human Services," *Hosp. & Comm. Psychiat.* 27 (1972): 566-73; "Massachusetts Mental Hospital Planning Project," *Community Mental Health and the Mental Hospital* (Boston, Mass.: United Community Services of Metropolitan Boston, 1973).
25. Psychiatric News, "Alabama Struggles."
26. Crane, G., "Clinical Psychopharmacology in its 20th Year," *Science* 181 (July 1973): 124-28.
27. Stotsky, B.A., "Social and Clinical Issues in Geriatric Psychiatry," *Amer. J. Psychiat.* (1972): 129; Kahn, N.A., "Geriatric Psychiatry," in P. Solomon and V. Patch (eds.), *Handbook of Psychiatry* (N.Y.: Basic Books, 1969).
28. Corsellis, J.A.N., *Mental Illness and the Aging Brain* (New York: Oxford University Press, 1962); National Association for Mental Health, "Reference Tables on Patients in Mental Health Facilities–Age, Sex, and Diagnosis," New York, N.Y., 1968.
29. Stotsky, "Social and Clinical Issues"; Kahn, N.A., "Report of the Office of Geriatrics," *Mass. Dept. of Ment. Hlth,* 1972.
30. Schulberg, "The Mental Hospital," 1972.
31. Broskowski, A.; Demone, H.W., Jr.; and Kaplan, H., "The Influence of State Regulatory Processes on Health Programs," *Human Service Reports* 88 (1973): 562-68.
32. Boggs, "The Mad Tea Party."
33. Oberleder, M., "A State Hospital Closes its Doors to the Elderly," *Gerontologist* 13 (1973): 45-49.
34. Stewart, A.; LaFave, H.; Grunberg, F.; and Herjanic, M., "Problems in Phasing Out a Large Public Psychiatric Hospital, *Amer. J. Psychiat.* 125 (1968): 82-88; Mosher, L. and Gunderson, J., "Special Report: Schizophrenia 1972, *Schizophrenia Bulletin* (1973): 7.
35. Broskowski, A. et al., "The Influence of State Regulatory Processes."

2

Trends and Projections in State Hospital Use
Earl S. Pollack and *Carl A. Taube*

In the 1940s and earlier, the state mental hospital was the primary resource for the treatment of the mentally ill, and, indeed in some states, the only resource. Since that time, the number of facilities that have served as alternatives to the state mental hospital increased rapidly. This trend, in addition to other factors, has produced a dramatic decrease in the size of the state mental hospital population nationwide. Further impetus in this direction was given in 1963 when the president, in his address leading to the community mental health center legislation, stated that, "It will be possible within a decade or two to reduce the number of patients now under custodial care by 50 percent or more. Many more mentally ill can be helped to remain in their own homes without hardship to themselves or their families. Those who are hospitalized can be helped to return to their own communities. All but a small portion can be restored to useful life. We can spare them and their families much of the misery which mental illness now entails."[1]

Nine years after that address, at year-end 1972, the resident population of these hospitals had already decreased 45 percent (from 504,604 to 275,995) and indications are that this decline will continue. This trend raises questions about how state mental hospitals are now being used and about the kind of care required by those who remain in the hospital. In this chapter the trend in the size and composition of the resident population of these hospitals will be analyzed and, based on this analysis, projections will be made to 1975. It may then be possible to form a clearer picture of the nature of the problems that mental hospitals might face so that alternative modes of care can be considered.

Source of Data

The data to be presented in this chapter, obtained annually through the national reporting program of the National Institute of Mental Health, pertain to the United States as a whole. Data on the movement of state and county mental hospital populations have been virtually 100 percent complete over the years and those on the characteristics of patients served by these hospitals have been over 90 percent complete. The data have been adjusted to allow for underreporting, thus, making it possible to estimate changes in the characteristics of these populations over time. Since county mental hospitals exist in only a few states[a] and function

---

[a]Michigan, New Jersey, and Wisconsin.

31

as though they were part of the state mental hospital system, the shorter term
"state mental hospitals" will be used throughout the paper.

Trend in the State Mental Hospital Population

Differences in the size of a resident patient population between two dates
is determined by the number of admissions to and removals from the population during the interval. Removals include the net releases (the number of discharges and placements on long-term leave less the number of returns from such
leave) and deaths. Therefore, the relationship between the trends in admissions,
net releases and deaths affects the trend in the number of resident patients.
Figure 2-1 and Table 2-1 present the number of resident patients, admissions,
net releases and deaths for state mental hospitals over the time period 1950-72.
The number of resident patients increased until 1955 and has been decreasing
ever since. Over the years there have been certain periods characterized by
relatively constant annual rates of change. Between 1950 and 1955 the number
increased by an average of 1.8 percent per year; from 1955-60 it decreased by
0.8 percent per year and from 1960-64 it decreased by 2.1 percent per year.
From 1964 onward, the number of resident patients did not decrease by a
constant rate, but rather by an accelerating rate that averaged 5.5 percent per
year between 1964 and 1972.

Between 1955 and 1964 the number of admissions increased by 6 percent
to 7 percent per year, while the number of net releases increased by 10 percent.
This excess of increasing net releases over increasing admissions resulted in the
decrease in number of resident patients. The average annual increase in both
admissions and net releases from 1964 to 1972 was lower than that for previous
periods because of an actual decrease in both of these measures between 1971
and 1972.

Age and Sex

The size of the resident population of the state mental hospitals changed in
different ways among the various age groups. As is evident from Figure 2-2,
the number in each of the age groups from 25 on has been decreasing since 1955,
with the most striking decreases occurring among females in the age groups
25-34 and 35-44. On the other hand, the numbers in the age groups under 15
and 15-24, which had been increasing, began to level off and decline in the late
1960s. If the number of resident patients is related to the number of individuals
in the corresponding age groups in the general population to obtain rates per
100,000 population, the decreases are even more striking, as indicated in Figure
2-3. The age group under 15 years of age is the only one showing constant
increases over the years.

Figure 2-1. Number of Resident Patients, Total Admissions, Net Releases, and Deaths, State and County Mental Hospitals, United States 1950-1972

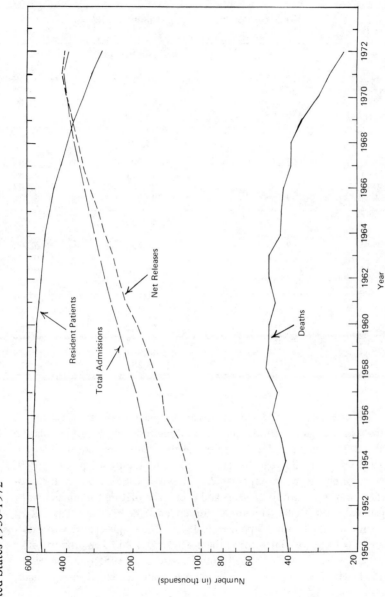

Table 2-1
Average Annual Percent Change in Number of Resident Patients, Admissions, Net Releases and Deaths, State and County Mental Hospitals, United States, 1950-55, 1955-60, 1960-64 and 1964-72

Time Period	Number at Beginning of Period	Number at End of Period	Average Annual Percent Change
	Resident Patients		
1950-55	512,501	558,922	+ 1.81%
1955-60	558,922	535,540	− 0.84%
1960-64	535,540	490,449	− 2.10%
1964-72	490,449	275,995	− 5.47%
	Admissions		
1950-55	152,286	178,003	+ 3.38%
1955-60	178,003	234,791	+ 6.38%
1960-64	234,791	299,561	+ 6.90%
1964-72	299,561	390,000	+ 3.77%
	Net Releases		
1950-55	99,659	126,498	+ 5.39%
1955-60	126,498	192,818	+ 10.49%
1960-64	192,818	268,616	+ 9.83%
1964-72	268,616	401,567	+ 6.19%
	Deaths		
1950-55	41,280	44,384	+ 1.50%
1955-60	44,384	49,748	+ 2.42%
1960-64	49,748	44,824	− 2.47%
1964-72	44,824	23,282	− 6.01%

The effect of these varying trends among age groups can be seen in the changes in the age distribution of the resulting resident patient population (Table 2-2). Among males, 14 percent of the resident patient population in 1971 was under 25 years of age, compared with only 4.5 percent in 1955. This major change was compensated by only modest decreases in the populations in the age group 25 years and over. The picture for females was considerably different. The proportion under 25 in 1971 was only 7.2 percent compared with 2.7 percent in 1955. The major change was a drop from 26 percent to 20 percent in the age group 25-44. The proportion of females 65 and over increased from 30 percent in 1955 to 35 percent in 1971, whereas the proportion in this age group decreased among males.

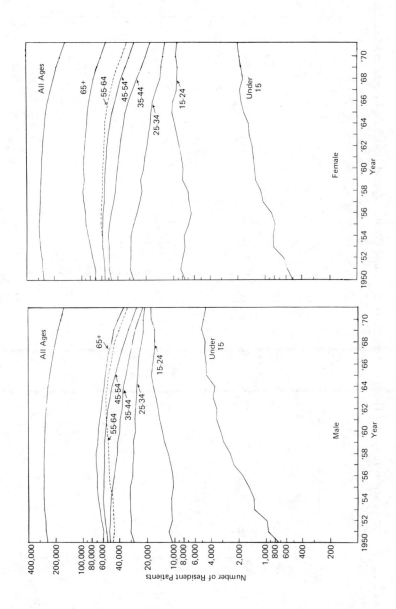

Figure 2-2. Number of Resident Patients, End of Year, State and County Mental Hospitals, by Age and Sex, United States, 1950–71

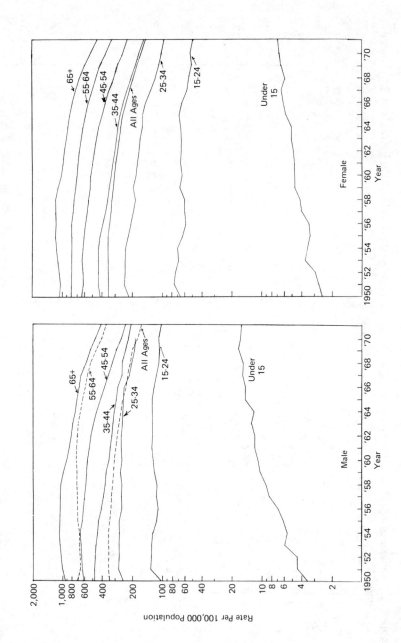

Figure 2-3. Resident Patient Rates per 100,000 Population, State and County Mental Hospitals, by Age and Sex, United States, 1950-71

Table 2-2

Percent Distribution of Resident Patients in State and County Mental Hospitals, by Age and Sex, United States, 1950, 1955, 1966, and 1971

Age and Sex	Year			
	1950	1955	1966	1971
Both sexes, all ages	100.0%	100.0%	100.0%	100.0%
Under 15	0.2	0.4	1.4	2.1
15-24	3.6	3.1	6.0	8.6
25-44	29.7	27.5	22.9	23.4
45-64	41.2	40.6	39.9	37.3
65 and over	25.4	28.3	29.8	28.6
Males, all ages	100.0%	100.0%	100.0%	100.0%
Under 15	0.3	0.6	2.0	2.8
15-24	4.2	3.9	7.8	11.2
25-44	31.2	28.9	25.6	27.0
45-64	40.3	40.6	40.4	36.4
65 and over	24.0	26.0	24.2	22.6
Females, all ages	100.0%	100.0%	100.0%	100.0%
Under 15	0.2	0.3	0.8	1.3
15-24	2.9	2.4	4.3	5.9
25-44	28.2	26.3	20.3	19.7
45-64	42.1	40.7	39.4	38.2
65 and over	26.7	30.4	35.2	34.9

Diagnosis

The diagnostic distribution of resident patients in state mental hospitals has been remarkable for its stability over time, as indicated in Table 2-3. Between 1955 and 1971, the proportion with schizophrenia has remained constant at 48 percent, the proportion with other psychoses has dropped from 12 percent in 1955 to 6 percent in 1971, and the proportion with diseases of the senium decreased only slightly. As one might expect, the proportion with central nervous system syphilis decreased from 6.5 percent in 1950 to 1.7 percent in 1971.

Geographic Changes

When the populations of the state mental hospitals first began to decrease nationwide, between 1955 and 1956, a detailed analysis of this reversal in the

Table 2-3

Percent Distribution of Resident Patients in State and County Mental Hospitals, by Selected Diagnoses, United States, 1950, 1955, 1966, and 1971

	Year			
Diagnosis	*1950*	*1955*	*1966*	*1971*
All diagnoses	100.0%	100.0%	100.0%	100.0%
Schizophrenia	45.3	48.0	48.2	48.2
Other psychoses	*	12.0	9.6	5.8
Diseases of the senium	12.4	13.2	12.4	11.4
Psychoneuroses	0.5	1.0	1.8	2.0
Personality disorders	1.1	1.5	2.3	1.9
Alcoholism	*	3.1	4.7	3.1
Brain syndrome with CNS syphilis	6.5	5.2	2.6	1.7
All other	*	16.0	18.4	25.9

*Categories not comparable with later years.

trend up to that point revealed that a decrease occurred in the mental hospital populations of 45 states.[2] The change, therefore, was not simply a reflection of decreases in the larger state mental hospital systems. Between 1960 and 1972 the populations of the state mental hospital systems decreased in every state without exception, with the size of decreases ranging from 11 percent to 84 percent. The change over that time period for the four major subdivisions of the United States is presented in Table 2-4. The decrease for the United States as a whole was 48 percent, with a low of 30 percent in the southern region and a high of 71 percent in the western region.

Trends in First Admissions

The number of first admissions to state and county mental hospitals for the years 1962, 1965, 1969, and 1972 and the corresponding rates per 100,000 population by age and sex are presented in Table 2-5. The number of male first admissions increased substantially between 1962 and 1969, then decreased

Table 2-4

Number and Percent Change of Resident Patients in State and County Mental Hospitals by Major Geographic Subdivision of the United States, 1960 and 1972

Geographic Area	1960	1972	Percent Change
Total U.S.	528,476	275,735	− 47.8%
Northeast	190,415	102,890	− 46.0%
North Central	148,741	65,786	− 55.8%
Southern	128,133	89,314	− 30.3%
Western	61,187	17,745	− 71.0%

slightly between 1969 and 1972. Female first admissions, on the other hand, increased only slightly between 1962 and 1969, then decreased by 31 percent between 1969 and 1972. These changes occurred differentially for the various age groups. For example, among both males and females, the number of first admissions increased most in the youngest age groups between 1962 and 1969 and decreased among those 65 and over. Among males, the number of first admissions continued to increase in the age groups under 25 between 1969 and 1972, while among females the numbers in these age groups dropped during that period.

The comparison of diagnostic distributions of first admissions over these same years reveals some striking changes (Table 2-6). In 1962 brain syndromes were the leading diagnostic category among first admissions, accounting for 26 percent of the total, but dropped to 10 percent of the total by 1972. Schizophrenia accounted for 21 percent of the first admissions in 1962, compared with only 14 percent in 1972. Alcohol disorders became the leading diagnostic category in 1972, increasing from 15 percent of the total in 1962 to 26 percent in 1972.

Projected Number of Resident Patients

The data presented above make it possible to estimate the future size and composition of the state mental hospital populations if certain assumptions are accepted. To make the estimates, three types of trend lines were fitted to observed data to determine which best describes past trends. The best fitting line was then projected into the future to estimate expected numbers of resident patients and first admissions in specific categories.

Each of these types of trend lines implies a certain assumption about the nature of the trend as follows: (a) the straight line assumes a constant annual

Table 2-5
Number of First Admissions to State and County Mental Hospitals and Rates per 100,000 Population, by Age and Sex, United States, 1962, 1965, 1969, and 1972

Age and Sex	Number of First Admissions				Rates per 100,000 Population			
	1962	1965	1969	1972	1962	1965	1969	1972
Both sexes, all ages	129,698	144,090	163,984	140,813	70.6	75.1	82.1	68.2
Under 15	3,460	4,510	6,553	7,661	6.0	7.5	11.0	13.5
15-24	19,473	25,878	37,507	35,111	76.9	88.6	114.4	95.1
25-34	22,761	25,625	26,614	27,767	105.1	118.5	111.4	103.8
35-44	23,146	25,669	30,779	24,069	96.0	106.6	134.3	107.2
45-54	19,243	21,205	24,676	19,618	91.2	96.6	106.8	83.3
55-64	13,280	14,597	18,264	12,097	82.4	86.1	100.3	63.3
65 and over	28,335	26,606	19,591	14,490	163.7	146.5	100.6	69.2
Males, all ages	72,663	82,536	98,885	95,755	81.4	88.5	102.7	96.0
Under 15	2,339	2,971	4,036	6,713	7.9	9.7	13.4	23.2
15-24	11,330	15,352	22,552	24,337	94.4	109.3	145.5	135.0
25-34	12,301	14,361	16,389	17,857	119.1	138.7	142.7	137.8
35-44	12,938	14,774	17,292	17,635	111.6	127.3	156.6	162.9
45-54	11,442	12,711	16,805	12,286	111.0	119.3	151.2	108.7
55-64	7,731	8,749	10,229	8,851	99.5	107.7	118.6	98.5
65 and over	14,582	13,618	11,582	8,076	188.8	171.7	139.6	93.1
Females, all ages	57,035	61,554	65,099	45,058	60.4	62.4	63.0	42.2
Under 15	1,121	1,539	2,517	948	3.9	5.2	8.7	3.4
15-24	8,143	10,526	14,955	10,774	61.2	69.4	86.5	57.1
25-34	10,460	11,264	10,225	9,910	92.3	100.0	82.4	71.9
35-44	10,208	10,895	13,487	6,434	81.5	87.4	113.5	55.3
45-54	7,801	8,494	7,871	7,332	72.2	75.2	65.7	59.9
55-64	5,549	5,848	8,035	3,246	66.5	66.2	83.8	32.1
65 and over	13,753	12,988	8,009	6,414	143.5	127.0	71.7	52.2

Table 2-6
**Number and Percent Distribution of Admissions with No Prior Inpatient
Psychiatric Care to State and County Mental Hospitals for Selected Diagnostic
Groups, United States, 1962, 1965, 1969, and 1972**

Selected Diagnostic Groups	1962	1965	1969	1972
	Number of First Admissions			
All diagnoses	129,698	144,090	163,984	140,813
Alcohol disorders*	19,406	24,380	42,078	36,788
Drug abuse disorders*	1,652	3,549	6,343	9,093
Brain syndromes	33,978	31,345	25,548	13,910
Schizophrenia	27,266	25,374	24,540	19,607
Other psychoses	9,662	9,683	10,132	4,573
Neuroses	12,191	15,821	19,806	17,406
Personality disorders	11,850	15,295	14,620	14,784
All other diagnoses	13,693	18,643	20,917	24,652
	Percent Distribution			
All diagnoses	100.0%	100.0%	100.0%	100.0%
Alcohol disorders*	15.0	16.9	25.7	26.1
Drug abuse disorders*	1.3	2.5	3.9	6.5
Brain syndromes	26.2	21.8	15.6	9.9
Schizophrenia	21.0	17.6	15.0	13.9
Other psychoses	7.4	6.7	6.2	3.2
Neuroses	9.4	11.0	12.1	12.4
Personality disorders	9.1	10.6	8.9	10.5
All other diagnoses	10.6	12.9	12.8	17.5

*
Includes those in the corresponding Brain Syndromes category.

change in the *number* of resident patients; (b) the straight line fitted to loga-
rithms of the observations implies a constant annual *percentage* change in the
number of resident patients; and (c) the quadratic implies a straight line trend
in the annual percent change over the period under consideration. It should
be emphasized that data do not fulfill the assumptions necessary for rigorous
mathematical application of these trend lines. For example, the assumption
that successive observations are independent of one another is not fulfilled
since the number of resident patients at the end of a particular year is not
independent of the number at the end of the preceding year. Nevertheless,
fitting these trend lines provides a convenient means of describing the data
and of raising questions about factors related to these trends.

The numbers of resident patients by age and by major diagnostic category
were available for each year 1961 to 1971. Data between the period 1961 to

1970 were used for the purpose of fitting trend lines, and the observed 1971 data were used for comparison against the 1971 projected estimates based on the fitted trend lines. In Table 2-7, the projected numbers of total resident patients at the end of 1971 and 1972 were estimated based on each of the three types of trend lines mentioned above and compared with the observed number of resident patients. Each of these three types of trend lines was fitted in turn to number of resident patients for successively longer periods of time during the ten-year period, beginning with the latest four years. Using only the latest four years, the fitted straight line provided the best estimate of 1971 and 1972 numbers, thus, indicating that perhaps for that four-year period and the two succeeding years the number of resident patients was decreasing by a constant annual number. However, if each of the types of trend lines is fitted to the entire ten years of observations, the quadratic provides by far the best estimates of the 1971 and 1972 values. This would seem to indicate that over the entire period the annual *percent change* in number of resident patients follows a straight line downward.

Table 2-7

Projected Number of Resident Patients in State and County Mental Hospitals at End of 1971 and 1972, Based on Three Types of Curves Fitted to Observations Over Varying Periods

Time Period of Observations	Year Projected or Observed	Observed Number of Resident Patients	Projected Number of Resident Patients		
			Straight Line	Straight Line to Logs	Quadratic
1967–70	1971	309,017	309,449	314,518	302,958
	1972	275,995	279,924	291,045	265,643
1966–70	1971	309,017	311,444	317,680	303,861
	1972	275,995	282,916	295,443	267,750
1965–70	1971	309,017	313,913	321,162	303,947
	1972	275,995	286,444	300,080	267,935
1964–70	1971	309,017	318,414	325,958	301,468
	1972	275,995	292,632	306,260	262,977
1963–70	1971	309,017	323,430	331,024	300,298
	1972	275,995	299,320	312,622	260,768
1962–70	1971	309,017	328,936	336,328	299,749
	1972	275,995	306,478	319,150	259,780
1961–70	1971	309,017	334,148	341,362	300,688
	1972	275,995	313,112	325,242	261,400

In Table 2-8 the projected numbers of resident patients by age and diagnosis for 1971, based on a fit of the quadratic curve to the 1961-70 observations, were compared with the corresponding observed numbers of resident patients. The projections overestimated the numbers in the age groups under 15 and 65 and over and consistently underestimated the numbers in the intermediate age groups. However, the differences were relatively small. The estimates also appeared to be relatively close to the observed values for each age group within the three selected diagnostic categories. Based on these fitted trend lines, then, the number of resident patients was projected to 1975 within each age-diagnostic category (Table 2-9). If the assumption is valid that the number of resident patients in each of these categories during the period 1961-70 follows a quadratic trend and that this trend will continue to 1975, there will be 125,286 resident patients in state and county mental hospitals at the end of 1975. This would be a 60 percent decrease from the actual number in these hospitals at the end of 1971. The expected percent changes between 1971 and 1975 within each age-diagnostic category is presented in Table 2-10 (p. 46). There would be an expected increase of just under 3 percent in the age group under 15 years, but an expected decrease of 80 percent in the age group 35-44.

Projected Numbers of First Admissions

The numbers of first admissions by age were available each year for the period 1962-68 as well as for 1969 and 1972. The same three types of trend lines mentioned above were fitted to the observed numbers of first admissions for the period 1962-68 within each age-sex group. Based on these trend lines, numbers of first admissions were projected to 1969 and 1972, respectively, and compared with the corresponding observed numbers. The results are presented in Table 2-11 (pp. 47-49). For both sexes combined in 1969, each of the trend lines provides a fairly good estimate of the number of each age group with the exception of the 65 and over group where the estimates are about 35 percent higher than the observed. For 1972 all of the estimates are much too high except for the number in the age group under 15.

The differences between observed and predicted numbers of first admissions were much greater for males than for females. This is undoubtedly accounted for by the fact that the trend in first admissions for each sex increased between 1962 and 1968, but the actual number of male first admissions decreased by 3 percent between 1969 and 1972, while the number of female first admissions decreased by 31 percent during that same period.

Discussion

The data presented above describe the change in numbers and selected characteristics of resident patients in and first admissions to state mental hospitals. It is

Table 2-8
Comparison of Projected and Observed Number of Resident Patients at End of 1971, by Age and Diagnosis, Where Projections are Based on a Quadratic Curve Fitted to 1961-70 Observations

Diagnosis		All Ages	Age							
			Under 15	15-24	25-34	35-44	45-54	55-64	65+
All diagnoses	projected	300,688	6,756	24,324	31,720	36,145	49,279	62,243	90,221
	observed	309,017	6,379	26,594	33,099	39,277	52,038	63,242	88,388
Schizophrenia	projected	143,360	1,534	9,193	17,792	20,462	27,246	34,048	33,086
	observed	148,842	1,466	10,849	18,819	22,439	29,259	34,161	31,849
Diseases of senium	projected	36,468						3,730	31,360
	observed	35,207						4,721	30,486
Other	projected	120,859	5,222	15,115	13,846	15,411	21,025	24,466	25,775
	observed	124,968	4,913	14,745	14,280	16,838	22,779	24,360	26,053

Table 2-9
Projected Number of Resident Patients in State and County Mental Hospitals at End of 1975, by Age and Diagnosis, Where Projections are Based on a Quadratic Curve Fitted to 1961–70 Observations

Diagnosis	All Ages	Under 15	15-24	25-34	35-44	45-54	55-64	65+
				Age				
All Diagnoses	125,286	6,548	17,800	23,200	7,819	13,641	17,126	39,151
Schizophrenia	53,431	879	4,036	11,816	2,700	3,835	10,629	19,535
Diseases of senium*	16,614						1,994	11,053
Other	55,241	5,668	13,721	11,171	4,414	7,201	4,503	8,563

*In computing projections, those with diseases of the senium who were less than 55 years of age were included in the 55–64 year age group, but for all diagnoses combined they were included in the appropriate age group. Therefore, for ages under 55, the numbers in the diagnostic categories do not add to the total for all diagnoses.

Table 2-10

Percent Change Between Number of Resident Patients in State and County Mental Hospitals at End of 1971 and Projected Number at End of 1975, by Age and Selected Diagnoses, United States

Diagnosis	All Ages	Under 15	15-24	25-34	35-44	45-54	55-64	65+
					Age			
All diagnoses	− 59.5	+ 2.6	− 33.1	− 29.9	− 80.1	− 73.8	− 72.9	− 55.7
Schizophrenia	− 64.1	− 40.0	≅ 62.8	− 37.2	− 88.0	− 86.9	− 68.9	− 38.7
Diseases of senium	− 52.8						− 57.8	− 63.7
Other	− 55.8	+ 15.4	− 12.9	− 21.8	− 73.8	− 68.4	− 81.5	− 67.1

Table 2-11a

Comparison of Projected and Observed Numbers of First Admissions for 1969 and 1972, by Age, Where the Projections are Based on Three Types of Curves Fitted to 1962-68 Observed Numbers

		Both Sexes		
			Projected	
Age	*Observed*	*Straight Line*	*Straight Line to Logs*	*Quadratic*
			1969	
All ages	163,984	168,673	170,051*	171,890
Under 15	6,553	5,881	6,091	6,161
15-24	37,507	34,047	35,216	34,685
25-34	26,614	29,941	30,181	31,071
35-44	30,779	30,016	30,252	29,990
45-54	24,676	24,948	25,158	25,503
55-64	18,264	17,437	17,596	17,610
65 and over	19,591	26,403	26,409	26,870
			1972	
All ages	140,813	186,256	191,891*	198,319
Under 15	7,661	7,027	7,932	8,072
15-24	35,111	40,345	45,131	42,734
25-34	27,767	33,216	34,271	37,455
35-44	24,069	32,958	33,874	32,864
45-54	19,618	27,591	28,452	29,671
55-64	12,097	19,318	19,961	19,970
65 and over	14,490	25,801	25,833	27,553

*Numbers for all ages were estimated independently; therefore, the total based on logs does not equal the sum of the numbers in the age groups.

important to review factors likely to have had an influence on these changes in order to assess the expected impact of future policies on the state mental hospitals.

The facts concerning the resident patient population of the state mental hospitals are quite clear. The number of resident patients increased at a constant rate from 1950 to 1955 and has been decreasing ever since, with this decrease accelerating rapidly since the early 1960s. The age composition has remained relatively constant over the years with the exception of an increase in the proportion under 25 years of age. The diagnostic composition has remained remarkably constant.

Table 2-11b
Comparison of Projected and Observed Numbers of First Admissions for 1969
and 1972, by Age, Where the Projections are Based on Three Types of Curves
Fitted to 1962-68 Observed Numbers

		Males		
		Projected		
Age	*Observed*	*Straight Line*	*Straight Line to Logs*	*Quadratic*
		1969		
All ages	98,885	100,522	101,684*	104,221
Under 15	4,036	3,850	3,970	4,033
15-24	22,552	20,915	21,747	21,583
25-34	16,389	17,877	18,135	18,923
35-44	17,292	18,084	18,304	18,520
45-54	16,805	15,416	15,570	16,163
55-64	10,229	10,938	11,085	11,240
65 and over	11,582	13,442	13,449	13,759
		1972		
All ages	95,755	113,074	118,019*	126,942
Under 15	6,713	4,564	5,080	5,248
15-24	24,337	25,067	28,558	27,570
25-34	17,857	20,431	21,595	24,354
35-44	17,635	20,330	21,237	21,966
45-54	12,286	17,271	17,946	20,070
55-64	8,851	12,362	12,973	13,495
65 and over	8,076	13,049	13,079	14,239

*Numbers for all ages were estimated independently; therefore, the total based on logs
does not equal the sum of the numbers in the age groups.

The data on admissions represent a more volatile picture. The number of
total admissions has increased steadily from 1950 to 1971 and then decreased
to 1972. The number of first admissions increased steadily until 1969 and then
decreased substantially between 1969 and 1972, particularly among females
and especially from age 35 onward. The diagnostic distribution of first admissions has changed drastically from 1962 to 1972 with alcohol disorders now by
far the most frequent cause of first admission to state mental hospitals.

Although the characteristics of patients admitted to the state mental hospitals have changed, the nature of the turnover has been such that the characteristics
of the residual population have remained virtually the same. The types of patients

Table 2-11c

Comparison of Projected and Observed Numbers of First Admissions for 1969 and 1972, by Age, Where the Projections are Based on Three Types of Curves Fitted to 1962-68 Observed Numbers

		Females		
		Projected		
Age	Observed	Straight Line	Straight Line to Logs	Quadratic
		1969		
All ages	65,099	68,151	68,442*	67,669
Under 15	2,517	2,031	2,124	2,128
15-24	14,955	13,132	13,483	13,102
25-34	10,225	12,064	12,091	12,148
35-44	13,487	11,932	11,967	11,470
45-54	7,871	9,532	9,587	9,340
55-64	8,035	6,499	6,522	6,370
65 and over	8,009	12,961	12,960	13,111
		1972		
All ages	45,058	73,182	74,300*	71,377
Under 15	948	2,463	2,865	2,824
15-24	10,774	15,278	16,659	15,164
25-34	9,910	12,785	12,900	13,101
35-44	6,434	12,628	12,755	10,898
45-54	7,332	10,320	10,528	9,601
55-64	3,246	6,956	7,051	6,475
65 and over	6,414	12,752	12,757	13,314

*Numbers for all ages were estimated independently; therefore, the total based on logs does not equal the sum of the numbers in the age groups.

who have become chronic in the hospital have not changed over the years. Half of the hospital population are schizophrenics, many of whom have been hospitalized for a long period. Planning for the future role of the state hospital must take this into account.

There appears to be no question that the sudden decrease in the state mental hospital population in 1956, after steady increases since World War II, was due to the widespread introduction of the psychoactive drugs into the mental hospitals.[3] This factor undoubtedly played a large role in the subsequent rapid increase in movement of the mental hospital populations. This increased movement can be seen by the rapid rise in admissions and net releases, noted above, during a period when the size of the hospital population has been decreasing rapidly. Further evidence of this increased turnover can be seen in a comparison of the probability of release among admissions to state mental hospitals at different points in time. A study of the probability of release among first admissions to eleven state mental hospital systems in 1954 found a range of 14 percent to 53 percent released within the first three months after admission and 29 percent to 68 percent within the first six months.[4] Although there are no comparable data on first admissions for the same states for a later period, a sample survey of total admissions to state mental hospitals in 1971 revealed that 75 percent were released within the first three months and 87 percent within the first six months.[5] Data for the State of Maryland, collected in a comparable fashion over a period of years, indicated that among those admitted to state hospitals in 1958, 11 percent were discharged in less than one month, compared with 41 percent among those admitted in 1968.[6]

The increase in use of other types of facilities as alternatives to the state mental hospital has resulted in a decreasing role of the state mental hospital in the total picture of care of the mentally ill. This change can be seen in Table 2-12, which presents the number of patient care episodes by type of psychiatric facility for 1955, 1965, 1968, and 1971. In 1955, 49 percent of the patient care episodes were in state mental hospitals, and this proportion decreased steadily to 19 percent in 1971. Concurrently, the proportion of patient care episodes in outpatient psychiatric services increased from 23 percent in 1955 to 42 percent in 1971. As the community mental health centers came into being, they began to assume a share of the patient care load, and by 1971 their proportion of total patient care episodes equaled that of the state mental hospitals.

The variation among age groups in the proportion of total patient care episodes accounted for by state mental hospitals is considerable, as seen in Table 2-13. In 1971, 5 percent of the patient care episodes among persons under 18 years of age were in state mental hospitals. This proportion increased with increasing age to 51 percent in the age group 65 and over. Although this latter figure represents a decrease from 60 percent in 1966, one-half of the patient care episodes in psychiatric facilities for those aged 65 and over were in state mental hospitals in 1971.

It should be emphasized that the data on patient care episodes given above pertain only to *psychiatric* facilities. They do not include other types of facilities that provide care for persons with emotional or mental problems. Part of the acceleration of the population decrease in the state and county mental hospitals in the 1960s was undoubtedly due to placement of long-term chronic patients into nursing homes. Of the 37,000 releases from state mental hospitals among those 65 and over in 1969, for example, 14,000 (38 percent) were referred to nursing homes or homes for the aged.[7] Surveys of nursing and personal care homes have been conducted to determine the number of residents

Table 2-12
Number and Percentage Distribution of Patient Care Episodes by Type of Psychiatric Facility, United States, 1955, 1965, 1968, and 1971

| Year | All Facilities | Inpatient Services | | | | | Outpatient Psychiatric Services | Community Mental Health Centers* |
		All Inpatient Services	State and County Mental Hospitals	Private Mental Hospitals	General Hospital Psychiatric Service	VA Hospitals		
			Number of Patient Care Episodes					
1955	1,675,352	1,296,352	818,832	123,231	265,934	88,355	379,000	N.A.
1965	2,636,525	1,565,525	804,926	125,428	519,328	115,843	1,071,000	N.A.
1968	3,380,818	1,602,238	791,819	118,126	558,790	133,503	1,507,000	271,590
1971	4,009,506	1,562,664	745,259	97,963	542,642	176,800	1,693,848	752,994
			Percent Distribution					
1955	100.0%	77.4	48.9	7.3	15.9	5.3	22.6	N.A.
1965	100.0%	59.4	30.5	4.8	19.7	4.4	40.6	N.A.
1968	100.0%	47.3	23.4	3.5	16.5	3.9	44.7	8.0
1971	100.0%	39.0	18.6	2.5	13.5	4.4	42.3	18.8

*Includes inpatient units of community mental health centers.

Table 2-13

Number of Patient Care Episodes in All Psychiatric Facilities and in State and County Mental Hospitals, by Age, United States, 1966 and 1971

| | | | Patient Care Episodes | |
| | | | State Mental Hospitals | |
Age	Year	All Facilities	Number	% of Total
All ages	1966	2,772,089	802,216	28.9%
	1971	4,038,143	745,259	18.5%
Under 18	1966	485,729	36,902	7.6%
	1971	771,874	39,196	5.1%
18-24	1966	334,422	53,748	16.1%
	1971	681,641	97,285	14.3%
25-44	1966	959,959	239,060	24.9%
	1971	1,433,133	236,337	16.5%
45-64	1966	678,965	283,985	41.8%
	1971	888,231	238,710	26.9%
65 and over	1966	313,014	188,521	60.2%
	1971	263,264	133,731	50.8%

of these homes who might be considered to have a diagnosis of mental disorder or senility. The results of such surveys in 1964 and 1969 are presented in Table 2-14.[8] The number of residents of these homes with mental disorders or senility was 607,000 in 1969, almost one and one-half times the number in 1964. Of these individuals in 1969, 542,000 were 65 and over, almost five times the number in that age group in state mental hospitals. Even if allowance is made for inaccuracy of diagnosis in nursing homes, it seems fairly certain that the entire range of purely *psychiatric* facilities cares for less than half of the aged mentally ill.

This rather widespread placement of patients in nursing homes undoubtedly contributed to changes in the length of stay distribution in the state mental hospitals. Table 2-15 shows a decrease of 35 percent in the state mental hospital population between 1960 and 1970, but decreases in the long-stay groups, 5-10 years and 10 years or more, were 54 percent and 39 percent respectively. These groups contributed heavily to the nursing home placements.

Conclusions

The factors that could potentially have an impact on the future role and use of the state mental hospital are many and diverse, ranging from the passage

Table 2-14

Number of Residents with Mental Disorders and Senility in Nursing and Personal Care Homes, by Age and Sex, 1964 and 1969

		Year	Percent Change
Sex and Age	May -June 1964	June -August 1969	1964-69
Both sexes, all ages	249,159	607,377	+ 143.8%
Under 65	34,956	65,623	+ 87.7%
65 and over	214,203	541,754	+ 152.9%
Males, all ages	83,630	184,650	+ 120.8%
Under 65	18,067	30,524	+ 68.9%
65 and over	65,563	154,126	+ 135.1%
Females, all ages	165,529	422,727	+ 155.4%
Under 65	16,889	35,099	+ 107.8%
65 and over	148,640	387,628	+ 160.8%

Source: U.S. Department of Health, Education and Welfare, National Center for Health Statistics. Prevalence of chronic conditions and impairments among residents of nursing and personal care homes. PHS Publication No. 1000–Series 12, No. 8, 1967.

U.S. Department of Health Education and Welfare, National Center for Health Statistics. Chronic conditions and impairments of nursing home residents, 1969. In press.

Table 2-15

Number of Resident Patients in State Mental Hospitals by Length of Stay, United States, 1960 and 1970

Length of Stay	1960	1970	Percent Change
Total	541,625	350,276	-35.3%
Less than 1.5 years	115,548	96,333	-16.6%
1.5-4.9 years	133,038	88.415	-33.5%
5-9.9 years	96,070	44,563	-53.6%
10 years or more	196,969	120,965	-38.6%

Source: U.S. Department of Commerce, Bureau of the Census, U.S. Census of Population 1960, Report PC(2)–8A, Inmates of Institutions, U.S. Government Printing Office, 1963 and unpublished data from the 1970 Census.

of federal and state laws to the changing of professional and public opinion. While it is beyond the scope of this chapter to try to list these potential events and their impact, a few illustrations are offered to demonstrate the complexity and diversity of the forces that affect the role of the state mental hospital.

Among other factors resulting in decreases in the state hospital population are deliberate policies or legislation on the part of the states to foster the use of alternatives to the state mental hospital. In California, for example, two major pieces of legislation, the Short-Doyle Act in 1957 and the Lanterman-Petris-Short Act in 1967, provided for state support to local communities for the provision of mental health services.[9] This undoubtedly played a major role in the dramatic decrease in California's state mental hospital population, which dropped by 76 percent between 1960 and 1972, the second largest decrease among the 50 states.

In New York State a selective admission policy for geriatric patients was introduced in 1968 whereby priority for admission to the state hospital among the elderly was given to those with a major psychiatric illness that responds well to modern treatment methods.[10] The expectation was that potential elderly patients with serious *physical* problems could best be treated in a general hospital and those who are mildly confused but without a family could be cared for in foster homes or homes for the aged. One year later the impact of this policy was beginning to appear in the form of a reduction in admission in those aged 65 and over from 1,964 in March-May, 1962 to 1,139 during the same three months in 1969, a decrease of 42 percent.

Of the 404,000 admissions to state hospitals in 1972, 169,000 were involuntary civil commitments. This category includes emergency and judicial commitments, civil commitments of alcoholics, drug addicts, sexual psychopaths, defective delinquents, juveniles, mentally retarded, and persons found not guilty of criminal charges by reason of insanity. State legislation requires that such involuntary civil commitments be to a state mental hospital in only ten states. The force of public and professional opinion to date, however, has resulted in the commitment of such persons to state hospitals in all other states as well. Failure to change these circumstances will presumably result in a similar irreducible number of such admissions annually to state mental hospitals.

Those with a primary diagnosis of alcoholism account for one-fourth of the total annual admissions to state mental hospitals. Several factors that have recently occurred or are currently developing may have a considerable impact on the use of the state mental hospital in the treatment of alcoholism.

1. Two states, Wisconsin[b] and Minnesota,[c] have passed laws recently requiring that all health insurance policies written within the state include

---

[b]Wisconsin, A.1348, 6/2/72.
[c]Minnesota, S.1895, 5/23/73.

benefits for the treatment of alcoholism. Similar bills have been proposed in eight other states. On the federal level, the passage of some form of national health insurance will undoubtedly have an effect on where alcoholism is treated.

2. As of August 1973, 17 states have adopted the Uniform Alcoholism and Intoxication Treatment Act or similar legislation, stating that alcoholics and intoxicated persons may not be subjected to criminal prosecution but should be afforded a continuum of treatment within the health or mental health system.[11] The locale of such treatment varies with the specific provisions of the law and the professional and public opinion regarding the alcoholic patient.

3. Legislation currently pending at the federal level (S.1125) would broaden the prohibition against discrimination by public or private general hospitals in admitting or treating alcohol abusers and alcoholics who are suffering from medical conditions solely because of their alcohol abuse or alcoholism.[d] Passage of such legislation could conceivably have an impact on the number of alcoholism admissions to state mental hospitals.

If reductions in the state mental hospital populations are to continue, they can occur either as a net result of forces already in operation or as a result of careful planning by directors of state mental health programs to prevent admissions to the hospitals, to reduce length of stay among those admitted and to find alternative settings for the care of the more chronic patients. Such planning can be carried out more efficiently if based on more specific quantitative information. Information of this type was obtained as part of a study of the needs of the patient population of the state mental hospitals in Texas in 1966.[12] The basic question under study was: If availability of facilities were not a factor, what is the most appropriate setting for the care of patients in the hospital as of July 1, 1966? A stratified random sample of patients was evaluated in relation to this question and was assigned to one of the eleven categories listed in Table 2-16. The results indicated that one-quarter were considered suitable for release from institutional care, almost one-third for transfer to some other form of institutional care and 43 percent were judged to be suitable for further care in state hospitals. A similar assessment of patients in St. Elizabeths Hospital, Washington, D.C., on May 31, 1970, revealed that only 32 percent were considered to be suitable for further care in the hospital, over one-half were deemed to be candidates for nursing home or foster home placement and almost 13 percent were considered able to live in independent settings outside the hospital (Table 2-17).[13]

While a further list of factors that would affect the future size of the state mental hospital population could be given, there is undoubtedly an irreducible

---

[d]U.S. Congress, Senate, S.1125, Comprehensive Alcohol Abuse and Alcoholism Prevention, Treatment, and Rehabilitation Act Amendments of 1973.

Table 2-16

Sample of Resident Patients in Texas State Mental Hospitals by Setting Judged Most Suitable for Care, July 1, 1966

Placement Category	Number	Percent of Total
Total in Sample	1,535	100.0%
Group I: Suitable for release from institutional care	386	25.1
Living outside on own	34	2.2
Outpatient psychiatric care	171	11.1
Halfway house, foster care	181	11.8
Outpatient medical and surgical care	0	0.0
Group II: Suitable for transfer to other institutional care	489	31.9
Nursing home, psychiatric support	361	23.5
Nursing home, medical support	18	1.2
Chronic disease hospital	5	0.3
Acute general hospital	6	0.4
Day or night hospital	99	6.4
Group III: Suitable for retention in mental hospital	660	43.0
Mental hospital—open ward	285	18.6
Mental hospital—closed ward	375	24.4

Source: Report of the Administrative Survey of Texas State Mental Hospitals, Mental Health Project Grant No. 09235-01 of NIMH.

number of individuals who will continue to require long-term care. Although this number is likely to be less than 150,000, careful plans must be made to afford them optimal care in the most appropriate setting.

Notes

1. President of the United States, message relative to mental illness and mental retardation, 88th Congress, February 5, 1963, House of Representatives, Document No. 58, Washington, D.C.
2. Kramer, M. and Pollack, E.S., "Problems in the Interpretation of Trends in the Population Movement of the Public Mental Hospitals, *Journal of the American Public Health Association* 48:1003-19, August 1958.

Table 2-17
**Recommended Placement of Patients Resident in St. Elizabeths
Hospital, Washington, D.C., on May 31, 1970**

Recommended Placement Category	Number of Resident Patients	Percent of Total
All patients	3,603	100.0%
Own home, apt., etc.	453	12.6
Foster home	1,248	34.6
Nursing home	745	20.7
Psychiatric hospital	1,157	32.1

Source: Preliminary Findings from the Psychiatric Inventory, unpublished study, St. Elizabeths Hospital, Washington, D.C., 1970.

3. Brill, H. and Patton, R.E., "Analysis of 1955-1956 Population Fall in New York State Mental Hospitals in First Year of Large-Scale Use of Tranquilizing Drugs," *Am. J. Psychiat.* 114, 6:509-17, 1957.
4. Pollack, E.S.; Person, P.H.; Kramer, M.; and Goldstein, H., "Patterns of Retention, Release and Death of First Admissions to State Mental Hospitals," DHEW Public Health Monograph No. 58, PHS Publication No. 672, 1959.
5. U.S. Department of Health, Education and Welfare, "Length of Stay of Admissions to State and County Mental Hospitals, United States 1971," Statistical Note 74, National Institute of Mental Health, February 1973.
6. _____ , "Length of Stay—State and County Mental Hospitals, Selected States," Statistical Note 20, National Institute of Mental Health, April 1970.
7. _____ , "Referral of Discontinuations from Inpatient Services of State and County Mental Hospitals, United States 1969," Statistical Note 57, National Institute of Mental Health, November 1971.
8. _____ , National Center for Health Statistics, "Prevalence of Chronic Conditions and Impairments Among Residents of Nursing and Personal Care Homes," PHS Publication No. 1000—Series 12, No. 8, 1967; , National Center for Health Statistics, "Chronic Conditions and Impairments of Nursing Home Residents, 1969, In press.
9. California Department of Mental Hygiene, "California Community Mental Health Service Programs," 1967.
10. Kobrynski, B. and Miller, A.D., "The Role of the State Hospital in the Care of the Elderly," *Journal of the American Geriatric Society* 18:3, March 1970.

11. National Conference of Commissioners on Uniform State Laws. Uniform Alcoholism and Intoxication Treatment Act, approved at 80th Conference, August 21-28, 1971, National Conference of Commissioners on Uniform State Laws, 1155 East 60th Street, Chicago, Illinois.

12. Texas Department of Mental Health and Mental Retardation, "Report of the administrative survey of Texas State Mental Hospitals," Austin, Texas, 1966.

13. U.S. Department of Health, Education and Welfare, National Institute of Mental Health, St. Elizabeth's Hospital, "Preliminary Findings from Psychiatric Inventory," unpublished study, Washington D.C., 1970.

**Part II
Outside Pressures for Change**

Introduction to Part II

Two major forces currently acting to bring about change in state hospitals are the judicial system and the consumer movement.

The law as a major element in the administration of state hospitals is a relatively recent development. Hardly more than ten years ago it would have been inconceivable that a judge would take seriously a suit by a patient in a state hospital, against the hospital, to improve conditions at the hospital or to provide damages for improper treatment. The limits of judicial involvement at that time were typically (1) the commitment of patients after relatively brief hearings at which the patients might not even be present; and (2) the rapid disposal of requests for writs of habeas corpus by patients who wished to be released from the hospital against the desires of their physicians.

For reasons that, in retrospect, are understandable but nontheless disturbing, it seemed hardly to occur to jurists or psychiatrists that patients were human beings with constitutional rights and that no matter how seriously ill, some of the things patients complained about made sense a good deal of the time. Even more startling is the recognition now that at the time when mental hospitals were far worse as treatment facilities than they are at present, and, in fact, where the typical hospital gave no treatment at all, thousands of patients were annually involuntarily incarcerated for nonexistent treatment. This incarceration, prescribed with the best of intentions, can only have damaged hundreds of thousands of innocent persons over the years.

Even now, there are many mental health professionals who resist legal attacks on the quality of care in state hospitals but yet who seem to offer no alternative means of improving quality. Even now there are few law schools offering courses so that attorneys will be sufficiently knowledgeable in the intricacies of mental health law and better able to defend the rights of state hospital patients.

But major progress has been made, nevertheless. Indeed, one of the striking discoveries of a review of all the papers presented at the 1973 conference on "The Future Role of the State Hospital" is that if case law already in existence in a number of the states were to be applied across the board in all states, state hospital systems would have to close. Clearly, cases such as *Lessard* v. *Schmidt* are incompatible with the current practice of admission to state hospitals.

In Chapter 3, Judge Franklin N. Flaschner, who is chief justice of the District Court of Massachusetts, reviews the law's new look at inpatient hospitalization. Judge Flaschner has been crucially involved in the development of Massachusetts' new mental health law, and for many years has been active in mental health concerns in Massachusetts. He has been a lecturer and a visitor on the national scene and is well aware of developments across the country. During his presentation at the conference, some of his purely descriptive statements were so shocking and annoying to mental health professionals in the audience that it seemed as if he personally was about to bear the brunt of their anger. As disturbing as it may be to some individuals, our own impression is that Judge Flaschner's presentation is quite moderate and is a conservative interpretation of what is happening.

In Chapter 4, Bruce Ennis, who for several years has been the full-time director of the Mental Health Law Project of the American Civil Liberties Union, describes his involvement in key cases that have changed the legal status of inpatient state hospital care. Mr. Ennis is one of the "new breed" of attorneys who have specialized in social welfare issues regardless of the fact that few of their clients could afford to pay for their services. Although Mr. Ennis' view will seem unsympathetic to some, he writes after perhaps having grown cynical from experience in dealing with state hospital systems.

In Chapter 5, Dr. Michael Peszke, who is one of the small group of psychiatrists specializing in the area of law and psychiatry, reviews the history and likely future course of legal aspects of the state hospital admission process. State hospitals have the advantage (or the torment, depending on one's point of view) of having all of their administrative decisions open to judicial review. With conditions as they currently are, it is very hard for a state hospital administrator to make a mistake and have it go unreversed for very long. Dr. Peszke indicates some of the reasons that this has come about.

In Chapter 6, William Carnahan discusses the newly enacted New York State Mental Hygiene Law, which is far in advance of provisions in other states in the ways in which it attempts to protect the rights of patients. Mr. Carnahan, trained through the Harvard Law School graduate course in law and psychiatry, specializes in mental health law and is co-author of a recent book on New York State mental hygiene law. This law, although a major step forward, is so complex that there are few individuals in New York State (quite likely including those who wrote the law) who understand all of its ramifications. Mr. Carnahan attempts to dissipate some of the mystery.

While some professionals do advocate patient review of programs, more often the issue of consumerism arises as the question of the proper role of citizen review and advisory boards. Among professionals this issue has come to have an importance that goes beyond the question of whether or not citizen boards can effectively promote better patient care. Since the 1960s, how an institution uses a citizen board has for some professionals become a measure of the effectiveness of a program. Certain professionals favor strong citizen boards as an article of faith. For this group, a strong board is a prerequisite to any effective treatment of the mentally ill. Proponents of strong boards argue that they must be vested with ultimate policy-setting powers and the authority to hire and dismiss all key program personnel. Armed with these powers, boards are to insure that programs remain innovative, responsive to their communities, and generally accountable. It is their responsibility to insure that the care given is humane and that professional interests do not come to predominate over the needs of the patients.

While the use of this kind of citizen board is generally seen as a basic tenet of the community mental health approach to care, it is difficult to find theoretical roots for this type of citizen involvement in the mental health literature much before the passage of the federal community mental health center legislation. Daniel Moynihan has traced the recent history of the citizen board movement in public services from its inception as an academic theory through its development in private philanthropic organizations such as the Ford Foundation to its eventual emergence as a keystone of the now defunct antipoverty programs of the Kennedy and Johnson administrations. The first mental health center legislation was drafted at the same time that the antipoverty programs were being developed. The legislation authorizing support of staff salaries in mental health centers marked the first time that the federal government offered direct funding of any form of health care for all citizens. There was major objection from various interest groups to this kind of federal involvement in health care. It was recognized early that the legislation could be passed only with strong support from the executive branch. In this atmosphere it was logical for those drafting the mental health center legislation to include in it proposals already known to be in favor with the administration, such as strong community control of the proposed programs, without too much consideration to the effect community control might have on the programs themselves.

There is a long history of citizen involvement in mental health and a strong argument can be made that most of the major changes in the care of the mentally ill have resulted from direct citizen input. The state hospital movement was spearheaded by Dorothea Dix, the mental health movement was led by Clifford Beers, a former mental patient, and the state hospital reform movement was the result of the muckraking efforts of newspaper reporter Albert Deutsch. However, the form of input proposed in the 1960s involves citizens going well beyond the role of program critics or advocates. It calls for citizen selection of the program staff and the content of the program. This raises serious questions about the functioning of the entire mental health system. There is no interlocking hierarchy of citizen boards corresponding to the different levels of government operation. The board responsible for a single local program is not itself accountable to a higher regional citizen board, which in turn must report to a citizen board with statewide policy responsibility. In the absence of such a hierarchy, it is unclear if the local board is accountable to anyone other than its own local constituency, which is itself ill-defined. In this setting, effective program planning by governmental authorities becomes difficult. Can a government official responsible for mental health programs on the regional or state level direct the activities of the local citizen boards and should he address himself to the board or to the local agency director?

On the other hand, should the local agency director follow the dictates of his local board or those of the government agency funding his program? Is the program that follows the directives of its local board more accountable than the one that responds through a chain of command to an elected office holder? Conflict between citizen boards and governmental agencies are becoming more common, with agency directors frequently caught between the conflicting parties. Points at issue in such contests often involve such basic questions as the selection of program goals, what activity can appropriately be considered legitimate for mental health programs, and what qualifications must personnel have to work and direct mental health programs. In this setting, the selection of citizens for membership on boards and panels at the local, state, and national level, has taken on new significance in as much as the selection process is one obvious route for structuring citizen input.

Dr. Noel Mazade, in conjunction with the University of North Carolina, has conducted a major study of citizen boards in that state, looking at the selection process and the functioning of these boards in the 1970s. In Chapter 7 he analyzes some of the effects emerging trends in health care are having on citizen boards.

In reaction to the more extreme claims made for citizen input in the operation of mental health programs, some professionals have declared that there is no role for citizens in directing mental health programs. Irving Blumberg, long active in the citizen movement and a nationally recognized advocate for improved care for the mentally ill, lays out a middle course for citizen input for the future in Chapter 8. He proposes strong citizen involvement in setting program goals and for acting in collaboration with professionals in operating mental health programs. Mr. Blumberg argues that the citizen is uniquely qualified to assist the professionals in reviewing his program. He warns that professionals cannot expect continued support for their programs by the public unless citizens are allowed to participate as equal partners in setting the goals and operating programs for the mentally ill in the future.

3

Constitutional Requirements in Commitment of the Mentally Ill: Rights to Liberty and Therapy

Franklin N. Flaschner

The major current trend in mental health, juvenile delinquency, and even in penology, is deinstitutionalization. Depopulating the state hospitals, the training schools and homes for juveniles, and even trying to do the same with jails and prisons is at the heart of human services' policies throughout the country. Substitutions, to the extent they may be necessary, are an amalgam of so-called community-based facilities, both residential and nonresidential, designed to divert at the earliest possible time the sick, the handicapped, the deviant, the alienated, and even the criminal from the cycle of institutionalization and reinstitutionalization. The hypothesis of this trend is rehabilitation rather than incarceration. The central theme is that rehabilitation is least likely to work in the most restrictive settings and is most likely to work on the basis of individual plans using the least restrictive alternatives.

Establishment of community mental health facilities was a stated purpose of the 1946 National Mental Health Act.[1] Its substantial implementation was assured by the 1963 Community Mental Health Centers Act.[a] Notwithstanding the rapid expansion of shifts from inpatient to outpatient, from state hospital to community, from public bureaucracy to purchase of private services, from patients committed involuntarily to those admitted on a voluntary basis, nevertheless, the civil libertarian and the antihospital forces are stronger today than ever before.

From a legal standpoint they maintain that the mentally ill and retarded have been deprived of the constitutional support given to the criminal defendant and to the juvenile in the 1950s and 1960s. As new legislation is enacted governing the commitment, admission, hospitalization, and discharge of the mentally ill and retarded, the major provisions speak to maximizing the patient's opportunities to stay out, to get out and, while in, to get the most out of it with a minimum of suffering.

The purpose of this chapter is to examine some of the significant new cases and types of statutes that reflect legal recognition of these forces.

---

[a]42 U.S.C.A. secs. 2681-87. The goal of this legislation was to reduce by one half the nation's public mental health residential population by the mid 1970s. It appears this goal will be met since this population has already decreased from 504,600 in 1963 to 308,000 as of June 30, 1971. Chambers, *Alternatives to Civil Commitment of the Mentally Ill; Practical Guides to Constitutional Imperatives,* MICH. L. REV. 70:1107, 1115 (1972). See BRAKEL AND ROCK, THE MENTALLY DISABLED AND THE LAW 9-13 (Am. Bar Foundation Study, 1971 ed.).

Since the United States Supreme Court has decided only a handful of cases involving the rights of the mentally ill or retarded, the constitutional questions currently being raised have not been definitively answered. There is one exception, and that relates to persons charged with crimes. In the 1966 case of *Baxstrom* v. *Herold*,[2] Chief Justice Warren, speaking for a unanimous Court, wrote a landmark opinion, the result of which is that no one can be committed to a mental health facility solely because he has been convicted of a crime or sentenced. The Court's holding was that the equal protection clause of the Fourteenth Amendment requires that the provisions of the civil commitment laws must be complied with irrespective of the status of the allegedly mentally ill person under criminal or penal laws.

While the *Baxstrom* case involved the necessity of a civil commitment procedure being afforded to a convicted defendant in a mental hospital when the term of his sentence had expired, logical extensions of *Baxstrom* have been applied in the following situations: (1) to a defendant's commitment by way of transfer from a penal institution;[3] (2) to a defendant's commitment in lieu of sentence following conviction as a sex offender;[4] (3) to a defendant's commitment after being found not guilty by reason of insanity;[5] and (4) to a defendant's commitment after being found incompetent or unfit to stand trial.[6]

In the case of one found incompetent to stand trial there is a special problem. If committed solely by reason of his status as a person incompetent to stand trial, is there any limit to the detention of one who predictably will never undergo any change in his capacity? An example is a twenty-seven-year-old deaf mute with the mental level of a preschool-age child, who cannot read, write, or otherwise communicate except by sign language, and who is charged with two separate robberies, one of $4.00 and the other of $5.00, of which the maximum sentence for each is twenty-five years. If his indefinite commitment were warranted solely by reason of his status of incompetency, he would be destined to spend the rest of his life in a state institution, whereas if he were not so charged he would be subject to a more stringent standard of commitment and a more lenient standard of release as either a mentally ill or a retarded person under the state's civil commitment laws. This was the situation in *Jackson* v. *Indiana,* decided by the Supreme Court in June 1972.[7]

Justice Blackmun, speaking for a unanimous Court, invoked both the equal protection and the due process clauses of the Fourteenth Amendment. This resulted in a holding that, without a finding of dangerousness, Jackson could be held only for a reasonable period necessary to determine whether there was a substantial chance of his attaining the capacity to stand trial, and that if the chances were slight or if he did not in fact improve, then he must be released. In Justice Blackmun's words: "At the least, due process requires that the nature and duration of commitment bear some reasonable relation to the purpose for which the individual is committed."[8]

Under the new Mental Health Code in Massachusetts no person can be committed other than pursuant to civil commitment procedures except a defendant pending trial or sentence[9] for an observational commitment that may not exceed forty days. In view of the new restrictive standards of commitment, it is entirely possible for a defendant, found incompetent to stand trial, also to be found noncommittable. In such an event his pending criminal case is continued, unless dismissed at the request of the prosecutor or by order of the court on the ground of no probable cause.[b] However, his release pending trial may be subject to conditions such as his periodic reporting to the probation department, the court clinic, or a community-based mental health facility.[c]

Dangerousness as a statutory standard of commitment is frequently subject to the criticism of vagueness. In the new Massachusetts code the statutory standard of "likelihood of serious harm" is defined as follows: (1) a substantial risk of physical harm to the person himself as manifested by evidence of threats of, or attempts at, suicide or serious bodily harm; (2) a substantial risk of physical harm to other persons as manifested by evidence of homicidal or other violent behavior and serious physical harm to them; or (3) a very substantial risk of physical impairment or injury to the person himself as manifested by evidence that such person's judgment is so affected that he is unable to protect himself in the community and that reasonable provision for his protection is not available in the community. (This is a far cry from the former Massachusetts statutory standard of involuntary commitment that was based on need of treatment and even included conduct "which clearly violates the established laws, ordinances, conventions or morals of the community.")

The new Massachusetts Mental Health Code eliminates indefinite commitments.[10] It requires periodic institutional reviews and limits initial commitments to ten days on medical certification and thereafter only by court order for six months initially and for one year on all subsequent commitments. These commitment proceedings are held in the local district courts where the hospitals are located. The hearings almost always take place at the hospitals.

---

[b]Mass. G.L. ch. 123, sec. 16(f) requires dismissal at "the expiration of the period of time equal to the time of imprisonment which the person would have had to serve prior to becoming eligible for parole if he had been convicted of the most serious crime with which he was charged in court and sentenced to the maximum sentence he could have received, if so convicted." Section 17(b) affords a defendant found to be incompetent to stand trial an opportunity for a probable cause hearing. "If after hearing such petition the court finds a lack of substantial evidence to support a conviction, it shall dismiss the indictment or other charges or find them defective or insufficient and order the release of the defendant from criminal custody."

[c]Most bail reform statutes establish a presumption for release on personal recognizance rather than bail. See Mass. G.L. ch. 276, sec. 58. Conditions of bail or RoR may include such reporting. Illinois Code of Corrections, sec. 1005-2-2(a) " . . . If the defendant is not ordered hospitalized in such hearing, the Department of Mental Health shall petition the trial court to release the defendant on bail or recognizance, under such conditions as the court finds appropriate, which may include, but need not be limited to requiring the defendant to submit to or to secure treatment for his mental condition."

The patient and his guardian or next of kin receive notice and a right to counsel (if indigent, paid for at public expense), as well as a right to request an independent psychiatric examination (also at public expense if indigent). There must be a hearing as a condition of either the initial six-month commitment or the first subsequent one-year commitment, and the patient has a right to a hearing on any petition for his commitment.

Before 1973 Massachusetts did not yet have statutory provision for a mental health information or advocacy service, as did New York since 1964[11] and more recently Maryland[12] and California.[d] Then, the Massachusetts Legislature did enact chapter 893 of the Acts of 1973, "An Act Providing for Legal Assistance to the Indigent Mentally Ill," pursuant to which a Mental Health Legal Advisors Committee is appointed by the Justices of the Supreme Judicial Court. This committee, if sufficiently funded, has the authority under this new legislation to render a significant service to the mental health patient population in Massachusetts.

Nevertheless, even before 1973 the new Code seemed to preclude any recurrence of the warehousing of forgotten men. The emptying out of Dannemora and Matteawan Hospitals for the dangerously insane in New York pursuant to the express mandate of *Baxstrom*[13] was followed in Massachusetts by the Bridgewater Release Project, which I had the privilege of heading.[14] In two years the patient population of the Bridgewater State Hospital for the Criminally Insane was decreased from 618 to 225. As in the New York experience, these depersonalized, overinstitutionalized patients were judicially determined not to require strict security[e] and were mostly transferred to open hospitals from which many of them have been discharged. According to follow-up studies, only a handful have fallen into trouble again, and none of them seriously.[15]

---

[d]The California statute only designates "the public defender or other attorney," Calif. Welfare and Institutions Code, sec. 5276, and while it does not mandate the appointment in every case of a person involuntarily hospitalized for seventy-two hours by medical certification under the Lanterman-Petris-Short Act, an administrative order for mandatory appointment has been approved by the decision in Thorn v. Superior Court, 1 Cal. 3d 666, 83 Cal. Rptr. 600 (1970). See Mandel, *Compulsory Counsel for California's New Mental Health Law,* U.C.L.A. L. REV. 17:851 (1970). Illinois imposes a legal obligation on judges of the county in which the facility is located to come in person to the facility to inform patients of their rights. Ill. Ann. Stat. ch. 91½, sec. 6-4. Patient Legal Services rendered by Cook County Legal Assistance Foundation, Inc. is an example of the valuable contributions being made in some metropolitan areas by certain public and private nonprofit legal services organizations.

[e]For commitment to Bridgewater, proof is required not only of "likelihood of serious harm" as defined above (see page 67), but also that the person "is not proper subject for commitment" to a conventional facility for the care and treatment of mentally ill or mentally retarded, and that "the failure to retain such person in strict custody would create a likelihood of serious harm." Mass. G.L. ch. 123, sec. 8(d). See Dixon v. Pennsylvania, 325 F. Supp. 966, 974 (M.D. Pa. 1971).

The whole concept of dangerousness has undergone a 180 degree change in the twenty-five years since I first studied commitment laws.[16] Right after World War II these laws were still permeated by the stigma of criminality inserted in their nineteenth century origins.[17] However, in the 1940s and 1950s most state legislatures ridded their commitment laws of procedures whereby allegedly mentally ill persons were arrested by a sheriff with a warrant, charged with dangerous insanity or lunacy, detained in a jail pending trail, remanded to jail pending a vacancy in the state asylum, and finally transported there by the sheriff.

In their place, legislatures tended to enact commitment procedures that acknowledged the therapeutic role of hospitalization. Authorizations were adopted for voluntary admissions.[f] The distinction was drawn between commitability or hospitalization on the one hand, and, on the other hand, adjudication of legal disability accompanied by appointment of a guardian. Whereas the latter constitutes a status involving the deprivation of rights, the former does not.[g] Moreover, post-World War II mental health reform laws started to set forth litanies of patients' rights while hospitalized.

By and large, however, involuntary commitment was still on an indefinite or indeterminate basis, subject to petitions for discharge in which patients not only bore the legal burden of proof, but also the unrealistic practical burden of obtaining legal assistance.[h] World War II and its aftermath made a sacred calf of psychiatry, and procedures were enacted for indefinite involuntary commitment solely on medical certification without court action. Commonly this certification attested to a statutory standard based not on dangerousness, but merely on a need for treatment.[i] The legal considerations in the commitment process were largely subordinated to the medical considerations.

---

[f]All states with the exception of Alabama now have statutes authorizing voluntary admission. From 1949 to 1968 voluntary admissions have increased from 10 percent to 40 percent of all admissions to state mental hospitals, Brakel and Rock, supra fn. a at 17.

[g]Brakel and Rock, supra fn. a at ch. 8; Flaschner, note 16 at 1188-90; A Draft Act Governing Hospitalization of the Mentally Ill, Public Health Serv. Pub. No. 51 (1951) 2; Ross, *Commitment of the Mentally Ill,* MICH. L. REV. 57:945, 980-95 (1957). One of the statutory inclusions of the mandatory quarterly review of each patient by the mental health facility in Massachusetts is "an evaluation of the legal competency of the person and the necessity or advisability of having a guardian or conservator appointed." Mass. G.D. ch. 123, sec. 4.

[h]While the traditional habeas corpus writ tests only the legality of the original detention, most states by statute or judicial decision have broadened the jurisdiction of the proceeding in the case of a mental patient to determine the status as of the time the petition is brought. Brakel and Rock, supra fn. a at 139-40.

[i]Ross, supra fn. g at 954-60; *Note, Civil Commitment of the Mentally Ill,* HARV L. REV. 79: 1288 (1966); *Comment, Due Process for All—Constitutional Standards for Involuntary Civil Commitment and Release,* U. CHIC. L. REV. 34:633 (1967); *Comment, Civil Restraint, Mental Illness and the Right to Treatment,* YALE L.J. 11:87

Starting in the sixties the pendulum has swung back to an emphasis on legal considerations relating the allegedly mentally ill person with the defendant in a criminal case. The emphasis, however, is not on fear of the devil, but on fair dealing. The legal principles in modern commitment reform laws are intended, as they have been in criminal law reform, to remove the shackles of raw state power and to replace them with a more humane and sensitive balance scale forged from the original Bill of Rights.

So we have a return to the standard of dangerousness, not prompted by an interest in protecting the community from the dangerously insane, but rather in protecting the mentally ill person from being involuntarily committed merely because a physician certifies that he is mentally ill and in need of treatment. So, too, we have a host of new constitutional claims of right by the mentally ill. In light of the unique legal problem attendant upon waiver by an allegedly mentally ill person,[18] it is probably more appropriate to consider these claims in terms of requirements rather than rights. Some of them are the following:

1. The requirement of effective legal representation at all significant stages of the commitment process[19]
2. The requirement of a judicial hearing as a condition of indefinite involuntary commitment and even as a condition of initial temporary or emergency commitment[20]
3. The requirement that the testimony at the hearing be transcribed and a transcript made available[21]
4. The requirement that the standard of proof be more stringent than by a preponderance of the evidence, such as by clear, unequivocal, and convincing evidence[22] or even by proof beyond a reasonable doubt[23]
5. The requirement to exclude from psychiatric reports, hearsay, and self-incriminating statements[24]
6. The requirement that no order depriving the allegedly mentally ill person of his liberty might be made unless it employs the least restrictive alternative[j]

(1967); Livermore, *Malmquist and Meehl, On the Justifications for Civil Commitment* U. PA. L. REV. 117:75 (1968). Even today only a small number of state statutes confine the standard of involuntary commitment to dangerousness. See Brakel and Rock, supra fn. a at 36. Ninety percent of all patients in mental hospitals, both public and private, were said to be harmless and 68 percent at St. Elizabeth's Hospital in Washington, D.C. *American Psychiatric Association Position Statement on Adequacy of Treatment,* AM. J. PSYCHIATRY 123:1458 (1967).

[j]Lake v. Cameron, 364 F. 2d. 657 (CCA D.C. 1966); *Covington v. Harris,* 419 F 2d 617 (CCA D.C. 1969); see Chambers, supra fn. a for a thorough discussion and review of authorities. Another of the statutory inclusions of the mandatory quarterly review of each patient by the mental health facility in Massachusetts is "a consideration of all possible alternatives to continue hospitalization or residential care including, but not necessarily limited to, a determination of the person's relationship to the community and to his family, or his employment possibilities, and of available community resources, foster care and

7. The requirement that a patient, if he wants it, receive treatment and even the particular treatment deemed most effective for his condition[25]
8. The requirement that a patient be free to refuse treatment if he chooses[26]
9. The requirement that no experimental treatment be permitted whatsoever[27]
10. The requirement that no mental health facility be permitted to function unless it conforms to minimum constitutional standards[28]

These are constitutional claims of the rights of the mentally ill. While the Supreme Court has yet to rule on them directly and definitively,[k] they are being litigated in lower courts with increasing intensity. Many of them are being recognized in the formulation of new state action by legislation and regulation. This leads to alternative court claims that the specific remedy sought in a particular case may be warranted by statutory interpretation rather than by constitutional mandate.[l] A review of the technical status of each of these claims is beyond the scope of this chapter, but some of them will be discussed in further consideration of the current shift in reliance from medical to legal authority.

Underlying this shift is the social revolution of the last two decades, with its emphasis on human rights, from the new frontier to the war against poverty.[m] Although advocacy for the rights of the mentally ill has been more difficult to marshall than for many other disenfranchised minority groups, the state mental hospital is among the most vulnerable of institutions. Located beyond the sight and convenient reach of population centers, these isolated compounds of stark buildings and sterile environments are hardly the appropriate settings for

---

convalescent facilities." Mass. G.L. ch. 123, sec. 4. See also Kesselbrenner v. Anonymous, 33 N.Y. 2d 161, 350 N.Y.S. 2d 889 (Ct. App. 1973) handed down after this chapter was originally prepared.

[k]"Considering the number of persons affected, it is perhaps remarkable that the substantive constitutional limitations on this power have not been more frequently litigated." Jackson v. Indiana, 406 U.S. 737. This list of constitutional claims is not intended to be complete. For instance, it does not include the litigation on behalf of mental patients asserting their rights not to work at mental hospitals, and to be paid for such work when they are so employed, nor the litigation on behalf of mentally handicapped persons asserting their rights to public education on a nondiscriminatory basis with those deemed not so handicapped. In both of these fields the constitutional significance of the claims has resulted in court decisions and legislation having broad social consequences.

[l]An example is the combined statutory and constitutional basis of petitioner's right to treatment in Rouse v. Cameron, supra note 25.

[m]The melting pot theory has been criticized as a rationalization for class distinction and has been eclipsed by a recognition of our pluralistic society. Disenfranchised groups have confronted and sought to change established values, conventions and institutions. See collection of papers compiled in IS LAW DEAD? EDITED BY EUGENE V. ROSTOW for the Association of the Bar of the City of New York (Simon and Schuster, 1971).

therapeutic communities.[n] Moreover, the staff professionals available and willing to work under these conditions are severely limited in number and qualifications.[o] Such a framework frustrates administrative reform and compromises even the purposes for additional appropriations. It is no wonder, therefore, that in 1961 it was reported that 50 percent of the patients in state mental hospitals were not under active treatment.[29]

Yet, many of the largest state facilities are still deplorably ill equipped to serve their patients. The most dramatic evidence of this is the class action in *Wyatt* v. *Stickney*[30] wherein Chief Judge Frank M. Johnson of the Federal District Court sitting in Montgomery, Alabama, assumed the responsibility for reviewing the ugly details behind that state's standing as fiftieth in the country in mental health expenditures per patient. Judge Johnson's orders amount to an entire restructuring of Alabama's mental health services. They include a comprehensive code of patients' rights to establish a humane psychological and physical environment and an elaborate set of rules addressed to patient labor, physical facilities, and nutritional standards. These orders also include standards for qualified staff in numbers sufficient to administer adequate treatment and staffing ratios in thirty-six categories. The ratio of employees to patients would be increased from 1 employee for every 3 patients to 1 employee for every 1.2 patients. The ratio of professional staff to patients would be increased over ten times. Judge Johnson's orders also include precise requirements for the establishment and maintenance of individualized treatment plans.[p]

The Circuit Court of Appeals for the Fifth Circuit heard the arguments on appeal early in 1973 and affirmed the decision (*Wyatt* v. *Aderholt*, 503 F. 2d 1305 [5th Cir. 1974]). It will be interesting to see how it rules on the legal question of whether each and every one of the hundreds of standards contained in Judge Johnson's orders actually qualify as "minimum constitutional standards

---

[n]"Once a patient has remained in a large mental hospital for two years or more, he is quite unlikely to leave except by death." Bloomberg, *A Proposal for a Community Based Hospital as a Branch of a State Hospital*, AM. J. PSYCHIATRY 116:814 (1960). See other authorities collected in HARV. L. REV. Case Comment, supra note 28 at 1291. See also GOFFMAN, ASYLUMS (Aldine Publishing Co. 1961).

[o]See much of the testimony and many of the articles and studies in *Constitutional Rights of the Mentally Ill, Hearings before the* Subcommittee on Constitutional Rights of the Senate Committee on the Judiciary, 91st Cong. 1st and 2nd Sess., 1969 and 1970. It is reported that in Massachusetts (and I daresay many other states) foreign medical graduates are authorized to practice in a state hospital, state school, or other mental health or retardation facility, though not qualified to practice "on the outside." Birnbaum, *A Rationale for the Right to Treatment*, GEO. L. J. 57:77, 95-96 (1969).

[p]The Fifth Circuit has sustained the holding "that the Fourteenth Amendment guarantees involuntarily civilly committed mental patients a right to treatment," Donaldson v. O'Connor (493 F. 2d 507 [5th Cir.], cert. granted,–U.S.–, 955 Ct. 171,–.L.Ed. 2nd–[1974]) and has affirmed Wyatt v. Stickney "on submission of proposed standards by defendants." See fn. 9 of Donaldson opinion. Moreover, the Fifth Circuit has not yet rendered a decision on Burnham v. Dept. of Pub. Health, 349F. Supp.

for mental institution."[31] Yet, what alternatives did the Judge have? When he made his initial findings in March 1971 he gave the state six months to produce specific plans for adequate and appropriate treatment. Subsequently he ruled that the state had failed to do so. While there are limits to judicial remedies in class actions to resolve all the injustices suffered by the class—obviously the judiciary cannot displace the other branches of government[32]—where might Judge Johnson have stopped once he made an ultimate finding that whatever treatment Alabama was prepared to provide was still constitutionally grossly deficient?

Wyatt v. *Stickney* represents a current high-water mark in the growing number of cases setting forth a constitutional basis for therapy as a condition to involuntary hospitalization.[33] Yet, in the commitment procedures themselves the accent is not on therapy, but rather on liberty. This has been activated not only by the vulnerability of state mental hospitals, but also by the fallibility of psychiatric judgment, at least as it is exercised in these hospitals.[34] The hospital psychiatrist may properly reply that his fallibility depends on how much is expected of him, and that the critics may be at fault for expecting too much. Both assessments, however, point up the need for downgrading the primacy of the psychiatrist's position in the judicial commitment process.

While the testimony of experts on the diagnosis of mental illness, its treatability and prognosis, is entitled to special weight, considerable doubt is now being raised as to the qualifications of experts of testify in conclusionary terms about dangerousness.[q] In any involuntary commitment where the statutory standard is defined in terms of dangerousness, this is the core question of the adjudication. It represents the making of a legal decision by a Judge or a jury that the public interest requires the imposition of forced confinement upon one who has not been convicted of a crime and who may not have been even charged with a crime.[35] The deprivation of liberty is a social, not a medical judgment. If treatment on an inpatient basis appears promising, its desirability

---

1325 (N.D. Ga. 1972) in which the District Court came to a conclusion contrary to that of the District Court in Wyatt v. Stickney. Wyatt and Burnham are class actions, while Donaldson is a damage suit against the patient's attending physicians, in which cause of action, as submitted to the jury, the constitutional right to treatment was an essential element. For definitive opinions after Wyatt and Burnham, but before the Fifth Circuit opinion in Donaldson, see Stachulak v. Coughlin, 364 F. Supp. 686 (N.D. Ill. 1973) and Welsch v. Likins, (D. Minn. No. 4-72-Civ. 451, Feb. 15, 1974), but see N.Y. State Assn. for Retarded Children Inc. v. Rockefeller, 357 F. Supp. 752 (E.D. N.Y. 1973).

[q]"Thus there is no justification for permitting psychiatrists to testify on the ultimate issue. Psychiatrists should explain how defendant's disease or defect relates to his alleged offense, that is, how the development, adaptation and functioning of defendant's behavioral processes may have influenced his conduct. But psychiatrists should not speak directly in terms of 'product' or even 'result' or 'cause'." Washington v. United States, 390 F. 2d 444, 456 (CCA D.C. 1967). See Cross v. Harris, 418 F. 2d 1095, 1100-1101 (CCA D.C. 1969). Rubin, *Predictions of Dangerousness in Mentally Ill Criminals*, ARCHIVES OF GENERAL PSYCHIATRY, 27:397 (1972); Steadman, supra note 13 (1973 paper); Goldstein and Katz, *Dangerousness and Mental Illness*, YALE L. J. 70:225 (1960).

is a separate issue. If dangerousness to self or others is an essential ingredient in the petitioner's case, its determination must not be substituted for or even confused by a consideration of treatability.

A parent's responsibility for custody of his child is not qualified by the prognosis of the child's becoming a responsible adult. Similarly, the state's responsibility for the custody of a dangerously sick person is not to be qualified by considerations of treatability. Even if there is an obligation to treat, the principle of parens patriae must apply as well to the untreatable.[r] It is up to the state to care for the mentally ill who are found by judicial process to be dangerous by reason of their mental illness, irrespective of their responsiveness to treatment. This would appear to be the primary obligation of the state as parens patriae. A further obligation may well be to administer treatment, particularly to all involuntarily committed patients who might benefit therefrom.

However, at all times during a patient's confinement the state should be prepared to satisfy a court that the patient cannot be discharged or even subjected to a substantially less restrictive confinement because of the likelihood of physical harm to himself or others by reason of his mental illness. Without some such rational basis for continued deprivation of liberty there would be no plausible distinction between involuntary commitment of the mentally ill and preventive detention.[36] Let the hospitals and their staffs be busy with those who voluntarily submit themselves to treatment,[s] thereby making the most of the hospital as a therapeutic community, and limit involuntary hospitalizatior to those whose refusal is judicially determined to constitute a threat of physical harm due to mental illness.

This rationale is at the heart of many of the recent decisions. The loss of liberty is said to be "an interest of transcending value."[37] As such it would appear to warrant legal support for its protection in the case of the mentally ill to no less an extent than in the cases of those charged with criminal and delinquent acts for which they may suffer a loss of liberty. The Supreme Court decisions in these fields, particularly those relating to juveniles—the

---

[r]Even the relief afforded by Jackson v. Indiana is ultimately subject to a judicial determination of dangerousness and civil commitment. Commitment as incompetent to stand trial under 18 U.S.C. secs. 4244 to 4248 now depends on finding of dangerousness. See United States v. Curry, 410 F. 2d 1372 (CCA 4th 1969) Gomez v. Miller, 337 F. Supp. 386, 392 (S.D.N.Y. 1971) and discussion in opinion of Jackson v. Indiana, 406 U.S. 715, 731-33 (1972).

[s]Extensions of constitutional rights to voluntary patients who are subject to being involuntarily committed if they give notice to leave the hospital are assuming importance. See Thorn v. Superior Court, supra fn. d; Matter of Buttonow, 23 N.Y. 2d 385 (1968); Spece, supra note 25 at 668; Gilboy and Schmidt, "Voluntary" Hospitalization of the Mentally Ill, NW. U.L. REV 66:429 (1971-72). The new code in Massachusetts creates two categories of voluntary patients as of the time of their admission: one who will be free to go at any time; the other who is subject to a three-day notice and a possible petition for his commitment. Mass. G.L. ch. 123, sec. 11.

Kent,[38] *Gault,*[39] and *Winship*[t] cases in 1966, 1967, and 1970, respectively—
had been relied upon by other courts as authorities for extending to allegedly
mentally ill persons the constitutional rights of counsel, notice, hearing, and
proof beyond a reasonable doubt as conditions of involuntary commitment.

Commitment proceedings, like juvenile cases, were always deemed to
be civil, not criminal, but as the Tenth Circuit Court of Appeals said in
Heryford v. *Parker*: "It matters not whether the proceedings be labeled
'civil' or 'criminal' or whether the subject matter be mental instability or
juvenile delinquency, it is the likelihood of involuntary incarceration—
whether for punishment as an adult for a crime, rehabilitation as a juvenile
for delinquency, or treatment and training as a feeble-minded or mentally
incompetent—which commands observance of the constitutional safeguards
of due process. . . . In our case the fundamental right to counsel is involved
and failure to have counsel at every step of the proceedings may result in
indefinite and oblivious confinement and work shameful injustice."[40]

In the wake of this movement to clothe the allegedly mentally ill person with all the rights of the defendant in a criminal case, any beneficial
effects of informal proceedings are subordinated to the principles of due
process. In 1951 when I helped write the Draft Act Governing Hospitalization of the Mentally Ill, it was thought that section 9(f) gave expression
to the reform tenor of those times when it stated: "The hearing shall be
conducted in as informal a manner as may be consistent with orderly procedure and in a physical setting not likely to have a harmful effect on the
mental health of the proposed patient."[41] The tenor of today's reform
may be reflected in the following comment of Justice Fortas in the
Gault case: "There is increasing evidence that the informal procedures,
contrary to the original expectation, may themselves constitute a further
obstacle to effective treatment of the delinquent to the extent that they
engender in the child a sense of injustice provoked by a seemingly all-powerful
and challengeless exercise of authority by judges and probation officers."[u]

In the highly influential 1972 decision of the United States District Court
for the Eastern District of Wisconsin in *Lessard* v. *Schmidt*[42] it was held that
the allegedly dangerously mentally ill person was constitutionally entitled

---

[t]In re Winship, 397 U.S. 358 (1970) (charges against juvenile must be proven beyond
a reasonable doubt). The Supreme Court stopped short of applying all constitutional
right of defendants in criminal cases to juveniles, when it held that a juvenile was not
constitutionally entitled to a trial by jury, McKeiver v. Pennsylvania, 403 U.S. 528 (1971).

[u]387 U.S. 1, 26. Yet, in 1952 a prominent jurist had the following to say about the
format of a commitment hearing: "The black robed figure of the judge on a bench
signifies a great deal to the patients, their friends and relatives. It conveys to them an
assurance of a day in Court, a priceless psychological reassurance, and for good reason. . . .
To the average American a day in Court presided over by a fair and experienced judge is
a pledge of the protection of his rights as an individual." Botein, Trial Judge, 269 (1952).

to a preliminary hearing within forty-eight hours of involuntary hospitalization and a full hearing within ten to fourteen days, the latter to be preceded
by advance written notice specifying with particularity the basis for the
proposed continued detention, the names of the experts who will testify in
favor of such detention and the substance of their proposed testimony. This
case also held that civil commitment cannot be justified upon mere preponderance of the evidence, but only upon proof beyond a reasonable doubt
that the person is mentally ill and dangerous, and even in such event, the
court should order indefinite involuntary hospitalization only as a last resort
upon the state's satisfying the court that less restrictive alternatives were
investigated and deemed not suitable. Finally, this case also held that counsel was required at least as early in the proceedings as the preliminary hearing, that counsel must have access to all reports that may be introduced, and
that no statement made by the proposed patient to an interviewer might be
introduced in evidence tending to prove either mental illness or dangerousness unless the patient had been advised in advance by the interviewer of
such possible use of his statement.

In the case of *In re Ballay*,[43] decided on May 31, 1973 by the United
States Court of Appeals for the District of Columbia, it was also held that
the standard of proof in a civil commitment is constitutionally required to
be proof beyond a reasonable doubt. In the opinion the court states: "There
can no longer be any doubt that the nature of the interests involved when a
person sought to be involuntarily committed faces an indeterminate, and,
consequently potentially permanent loss of liberty and privacy, accompanied
by the loss of substantial civil rights (the loss of which frequently continues
even if his liberty is restored) is one within the contemplation of the liberty
and property language of the Fourteenth Amendment."

Quoting from a criminal case involving the rights of parolees decided by
the Supreme Court in 1972,[44] the Circuit Court in *Ballay* reminds us that:
"Due process in flexible and calls for such procedural protections as the particular situation demands." It seems, therefore, that all the arguable remedies
of the Bill of Rights may now be considered by the courts to establish protection for the mentally ill against unfair deprivation of liberty. This will have
continued impact not only in commitment proceedings, but also in the environment and the therapy to which committed patients are subjected.[v]

As the modern administration of justice for the mentally ill unfolds, there
is a vital need that is as of now totally unmet. That is the development of

---

[v]See development of constitutional bases for right to treatment in articles referred to
in notes 26 and 28. In addition to equal protection and due process, there is cruel and
unusual punishment—see Robinson v. California, 370 U.S. 660 (1962) and United States
v. Johnston, 317 F. Supp. 66 (S.D. N.Y. 1970)—and right to a speedy trial in the case of
criminal defendants. See also Chambers, supra note 21 for development of constitutional
rights to the least restrictive alternative.

experienced attorneys to represent the mentally ill.[45] Judges, too, need education and experience in this field, but the major challenge is on the practitioner to implement effectively the new primacy of legal considerations in the hospitalization of the mentally ill.

The court will not be persuaded to disagree with the state's psychiatrists unless the respondent is represented by an advocate who is at home in his role and who has the feel for the proper reach and the proper limit of his advocacy in any given case. This cannot be accomplished by court-appointed counsel or public-agency counsel so long as their assignments are accepted in subordination to the rest of their practice.[w] On this basis they will do no more than "walk through" their steps of representation and they will be unwittingly merged in the paternalistic approach to the mentally ill person usually evidenced by all the other professionals in the case, particularly the hospital psychiatrist and the judge.[x]

Criminal lawyers know how to represent their clients with comprehensive investigation, pretrial practice and preparation for both direct and cross-examination. The better of them know how important it is to be prepared also on the issues of deposition if their clients are found guilty. Sometimes they will help the court determine a less restrictive alternative than jail by the formulation of a plan involving the defendant with community resources and implemented by conditions of probation.[y]

These are the techniques the mental health lawyers will have to learn. They will have to be as adept in cross-examining hospital psychiatrists as criminal lawyers are in cross-examining police officers. They will have to spend time investigating their clients' records and all the circumstances that may be relevant to the ultimate questions of fact, such as mental illness and dangerousness. They will have to challenge the state's evidence on dangerousness,

---

[w]"For some attorneys the $300 or $400 received once or twice a year for at most a few hours 'work' is a windfall not to be regarded lightly." Cohen, supra note 45 at 448.

[x]Paternalism may also be seen as "a cover" for professional conservatism. In the case of the psychiatrist the so-called "type-2 error" identifies his tendency to diagnose on the side of illness rather than on the side of health. Christiansen and Ostberg, supra note 45 at 97-104. The best the Rosenham pseudo-patient schizophrenics came away with when discharged was the label "in remission." Rosenham, supra note 34 at 252. In the case of the judge: "Little acclaim will come to him for ten aggressive patients successfully treated in the community and little condemnation for ten harmless patients needlessly confined, but condemnation (and guilt) may hound him for one ill person released to the community who commits a serious assault." Chambers, supra note 21 at 1123.

[y]Notwithstanding the statement of the dissent in Lake v. Cameron, supra fn. j, by the then Circuit Court Justice Warren Burger to the effect that a district court in our legal system is not set up to initiate inquiries and direct studies of social welfare facilities or other social problems, what difference is there between this initiative in the case of a mentally ill person and that being taken increasingly by federal, state, county, and municipal trial courts through their probation departments and court clinics to investigate and make the most of community facilities and resources in lieu of incarceration in the cases of juveniles and even adult offenders?

so that no affirmative finding can be made unless it is based on overt conduct
causally related to mental illness.[z] They will have to become familiar with
the jargon of psychiatrists, psychologists, and social workers and the environment of hospitals, clinics halfway houses, and other community facilities.
Finally, they will have to regard the allegedly mentally ill person as a client
to whom they can relate comfortably, as a client whom they can accept with
his peculiar problems as a whole person, as a client with real, live, third-party
relationships to be understood and assessed.[aa] Without the development of
a mental health bar, the development of the rights of the mentally ill will
still be meaningless litany in altogether too many instances.

Senator Sam Ervin summarized the matter best in his remarks opening the
hearings on November 4, 1969, before his sub-Committee on Constitutional Rights
of the Committee on the Judiciary: "Mental illness and the laws governing it are
the concern of all of us. The truth of the matter is that when we tolerate arbitrary acts, vague standards, administrative and legislative lethargy, which
deprives others of their right to health and to effective exercise of their freedom,
then we tolerate a breakdown in our constitutional form of government."[bb]

Notes

1. 42 U.S.C.A. sec. 201 *et seq.*
2. 383 U.S. 107.
3. Schuster v. Herold, 410 F. 2d 1071 (CCA 2nd 1969).
4. Humphrey v. Cady, 405 U.S. 504 (1972).
5. Cameron v. Mullen, 387 F. 2d 193 (CCA D.C. 1967); Bolton v. Harris, 395
   F. 2d 642 (CCA D.C. 1968); People v. Lally, 19 N.Y. 2d 27 (1966).
6. Commonwealth v. Druken, 356 Mass. 503 (1969).
7. 406 U.S. 715.
8. 406 U.S. 715, 738.

---

[z]Examples of psychiatric testimony in hearings at Bellevue Hospital, even when New
York Mental Health Information Service is appearing for the patient: "So I think the index
of suspicion of potential violence here would be quite high." "She is a very nice and peace-
ful person, but when you are dealing with a paranoid person, you never know how she will
react." Kumaska and Gupta, supra note 45 at 7.

[aa]The paternalism of the attorney for the patient may be discerned by his referral to
the person not as "my client" but as "the patient." Cohen, supra note 45 at 445.

[bb]*Constitutional Rights of the Mentally Ill,* supra fn. o at 1. Perhaps the most often
cited quotation in modern writings on the rights of the mentally ill is taken from Justice
Brandeis' dissent in Olmstead v. United States, 277 U.S. 438, 479 (1928): "Experience
should teach us to be most on our guard to protect liberty when the government's purposes
are beneficent. . . . The greatest dangers to liberty lurk in insidious encroachment by men
of zeal, well-meaning but without understanding."

9. Mass. G.L. ch. 123, 15(b), 15(c).
10. Mass. G.L. ch. 123, secs. 4, 5, 6, 7, 8, 12.
11. MCKINNEY, CONSOL. LAWS OF N.Y., vol. 34A, sec. 88; Gupta, *New York's Mental Health Information Service: An Experiment in Due Process*, RUTGERS L. REV. 25:405 (1971); Kumaska and Gupta, *Lawyers and Psychiatrists in Court: Issues on Civil Commitment*, MD. L. REV. 40:6 (1972).
12. Ann. Code of Md., art. 59, sec. 54.
13. Hunt and Wiley, *Operation Baxstrom After One Year*, AM. J. PSYCHIATRY 124:974 (1968); Steadman and Kevelles, *The Community Adjustment and Criminal Activity of the Baxstrom Patients*: 1966-1970, AM. J. PSYCHIATRY 129:3 (1972); Steadman and Halfon, The Baxstrom Patients: Background and Outcomes, Seminars in Psychiatry (Aug. 1971); Steadman, Implications from the Baxstrom Experience, excellent paper presented in March, 1973 (Mental Health Research Unit, N.Y. State Department of Mental Hygiene, Albany, N.Y.).
14. Flaschner, *Florida's New Mental Health Law*, FLORIDA BAR JOURNAL 46:344, 348 (June 1972).
15. See study by Dr. A. Louis McGarry, Director of Division of Legal Medicine, Mass. Dept. of Mental Health, Boston, Mass.
16. Flaschner, *Analysis of Legal and Medical Considerations in Commitment of the Mentally Ill*, YALE L. J. 56:1178, 1185-86 (1947).
17. DEUTSCH, THE MENTALLY ILL IN AMERICA, 2nd. ed., Ch. 19 (New York: Columbia University Press, 1949).
18. See Pate v. Robinson, 383 U.S. 375, 384 (1966); Rees v. Peyton, 384 U.S. 312; Virgin Islands v. Niles, 295 F. Supp. 266 (D.V.I. 1969); Thorn v. Superior Court, supra fn. d.
19. Heryford v. Parker, 396 F. 2d. 393 (CCA 10th 1968); Lessard v. Schmidt, 349 F. Supp. 1078, 1097 (E.D. Wisc. 1972).
20. Lessard v. Schmidt, supra note 19 at 1090; In re Barnard, 455 F. 2d 1370 (CCA D.C. 1971); Dixon v. Pennsylvania, supra fn. e; Anderson v. Solomon, 315 F. Supp. 1192 (D. Md. 1970); Specht v. Patterson, 386 U.S. 605 (1967); but see Fhagen v. Miller, 29 N.Y. 2d 348 (1972).
21. Dixon v. Pennsylvania, supra fn. e at 974. See Roberts v. LaVallee, 389 U.S. 40 (1967).
22. Woodby v. Immigration and Naturalization Service, 385 U.S. 276 (1966); Tippett v. Maryland, 436 F. 2d 1153, 1165-66 (CCA 4th 1971) (opinion of Sobeloff, J.); Dixon v. Pennsylvania, supra fn. e at 974.
23. Murel v. Baltimore City Criminal Court, 407 U.S. 355, 358 (1972) (dissenting opinion of Douglas, J.); Lessard v. Schmidt, supra note 19 at 1093; In re Ballay, No. 71-2023 (CCA D.C. May 31, 1973).
24. McNeil v. Patuxent Institution Director, 407 U.S. 245, 252 (dissenting opinion of Douglas, J.); Lessard v. Schmidt, supra at 1100 and 1102; but see Tippett v. Maryland, supra note 22, Sofeloff, J. opinion at 1160-61.

25. Rouse v. Cameron, 373 F. 2d 451, 453 (CCA D.C. 1966); Whitree v.
    State, 290 N.Y.S. 2d 486 (1968); Nason v. Bridgewater, 353 Mass. 604
    (1968); Comment, Civil Restraint, Mental Illness and the Right to Treat-
    ment, supra fn. i; Note *The Nascent Right to Treatment,* VA. L. REV.
    53:1134 (1967); *Symposium on the Right to Treatment,* GEO. L. J.
    57:673 (1969); Bazelon, *Implementing the Right to Treatment,* U. CHIC.
    L. REV. 36:742 (1969); Spece, *Conditioning and Other Technologies
    Used to "Treat?" "Rehabilitate?" "Demolish?"—Prisoners and Mental
    Patients,* SO. CALIF. L. REV. 45:616 (1972).
26. New York City Health and Hospitals Corp. v. Stein, 70 Misc. 2d 944,
    335 N.Y.S. 2d 461 (1972) (patient's right to refuse EST upheld notwith-
    standing mother's consent); Winters v. Miller, 446 F 2d 65 (CCA 2nd 1971)
    (patient's right to refuse supports claim for damages where treatment
    administered over objection and no effort made to have patient judicially
    declared incompetent); Stowers v. Wolodzko, 386 Mich. 110 (1971) (same,
    at least during period of temporary hospitalization). See Spece, supra note
    25 at 655; Katz, *The Right to Treatment—An Enchanting Legal Fiction?*
    U. CHIC. L. REV. 36:755 (1969); Morris, *"Criminality" and the Right to
    Treatment,* U. CHIC. L. REV. 36:784 (1969).
27. Kaimowitz v. Dept. of Mental Health, C.A. No. 73-19434-AW (Circuit
    Court for Wayne County, Michigan, July 10, 1973) (informed consent
    by involuntarily detained mental patient may be given to accepted, but
    not to experimental neurosurgical procedures. The Massachusetts
    Supreme Judicial Court approved rare bone marrow transplant in desper-
    ate move to save life of victim, the transplant being taken from retarded
    brother of victim not able to give infomed consent.) BOSTON GLOBE,
    Sept. 7, 1973. See Spece, supra note 25 at 667.
28. See discussion below of Wyatt v. Stickney and excellent recent Case Com-
    ment, Wyatt v. Stickney and the *Right of Civilly Committed Mental
    Patients to Adequate Treatment,* HARV. L. REV. 86:1282 (May 1973).
    See also *Note, Guaranteeing the Right to Treatment,* MD. L. REV. 40:42
    (1972).
29. Hearings Before the Subcommittee on Constitutional Rights of the Senate
    Committee on the Judiciary, 87th Cong., 1st Sess. pt. 1 at 23 (1961).
30. 325 F. Supp. 781 (1971); 334 F. Supp. 1341 (1971); 344 F. Supp. 373,
    387 (1972).
31. 344 F. Supp. 373, 379; 344 F. Supp. 387, 395.
32. See Swan v. Charlotte-Mecklenberg Board of Education, 402 U.S. 1 (1971);
    Katzenbach, *A Plea for Diffusion of Responsibility,* MASS. L. Q. 57:7
    (1972).
33. Saville v. Treadway, C.A. No. 6969 (M.D., Tenn. filed April 10, 1973);
    Ricci v. Greenblatt, C.A. No. 72-469F (D. Mass. filed Feb. 11, 1972);
    Lebanks v. Spears, C.A. No. 71-2897 (E.D. La. 1972). See parallel class

actions brought to humanize jails and prisons: Holt v. Sarver, 309 F. Supp. 362 (E.D. Ark. 1969) aff'd 442 F. 2d 304 (CCA 8th 1971); Collins v. Schoonfield, 344 F. Supp. 257 (D. Md. 1972); Inmates of Suffolk County Jail v. Eisenstadt, C.A. No. 71-162-G (D. Mass. June 20, 1973).

34. The most dramatic evidence in Rosenham, *On Being Sane in Insane Places,* SCIENCE 179:259 (1972). See also Scheff, *The Societal Reaction to Deviance: Ascriptive Elements in the Psychiatric Screening of Mental Patients in a Midwestern State,* SOCIAL PROBLEMS 11:401 (1964).

35. *Constitutional Rights of the Mentally Ill,* supra fn. o, prepared statement of Bruce J. Ennis at 271; Dershowitz, *The Psychiatrist's Power in Civil Commitment: A Knife That Cuts Both Ways,* PSYCHOLOGY TODAY (Feb. 1969).

36. See authorities collected in HARV. L. REV. Case Comment, supra note 28 at 1289-90.

37. In re Ballay, supra note 23 at 41.

38. Kent v. United States, 383 U.S. 541 (1966) (waiver of juvenile proceedings and transfer to adult session cannot take place without notice of reasons, hearing, and effective assistance of counsel).

39. In re Gault, 387 U.S. 1 (1967) (defendant in juvenile proceeding entitled to notice of charges, counsel, confrontation, cross-examination, and protection against self-incrimination).

40. 396 F. 2d 393, 396-97 (1968).

41. A Draft Act Governing Hospitalization of the Mentally Ill, Public Health Serv. Pub. No. 51 (1951) 2.

42. Lessard v. Schmidt, 349 F. Supp. 1078, 1097.

43. In re Ballay, No. 71-2023 (CCA D.C. May 31, 1973) 14-15.

44. Morrissev v. Brewer, 408 U.S. 471, 481 (1972).

45. Cohen, *The Function of the Attorney and The Commitment of the Mentally Ill,* TEX L. REV. 44:424 (1965); Gupta, *New York's Mental Health Information Service: An Experiment in Due Process,* RUTGERS L. REV. 25:405 (1971); Kumaska and Gupta, *Lawyers and Psychiatrists in Court: Issues on Civil Commitment,* MD. L. REV. 40:6 (1972); Christiansen and Ostberg, Civil Commitment in Massachusetts, unpublished Harvard Law School student paper submitted to Professor Ely (April 1972). The effectiveness of representation by counsel is demonstrated as well as advocated by by these articles. See also study reported by Lewin, *Disposition of the Irresponsible: Protection Following Commitment,* MICH. L. REV. 66:721, 725 (1968).

4

The Impact of Litigation on the Future of State Hospitals
Bruce Ennis

Courts have always been concerned to some extent with the legal rights of persons facing involuntary commitment to a state institution for the mentally ill or the mentally retarded. But until very recently courts have refused to look behind institution doors. It is, literally, only in the past five years that courts have begun to consider the rights that patients retain inside such institutions once they are there lawfully. The rights that have become the focus of that examination include the following: the right to treatment; the right to refuse treatment; the right to protection from harm; the right to be paid for institution-maintaining labor; the right to be treated in the least restrictive setting and in the least restrictive and intrusive manner; the right to a free lawyer to resolve problems resulting from and problems separate from institutionalization; the right to a nonrenewable limitation on the permissible period of involuntary institutionalization; the right to decent living conditions—including the right to regular outdoor exercise, adequate clothing, and adequate medical care; the right to a public education regardless of the degree of mental handicap; and the right to meaningful notice—not just notice, of these and other rights.

Not one of these rights has as yet gained nationwide acceptance, much less nationwide implementation. But it is fair to say that through court decisions and, less frequently, through revised statutes and administrative regulations, each of those rights has been recognized as an enforceable right, a right with teeth, across substantial portions of this country. Moreover, there are strong indications that the United States Supreme Court will place its stamp of approval on many if not all of these rights in the next year or so. As the rights of patients expand, the power and the discretion historically assumed and exercised by mental hospital professionals and administrators will of necessity contract. With this expansion of patients' rights will come the end, not just the reform, but the end of the state hospital as we know it.

The Rights to Treatment

One of the most significant of the newly emerging rights is the so-called right to treatment, which is, in fact, a misnomer, since there is nothing in the United States Constitution that refers to such a right. The right to treatment is in effect a shorthand phrase covering a host of other constitutional rights,

primarily the right to liberty. The thesis is simple: If a person has been deprived
of liberty on the premise that he needs treatment the justification for depriving
him of his liberty disappears if he is not given treatment, and he is, therefore,
deprived of his constitutional right to liberty.

It is really more accurate at the present stage of litigation to refer to a right
to "treatment or release." Most of the so-called right-to-treatment cases developed thus far have been limited to the rights of involuntarily institutionalized
patients, for example, the Alabama case of *Wyatt* v. *Stickney*.[1] The significance
of this decision, if it is confirmed on appeal and is followed in other states, is
that it, literally, will force the closing of most state mental hospitals in the
country because states will not be able to afford the extra psychiatrists, psychologists, social workers, and attendants needed to adhere to the ruling.

This case is not simply a radical idea by a group of activist lawyers. In fact,
it represents the opinion of several quite "establishment-oriented" organizations
including the American Psychiatric Association, the American Psychological
Association, the American Orthopsychiatric Association, and the American
Association on Mental Deficiency, all of which have joined either at the trial
or appeal level in supporting the *Wyatt* v. *Stickney* decision and its standards.

There are many other right-to-treatment cases patterned after *Wyatt* pending around the country at this time. One of these, *Donaldson* v. *O'Connor*[2]
may prove almost as important as *Wyatt* v. *Stickney* in its overall impact. It,
too, is a right-to-treatment case, but with a difference, resulting in a former
mental patient being awarded $38,500 in damages for being held in a Florida
State mental hospital for fifteen years without adequate treatment. It was not
disputed that he obtained adequate and decent custodial care; the institution
was clean; he got good meals and fresh change of linen. But he did not get
an affirmative psychiatric treatment program, and the judge instructed the
federal jury that patients involuntarily committed have a constitutional right
to receive more than mere custodial care.

The important point of this case is that the money damages, more than
$40,000, came out of the pockets of the hospital director and the staff psy-
chiatrist in charge of that patient, not from the state of Florida. If the case
is confirmed on appeal and is followed in other states it will mean that in the
future, hospital directors and psychiatrists must either provide treatment to
their involuntary patients, or, if that is not possible, let them go or convert
them to voluntary status.

Along with the right to treatment goes the right to refuse treatment.
Somewhat less attention has been given to that facet, but brief mention will
be made of a few important cases in the area. In *Wyatt* v. *Stickney* the court
found that patients retain the right to refuse shock treatment, lobotomy,
and major surgery. In *Winters* v. *Miller*[3] the Second Federal Court in New
York ruled that Christian Scientists retain the right to refuse thorazine, or

any other kind of medication or physical treatment, on religious grounds even though they are hospitalized lawfully. In the case of *New York City Health and Hospitals Corporation* v. *Stein*,[4] a New York State case, the court ruled that a patient committed lawfully retained the right to refuse shock treatment. On the further fringes of this same subject is a strange case—*Kaimowitz* v. *Dept. of Mental Health*[5]—in which a Michigan court ruled just a few months ago that a patient confined involuntarily would not be permitted to consent to psychosurgery. The patient himself had consented to psychosurgery, but the court had found that the pressures of involuntary hospitalization were so great that such consent should be disregarded and psychosurgery not permitted on any patient confined involuntarily.

The Right to Protection from Harm

The constitutional right to protection from harm is another concept that is beginning to take shape along much the same lines as the right to treatment but is different from it in one important respect: Where the right to treatment is essentially an affirmative right, altering the status quo of a patient for the better, the right to protection from harm simply assures that the patient will be preserved in at least the same condition in which he entered the institution. It, unfortunately, is true that in almost all institutions for the retarded, as well as in a great many of the institutions for the mentally ill, patients deteriorate through the institutionalization process. It is now well recognized that long-term hospitalization is antitherapeutic. People have a right not to be exposed to the kind of psychological, mental, and physical deterioration that it entails, nor, moreover, to the danger of injury that is very real in many state institutions.

In the Willowbrook State School in New York State, for example, in one ten-month period there were 1,400 physical assaults and injuries on residents sufficiently severe to require an incident review committee investigation. In the brief that I wrote in the *Willowbrook* case,[6] I began by saying (not at all facetiously) that there is probably no more dangerous place to live in all of New York City than the back wards of the Willowbrook State School. We talk a lot about law and order in the streets, perhaps we should pay more attention to law and order in institutions. It is a tragic thing to walk through an institution corridor and find a mentally retarded child tied to a chair so that he or she cannot move, and have other children hitting that child on the head with a shoe because there are not enough attendants around to stop them.

The presiding judge in the *Willowbrook* case, Judge Judd, determined to put an end to such disasters and ordered the state of New York to hire at least one attendant for every nine residents, in other words, to hire enough additional attendants so that one attendant would actually be present on duty each of the daytime shifts for every nine residents. He also ordered other steps that he considered necessary to protect residents from harm, for example, an end to the use of seclusion and isolation rooms. We found mentally retarded children in Willowbrook who had been locked in seclusion rooms without beds, without anything but a vinyl mat on the floor, without linen or blankets, without toilet facilities, without water or books or anything at all, but a bare twelve-foot by twelve-foot concrete room where they were forced to lie in their own feces on the cold floor often for long periods. We found people who had been locked in solitary confinement at Willowbrook for periods of seven to eleven years. That is over now, and it is going to be over in hospitals for the mentally ill in the very near future.

Also included in the right to protection from harm in Judge Judd's *Willowbrook* decision was a right to outdoor exercise at least five days a week and a right to adequate medical care. Willowbrook's so-called hospital had never been accredited as a hospital and Judge Judd ordered the state to close it and either provide an accredited hospital or to contract with an accredited hospital for medical care. The state has chosen to contract with a medical hospital. This is going to happen in most state institutions. It is no longer going to be possible to give second class medical care to residents.

An important point to remember about the "right to protection from harm" is that although it does not go as far as the right-to-treatment argument it includes a much greater number of persons. Judge Judd explicitly ruled that the constitutional right to protection from harm, unlike the right to treatment, applies whether the patient is involuntary or voluntary. Even voluntary patients have this right to protection from harm. That is an important point to bear in mind in light of the forecast made elsewhere in this volume of a tremendous shift from state hospitals to nursing homes and other facilities that are generally voluntary. This same right applies in those situations also.

The Right to Legal Representation

One of the major principles that will be widely recognized in the near future is the right of patients in a mental hospital to have legal representation for problems that are not directly connected with institutionalization. Many people in mental hospitals continue to have legal problems. They may be in the process of being evicted from their homes. Perhaps they are faced with divorce actions or child custody suits. In many cases property that has been purchased on the installment plan is in danger of being repossessed. If they were not confined, people facing such problems could readily get redress by contacting the neighborhood legal aid organization for an attorney's services free of charge. There is little justification for depriving patients simply because they are in a hospital of the rights they would be entitled to if they were out

in the community. It appears very likely that in the near future states will be
forced to provide hospitalized patients with a massive range of legal services.

One other point that has been mentioned elsewhere in this volume is the
newly developing right to an outside time limit on involuntary institutionalization. As Dr. William B. Beach points out in Chapter 15, in California some
people cannot be committed for more than a set period. Persons who are committed because they are suicidal get out in a month or less. For the most part,
persons who are committed because they are considered dangerous to others
get out in ninety days or less. In fact, the average period of hospitalization in
California for those two classes is now only thirteen days, according to the
latest figures available.

The United States Supreme Court's interest in this principle is reflected
in two cases that do not directly involve the rights of hospitalized patients.
One is *Jackson* v. *Indiana*[7] that involves the rights of incompetent defendants;
the other is *McNeil* v. *Director of Patuxent Institution,*[8] that involves the rights
of persons committed for observation, not for treatment. In these cases the
Supreme Court imposed absolute outside time limits on the length of time
the principals could be confined in institutions. Since they were both unanimous Supreme Court decisions, it appears quite likely that in the next year or
so the Supreme Court will impose an outside time limit on the permissible
period of commitment for treatment. What that limit is likely to be is any
one's guess, but it seems likely it will be somewhere within the range of two
years to six months. As Dr. Beach points out, once this concept of a time
limit on involuntary hospitalization gains wider acceptance, it is going to
force a reevaluation of the whole conception of mental illness and how to
deal with it. Today, when a patient is brought to a hospital by relatives, he
is accepted with no questions asked. In the future, when a prospective patient
is brought to a hospital by relatives the authorities are going to require them
to be prepared to take him back home within a specified time. That is going
to change expectations very considerably.

The Right to Meaningful Notice

Unfortunately, most of the rights that patients have are, even now, only
paper rights; they are seldom exercised or practiced in part because patients
are not aware of them or how to go about obtaining them. A case in point
is the right to meaningful notice. A recent issue of the *New York Law Journal*
included a case known as *Dale* v. *Hahn*[9] in which the Second Circuit Federal
Court of Appeals made a very important ruling. It ruled that even though a
patient in a New York State mental hospital had been given personal notice
that he was going to be subjected to a separate proceeding to find him mentally
incompetent—as well as mentally ill, the basis for hospitalization—with the
result that all his personal assets would be taken away, personal notice was

not enough. The court did not indicate what would be enough, but it hinted very strongly that in such a case giving notice to the patient was insufficient, that the hospital should also give notice to a court-appointed guardian or lawyer who could then act on the patient's behalf.

Basic to these developments is the concept that whenever state actions appear to interfere significantly with the life of a person alleged to be under mental disability, simply informing that person of his/her right to protest is meaningless. Increasingly, the state will be forced to assume responsibility for appointing lawyers or guardians in each case. The ramifications of this are endless. If New York State literally set out to appoint a lawyer for every involuntary patient the whole system would collapse; at the moment only the very minimum are given court-appointed attorneys.

It seems reasonably certain that the rights discussed above are going to be implemented in major portions of the country within the next few years. For three or four years, the present writer was the only lawyer in the entire United States employed full time to bring test case litigation for the mentally handicapped. Things are now changing rapidly. There are at present several organizations specializing in this kind of litigation, besides the Mental Health Law Project of Washington D.C. with which the writer is associated.

As an indication of the way things are accelerating, this project, started in 1972 with a total beginning budget of about $17,000, now operates to the tune of nearly half a million dollars in annual expenses. This much money was contributed by concerned citizens and foundations because it was an idea for which its time had come. It is long overdue that people in mental hospitals be given at least the same rights as those in general hospitals, and that, essentially, is what will occur in the future. At present there are only thirty major test cases pending around the country; within a year from now there are more likely to be 300. Whatever pressure there has been from the judicial process in right-to-treatment and right-to-payment-for-labor cases up to now will be increased enormously in the near future.

There are also going to be many more lawyers in the field. The Mental Health Law Project is sponsoring with the Practicing Law Institute a series of training seminars for lawyers on the legal rights of the mentally handicapped, scheduled to take place in the first six months of 1975 in four different cities. We expect to reach a potential 1,000 lawyers who previously have not been involved actively in this area and train them to bring these kinds of cases.

Thus, the statistical predictions made elsewhere in this volume about the rate of deinstitutionalization are probably conservative, because whatever factor judicial pressures bring to bear on deinstitutionalization is likely to augment those rates. By 1975, instead of the estimated 125,000 in state and county mental hospitals, we might very well have only half that number, with further decreases to come.

The significance of these trends for the future role of the state mental hospital consist of various factors. First, it is probable that there will be a real shift in the percentage of involuntary as opposed to voluntary patients. Most of the patients in state mental hospitals in the future will be at least ostensibly voluntary. This will bring with it a concomitant need to investigate voluntary admissions to assess their true nature. New York State has taken some progressive steps in that regard in its recent Mental Hygiene Law,[10] which requires the Mental Health Information Service to investigate every voluntary admission to discover whether it is in fact truly voluntary.

Second, it is probable that in the near future there will be the establishment of absolute time limits on the permissible period for which a person can voluntarily enter a mental hospital; after six months or a year a court will have to approve even the supposedly voluntary admissions and the process will have to explore whether less drastic alternatives can be utilized.

Third, it seems likely that with the decline in populations there is going to be a decline in the relative percentage of professionals in state mental hospitals as they move into community facilities, and a relative increase in the percentage of paraprofessionals and social workers. Mental hospitals, if they survive at all (and that is seriously questionable), are going to become human service centers at which legal services and social work services will be brought to bear on the social problems of persons who come to these institutions. Several recent studies have shown that psychiatric patients do as well or better in general hospitals as they do in mental hospitals, and it is likely that general hospitals will treat increasing numbers of psychiatric patients.

In short, the mental hospital system is dying, and there are those of us who believe its death is overdue.

Notes

1. *Wyatt* v. Stickney, 344 F. Supp. 373 (M.D. Ala. 1972).
2. Donaldson v. O'Connor, 493 F.2d 507 (5th CIR.), Cert. granted, –U.S. –, 955.Cr.171, –. L. Ed. 2d–(1974).
3. Winters v. Miller, 446 F. 2d 65 (2d Cir. 1971).
4. N.Y. City Health and Hospitals Corp. v. Stein, 70 Misc. 2d 944, 335 N.Y. S. 2d 461 (1972).
5. Kaimowitz v. Dept. of Mental Health, C.A. No. 73-19434-AW (Circuit Court for Wayne County, Michigan, July 10, 1973).
6. N.Y. State Assn. for Retarded Children v. Rockefeller, 357 F. Supp. 752 (E.D.N.Y. 1973).
7. Jackson v. Indiana, 406 U.S. 715, 92 S.Ct. 1845, 32 L. Ed. 2d 435 (1972).
8. McNeil v. the Director, Patuxent Institution, 407 U.S. 245 92 S. Ct. 2083, 32 L. Ed. 2d 719 (1972).
9. Dale v. Hahn, 440 F. 2d 633 (2d Cir. 1971).
10. N.Y. Mental Hygiene Law, Sect. 31.25 (McKinney Supp. 1974).

5

Psychiatric Admissions: A Medical Viewpoint

Michael Alfred Peszke

The dream and the goal of medical men and women since time immemorial has been utopian—the relief of suffering and the cure of illness. In the area of mental illness, however, the attorney has set as his professional goal the upholding of the constitution and the spirit of John Stuart Mill's words: "The only purpose for which power can be rightfully exercised over any member of a civilized community, against his will, is to prevent harm to others. His own good, either physical or moral is not a sufficient warrant."[1] The average physician and psychiatrist would probably agree with this remark, and the acrimony about psychiatric admissions, particularly those that are involuntary, has to do with the problem of whether a mentally sick individual is, indeed, able to exercise his will.

It would be a mistake to see progress as a uniform and always benevolent progression of understanding and of humanitarian and ethical concern on the part of medicine. There were many vicissitudes, with cruel regressions, and often the interest and good intentions of the physicians were either contaminated by professional and traditional guild interests or by ideological attitudes that were carried to a fanatical extent. It is quite obvious that society has always shown marked ambivalences in its attitude and treatment of the mentally ill. While the sixteenth century saw such an independent thinker as John N. Weyher, whose writings on psychiatry have entitled him to be considered the founder of modern psychiatry, in the same period the father of modern surgery, Ambroise Pare, urged the King of France, his royal master, to execute all witches, quoting the biblical injunction, "Thou shalt not suffer a witch to live." Also the age of moral treatment in the eighteenth century initiated by Philippe Pinel and Daniel Hack Tuke was followed by the tragic abuses described in the reports of the Madhouse Commission in Britain during the nineteenth century.[a] But Virchow said that "physicians of other centuries have been the attorneys and caretakers of the poor."[2] This succinctly describes many of the pursuits, interests,

---

[a]For details of this, Zilboorg, G. and Henry, G.W.,eds.: *A History of Medical Psychology,* New York, Norton, 1941. Also, Rosen, G.: *Madness in Society,* London Routledge, Kegal, Paul, 1968; and Hunter and MacAlpine: *Three Hundred Years of Psychiatry: 1535-1860,* London, Oxford University Press, 1963. Benjamin Rush advocated in *Medical Inquiries and Observations upon Diseases of the Mind,* Philadelphia, Kimber and Richardson, 1812: "For refractory patients pouring cold water under the sleeve, so that it may descend into the armpits and down the trunk of the body." He also recommended deprivation of food and threats of death.

and professional commitments of the physician who only in the nineteenth century developed a so-called scientific background as a result of his better and more scientific understanding of natural biological disease. The tradition of the sage, of the shaman, witch doctor, and religious guide is still strong in the medical profession and probably more so in psychiatry, and only in recent history has medicine become separated from the general pursuit of natural sciences. Psychiatry, the treatment of the mad or of the alienated, is a direct result of these many and multiple historical antecedents. It is impossible to put a date to the time when psychiatry really became a distinct specialty. To this day, in the veterans' and United States military hospitals, it is still referred to as neuropsychiatry. Only in the last fifty years have medical schools established separate departments of psychiatry. However, universal credit has been given to Weyher for being the first "modern" psychiatrist. Yet, this is an academic issue, since for many centuries some physicians were more adept and more interested in the care and the treatment of those conditions that are now loosely described as mental illness. As a matter of fact, during the late medieval ages in England, there were licences issued to specialists of medicine both for the practice of midwifery and those who treated the melancholic and distracted.[b]

The scientific revolution highlighted the disparity between psychiatry and medicine. As the etiology of illness became better understood, the treatment more specific and successful, and the results more predictable, so psychiatry fell by the wayside and became the "Cinderella" of medicine. Unfortunately, rather than doing what they had a chance of doing well, many practicing psychiatrists forgot their traditional humanitarianism and turned their backs on the successful but time-consuming moral treatments as advocated by Pinel in France and Tuke in England and became frustrated custodians indulging themselves and exposing their patients to numerous and, at times, irresponsible and, in retrospect, ridiculous procedures.[c] This attempt to continue their medical identity by indulging in active therapeutic endeavors was only brought to a partial halt by the advent of the psychoanalytic movement when listening and compassion once again became legitimate and respectable and, at times, the sole treatment modalities of the psychiatrist.

Scientific medicine has, as its goal, the eradication of disease either through preventive measures or through the rational scientific application of therapeutic skills. The logical development of the medical model in psychiatry has been the

---

[b]Many centuries prior to Weyher, the diocesan bishops of England by an Act of Parliament (1511) were empowered to recognize and grant licenses to two kinds of medical specialists, those treating the distracted and the melancholic and those practicing midwifery. See Hunter and MacAlpine's *Three Hundred Years of Psychiatry: 1535-1860,* supra footnote a.

[c]For a general discussion of the problem, see the books on the history of psychiatry, supra footnote a, particularly P. Pinel, *Traite Medico-philosophique sur L'alienation Mentale,* Paris, J.A. Broson, 1801.

application of these same concepts to psychiatric problems. If historically the asylums were havens for the sick and the inadequate, so also did they become places for custodial care of those whose psychosocial disabilities prevented them from adapting to the challenge of their everyday life or "expectable environment." The challenge of the growing number of inmates and the inchoate but atavastic conviction in all European and European-derived civilizations that these problems were in fact medical led in growing ways to the application of treatability as a reasonable condition for admission to these institutions. While historically only those who had been unable to take care of themselves and who were charges to the family or to the local community were allowed to seek refuge in these havens, so did the nineteenth century see the emergence of what has been described by some with pride and by some with derision as the therapeutic state. In 1845 the judge of the Supreme Court of the state of Massachusetts ruled on a case brought for habeas corpus by one Josiah Oakes, who argued that he had been illegally committed by his family. Judge Shaw held him lawfully committed and made a ruling that, in the United States, is still the foundation for many of the commitment laws as well as the bone of acrimony between the psychiatric profession and many attorneys:

> The right to restrain an insane person of his liberty is found in that
> great law of humanity which makes it necessary to confine those
> who going at large would be dangerous to themselves or to others.
> And the necessity which creates the law creates the limitations of
> the law. The question must then arise in each particular case whether
> a patient's own safety, or that of others, requires that he should be
> restrained for a certain time, and whether restraint is necessary for
> his restoration, or will be conductive thereto. The restraint can con-
> tinue as long as the necessity continues. This is the limitation and
> the proper limitation.[d]

As is the case with many court decisions, it neither became accepted by all nor did it represent necessarily a unanimous legal consensus. Neither was it a completely new innovation because for many years prior to that ruling, physicians committed patients to hospitals on a mere scribbled signature with a statement that John Doe is a fit subject for confinement in the asylum.[e] That "fit

---

[d]Both Deutsch, A.: *The Mentally Ill in America,* New York, Columbia University Press, 1949 (2nd edition) as well a Kittrie, N.N.: *The Right to be Different,* Baltimore, Johns Hopkins Press, 1972, discuss this problem from slightly different historical and philosophical viewpoints.

[e]Deutsch, ibid, makes reference to the informality of admitting an individual to an asylum during the early days of this country. A couple of scribbled words on a piece of paper to the effect that "an individual is a proper patient for the hospital" were sufficient.

subject" concept represents a potential variety of both innovative and progressive ideas as well as of intellectual, medical, and legal ineptitude. The
decision, however, reflected a judicial sanction of a practice that had been
underway in America and in Europe for many years, if not centuries. The
decision, therefore, *reinforced* the application of this practice and of this
philosophy.

The end of the nineteenth century and the first part of the twentieth
saw the optimistic and growing application of various statutes and regulations
pertaining to the treatment, albeit involuntary, of the mentally ill. At no
time did society through its elected officials or judicial officers who administered these regulations ever give up the conviction that the final arbitrator
and decision-making agents in situations where citizens may be deprived of
liberty for whatever good reason or cause should be the judges.[f] Society continued in the words of Dr. G. Alder Blumer to express considerable anxiety
about the potential for an innocent citizen to be locked up, about abuse and
about the possibility of "railroading" into a setting where exposure to the
mentally ill would deprive even the most sane of his reason.[g] Unfortunately,
as we know from our own clinical work, the paranoia of an individual usually
has a core of realistic concern, so abuses, though infrequent, have at times
been documented and "fire" these concerns. Most often these abuses result
from carelessness or negligence and not maliciousness; yet, they exist and
exacerbate acrimony. While society continues to view involuntary psychiatric
hospitalization as being so serious a step as to preclude it from being merely
a medical matter, so most psychiatrists urge that hospitalization, whether
voluntary or involuntary, is purely a medical issue. Physicians' statements
are often made that the various "rigamaroles" of legal interventions should
be minimized or abolished in the best interest of the patient. Overholser

---

[f]The concern for individual liberties was not a uniquely legal monopoly. Dr. Theodore Diller, in his article "Commitment of the insane in the United States," *Illinois
Medical Journal,* 26:322-24, 1914, wrote, "No one should be deprived of his liberty for
any cause whatsoever except by due process of law and by action of the court and this
should apply to the deprivation of liberty on account of insanity as well as crime."
Dr. Diller was particularly concerned at the looseness of the Pennsylvania statutes, which
were still as informal in his time as they had been in the days of Dr. Benjamin Rush. See
supra footnote e.

[g]The medical side of the question was well presented by Dr. Blumer in his presentation at the International Congress of Charities, Correction and Philanthropy, Chicago,
1893 (published 1894 by Johns Hopkins, Baltimore). Addressing himself to the issue of
commitment, detention, care, and treatment of the insane in America, he stated, "Too
much of our legislation seems to be based on the assumption of improper motives on the
parts of friends and relatives as if it were to be expected that cruelty and inhumanity
instead of being the rare exception should be the normal rule in state of things in civilized
society." In more recent years in the same vein, Professor Ralph Slovenko assessed the
current situation in the United States in "Civil Commitment in Perspective," *Journal of
Public Law,* 20:3-32, 1971.

and Weihofen, for example, concluded their review and plea for a less judicially determined commitment procedure by quoting Isaac Ray:[3]

> In the first place, the law should put no hindrance in the way of the prompt use of those instrumentalities which are regarded as most effectual in promoting the comfort and restoration of the patient. Secondly, it should spare all unnecessary exposure of private troubles, and all unnecessary conflict with popular prejudices. Thirdly, it should protect individuals from wrongful imprisonment. It would be objection enough to any legal provision that it failed to secure these objects in the completest possible manner.[4]

Most physicians are convinced that the citizen's liberties are adequately protected by the possibility of initiating a habeas corpus proceeding or a suit for professional negligence, while his medical condition is assured of treatment appropriate to the needs.

In April 1948 the Group for Advancement of Psychiatry (GAP) issued a report (No. 4) on commitment procedures. In this they very strongly urged the least restrictive and most medical approach to the problem. However, it is interesting that by 1973 the American Psychiatric Association issued a position statement on involuntary hospitalization of the mentally ill (reported in *American Journal of Psychiatry,* 130:3, 1970). This position statement once again accepted the idea of jury trial to determine need for hospitalization should that be requested by a patient or by his legal advisor. One can only assume that the change in philosophy on the part of the psychiatric profession towards acceptance of the need for involuntary hospitalization being determined by lay people had to do with the concern about the political situation in the United States in the late 1960s and early 1970s, as well as being a reflection of concern arising from reports that in the Soviet Union political dissidents are being hospitalized in a Soviet political psychiatric institute.[h] It is also a reflection of the ideological position and political climate that when in the early 1960s the mental health movement was being assaulted by the extreme right as a form of atheistic and Communist-controlled conspiracy, the reaction of the majority of psychiatrists was one of amusement.[i]

---

[h]For a review of that specific problem, see Chodoff, P.: "Involuntary Hospitalization of Political Dissenters in the Soviet Union," *Psychiatric Opinion,* 11:5-19, 1974. Also, Report of U.S. Senate Judiciary Committee, *Abuse of Psychiatry for Political Repression in the Soviet Union,* New York: Arno; Warminster, Wiltshire: Aris and Phillips, 1973.

[i]See Branch, C.H.H.: "Legal Problems Related to the Care of the Mentally Ill," *New England Journal of Medicine,* 269:137-42, 1963. Dr. Branch quotes a letter he received: "Caesar had his arena, Hitler his gas ovens, Russia her slave labor camps and the Kennedy Administration its mental health institutions." The concern now is from the liberals and the concern is closer to home for most psychiatrists. This ideological

The growth of the medical model and the growth of the therapeutic optimism that was particularly exuberant in the decades following World War II did
not, however, see a commensurate or acceptable improvement in the treatment
modalities or the treatment facilities. It is not the intention of this chapter to
review in depth all the problems confronted by state psychiatric facilities, but
some mention has to be made of the general problems. The change of name
from "lunatic asylum" or "institutions for the insane" to "psychopathic hospitals" and "psychiatric state hospitals" and now as in New York State to "psychiatric centers" did not change the internal physical plant materially or in any
meaningful way, improve the budget, or raise the quality of the staff. These
centers continued to be seen by society as the end of the road for the alcoholic
or as the houses for the mad. Their physical isolation led to disruption of the
social and family contact of the patient and encouraged a parochialism in the
staff. The low prestige of state employees in this country compared to Europe
also vitiated against the recruitment of better professional staffs.

There is a distinct difference in attitudes between the United States and the
majority of European countries, particularly the continental ones, about the
status of civil employees and those in private practice. While consultation or
employment in the Federal Civil Service may have a certain amount of prestige
in the United States, it is quite clear that employees of state governments are
often seen as people of dubious character and integrity or of second-rate competence. I do not in any way mean to imply that this is necessarily the case, but
I think it is a fair reflection of general public opinion. In Europe, by and large,
employment by the state or consultation for the state is a reward for competence and seen in that light. Furthermore, a significant number are foreign-
trained. R. Stevens, and J. Vermenlon, present the following statistics: 23
percent of all psychiatrists are foreign-trained, but in staff salaried positions
40.5 percent are foreign-trained. However, while the weakness in training
of the foreign-trained physician is all too often documented, the following
should also be noted: 20 percent of all research and full-time academic positions in psychiatry are occupied by foreign trained physicians.[5]

As recently as 1948 a GAP study documented that a number of states
did not allow voluntary admission to their psychiatric state facilities.[6] Whether
this was a natural development of the premise argued by Dr. Theodore Diller
that it is illogical to allow the insane to exercise judgment about voluntary
admission, or whether it was a result of the legislative concern that state facilities might be abused by individuals looking for an easy way of life is difficult
to determine. In "Commitment of the insane in the United States" (footnote
f) Dr. Diller makes the interesting point that voluntary commitment of

concern is expressed in the language of the ACLU Memo. No. I, December, 1969:
"Proponents of civil confinement of the mentally ill quite correctly argue that abolition
of involuntary confinement would cause much human degradation and social harm but
less, perhaps, than its retention."

insane persons by themselves is an anomoly and cannot stand logical and legal scrutiny. A man who is sound mentally may make a reasonable contract, but if a man is insane it is a farce and against all rules of logic to permit him to make a written contract depriving himself of his liberty. The New York amended statutes for voluntary admissions also make a specific condition that the individual seeking voluntary and informal admission to a psychiatric hospital, state or private, has to understand what he is doing and that he is seeking admission to a hospital for the mentally ill.[j] At the date of writing, all states allow voluntary admission, although it is likely that some states or institutions will tend to discourage such practices. Even within the state of Connecticut the number of voluntary admissions in the three state facilities varies considerably.

Various philosophies and practices appear to account for such disparities. Some institutions allow the senile patients to sign in voluntarily; others argue that these patients are unable to exercise such informed consent. Voluntary admission, the preferred route by all, is still not easily implemented. Many state facilities are so crowded with committed patients that they discourage such voluntary admissions and in many of these facilities the conditions are such that people would rather do without treatment than seek a voluntary entry. Furthermore, the state psychiatric facilities are still in the predicament of not being accepted as a legitimate part of the medical system, but are perceived as the end of the road for the indigent, the inadequate, and the criminal. The failure of most insurance programs to reimburse patients in psychiatric state facilities, furthermore, also aggravates as well as accentuates the feeling that state psychiatric centers are not quite legitimate. In fact, insurance companies continue to balk at payments for psychiatric treatment where an agressive so-called prescriptive approach is not applied.[k]

This chapter will not review the medical or psychiatric indications for hospitalization as opposed to ambulatory treatment. It will confine itself to discussing the current situation and the problems of the physician and his responsibilities as well as discuss some of the challenges and criticisms that have been made of the practice. Even some of the most critical and acerbic

---

[j]The problem of individuals seeking relief from outside stresses in psychiatric centers has been touched on by Braginsky, B.N. and Braginsky, D.P.: "Mental Hospitals as Resorts," *Psychology Today*, March, 1973.

[k]As a member of the Peer Review Committee for the Connecticut State Psychiatric Society, 1972-1974, I was privy to a number of issues that were delegated to our committee. These situations, more often than not, stemmed from insurance companies being unwilling to honor accounts presented to them for long-term psychiatric treatment. The insurance companies felt that custodial treatment, milieu therapy treatment were not within the province of medical therapeutics as it is currently understood in this day and age. This is not a finally settled question, and it is my impression that it will be resolved through a compromise that will protect the insurance companies, the patients, as well as the hospitals, but it does point up the ongoing problem and has led to a position statement by the American Psychiatric Association arguing the need to keep some long-term psychiatric facilities, *American Journal of Psychiatry*, 131:745, 1974.

statements that would be more in place in a *Harvard Lampoon* than in professional or judicial journals have enough truth in them for the medical profession
to pause and take heed.

A representative of the Civil Liberties Union, Mr. Chris Hanson—an attorney
for the Mental Health Law Project—states:[1] "They are (that is the discharged
chronic patients) better off outside of a hospital with no care than they are
inside with no care. The hospitals are what really do damage to people. If
psychiatrists think that patients would be better off inside, they are deceiving
themselves, and psychiatrists are less capable of predicting dangerous behavior
than grocery clerks. Besides you can't lock people up for what they might do
in the future". Unfortunately, language like this is exactly the style that psychiatrists have learned to associate with the so-called truth-seeking aspect of the
adversary proceeding. If one analyzes the statement, it is based on unsubstan-
tiated statements and on acerbic innuendo. The fact the psychiatrists *are* unable
to predict dangerousness is probably well accepted at this point.[m]

The question of voluntary admission appears so simple. The physician-
psychiatrist and his patient agree that inpatient treatment is required and the
appropriate steps are then followed. Yet, the psychiatrist is confronted in the
1970s with two developing concerns that prey on him as Scylla and Charybdis.
On the one hand, he now has to justify to a review committee the need for
inpatient treatment of his patient, since even sick individuals can, in fact, be
successfully treated in an ambulatory setting and since custodial or milieu treatment in itself is not an indication for hospitalization. On the other hand, it is
probably true to say that patients are often psychologically coerced into signing
in as voluntaries. I am sure that the practice of confronting a patient with the
choice of either going in committed to making no waves and signing in has been
and is quite common. The warning signals are out to the medical profession,
however, and treatment under coercion of any kind is going to be seen as infring-
ing on the patients' rights of informed consent. In fact, attorneys are advising
physicians that in *any* situation when a patient balks at treatment he should not
be made or persuaded to follow it, but the medical patient/physician contract
should be terminated. Informed consent requires full knowledge, competency

---

[1]In an article on the discharged chronic mental patient in *Medical World News*,
15:47-57, 1974.

[m]See Rubin, B.: "Prediction of Dangerousness in Mentally Ill Criminals," *Archives of
General Psychiatry*, 27:397-407, 1972, and Stedman, H.J.: "Some Evidence of the Inadequacy of the Concept and Determination of Dangerousness in Law and Psychiatry," *Journal
of Psychiatry and Law*, 1:409-26, 1973. But the problem of chronic patients discharged to
the world at large is a human tragedy and travesty of justice. See also, Robbins, E. and
Robbins, L.: "Charge to the Community: Some Early Effects of a State Hospital System's
Change of Policy," *American Journal of Psychiatry*, 131:641-45, 1974. Also Reich, R.
and Siegel, L.: "Psychiatry Under Siege: The Chronically Mentally Ill Shuffle to Oblivion,"
Psychiatric Annals, 3:35-55, 1973.

to make decisions, and voluntariness! Coercion may be argued as taking away the voluntariness of the decision-making process.

If voluntary admission already raises such problems, it is quite clear that involuntary commitment raises more serious legal and ethical issues. The variety of practices and procedures in the implementation and interpretation of the rules governing involuntary hospitalization defies a reasonable synthesis or even a reasonable explanation. Various states have approached this problem in a chaotic manner. Guided by pressure groups, previous experiences and possibly the model draft act, their rules are hard to understand because the implementation is by medical rather than legal personnel.[n] A good example of that is the Connecticut statute (Section 17-183 of the Connecticut General Statutes), which states: "Prior to hospitalization under the provision of this section, any person shall have the right to be examined by a physician of his own choosing, and if such physician concludes from his examination that such person is not mentally ill or acutely drug dependent, such person shall not be admitted or detained in a hospital for mental illness under the provisions of this section." I have talked to many attorneys and physicians about this and none has offered a reasonable explanation as to how it should be implemented with the exception of some attorneys who argue that it should be read like a "Miranda" warning to the patient. The possibility of doing this at night in the emergency room to a psychotic patient defies the imagination.

Furthermore, these laws and statutes change frequently, due to pressure from the community, from the advocates for the rights of the mentally ill, and through lobbying by various mental health groups. At times they are affected by specific or threatened court action. Unfortunately, there currently appears to be if not an alliance then at least mutual encouragement and collusion between those who wish to protect societal rights to freedom and legislators who are interested in saving money by cutting down the number of inmates and limiting the services offered by state psychiatric facilities. For a comprehensive review of the language of the different rules and regulations in the various jurisdictions of this country, you are referred to S.J. Brakel and R.S. Rock's comprehensive and definitive study, *The Mentally Disabled and the Law.*[7]

Most jurisdictions make provision for an emergency detention of a mentally ill individual. Also most make provision for legal court-adjudicated commitment. A number of states, at this point, still insist on or give the option to the patient for a jury trial. In what has been a most distinct reversal of many decades of

---

[n]A draft act governing hospitalization of the mentally ill was prepared by a group of the National Institute of Mental Health and the Office of General Council of the United States. It was issued as Public Health Service Publication No. 51, U.S. Government Printing Office in 1952, and is reprinted in full as Appendix A in Brakel, S.J. and Rock, R.S.: *The Mentally Disabled and the Law,* rev. ed., University of Chicago Press, Chicago, 1971 (the original edition was edited by Lindman, F.T. and McIntyre, D.M., Jr. in 1961).

policy, the American Psychiatric Association recently stated that jury trials should be permitted to adjudicate the need for psychiatric involuntary hospitalization.[8] Emergency detentions are usually initiated either by physicians or by public health agencies such as the police or welfare. In most instances such emergency detention is temporary and subject to various scrutinies and a system of examinations that can either limit or undo the original certification. Most jurisdictions follow this emergency detention by some kind of court adjudication either through a form of mental health tribunal, a magistrate's court, a probate court, or in New York by a branch of the Superior Court. This particular procedure is more often than not referred to as the "commitment." However, the terms applied are interchangeable and commitment in one jurisdiction may not mean exactly the same as in another.[o]

The language, the definition, the looseness, and the variety of procedures all reflect the inchoate thinking of the medical profession in this area, the disinterest of the legislature, as well as the perplexity of the legal profession. The recovered mentally ill, with few historical exceptions such as Clifford Beers,[9] do not act as advocates to improve facilities. The chronic sick have no credibility, while too often psychiatrists have accepted the status quo and have been perceived as deriving a financial advantage from the practice. Society has always recognized deviant behavior and over the centuries has acted either to expunge it, to ridicule it, to sequester it, or to repress it. As forms of deviant behavior became differentiated and as some became recognizable as falling within the scope of the medical profession, the attorneys have continued to approach the problem of commitment with two legal philosophical precepts: (1) the *parens patriae* philosophy of taking care of those who are unable to take care of themselves and (2) invoking the police power of the state to prevent citizens from hurting others or the property of others.[p] Attorneys recognize the need to incarcerate for dangerousness, since this deals with conduct. Physicians continue to be concerned with sickness and they wish to cure. It is this preoccupation with dangerousness and with the old concepts of madness that results in the statutory language of many states being so archaic. On the other hand, psychiatric texts make no provision

---

[o] *Black's Law Dictionary*, 4th ed., 1951, defines commitment as "The warrant by which a court directs an officer to take a person to prison and a proceeding for the restraining and confining of insane persons for their own and public's protection." With such a definition, a number of statutes have tried to omit such language and the Draft Act avoids the use of the word "commitment," speaking about various kinds of hospitalization.

[p] An excellent legal analysis of the problem is contained in Ross, H.A.: "Commitment of the Mentally Ill: Problems of Law and Policy," *Michigan Law Review*, 57:943-1007, 1959. A very scholarly but legalistic review article is the one by Livermore, J.M., Malmquist, C.P., and Meehl, P.E.: "The Justifications for Civil Commitment," *University of Pennsylvania Law Review*, 117:75-96, 1968.

for instructing the physician or the psychiatrist in the criteria for emergency commitment.

For example, one of the major textbooks of psychiatry has this to say about emergency commitments:

> Interestingly, however, the behavioral sciences have not yet been able to evolve simple and operational definitions of eccentricity or of dangerousness. As therapuetic interventions increase in intensity and scope, they more frequently encounter the question of a person impulsively leaving treatment where there appears to be a good chance that he could further improve his status and diminish his self-destructive behavior. Without some element of restraint, such a person might not have received therapeutic help at all. Nonetheless, it is probably best, both for society and for the therapy of the patient, that coercion be restricted to the minimum necessary for the protection of life.[10]

In another, the section on forensic psychiatry states: "In fact, however, for the lawyer a commitment is a mittimus, a warrant for imprisonment. On the other hand, for the psychiatrist the term denotes a helpful procedure, in that it facilitates the hospitalization and appropriate treatment of a patient as mentally ill."[11]

The late Dr. Henry Davidson, a distinguished forensic psychiatrist, described the variety and confused aspect of state requirements for commitments. He also gave general warnings to physicians and psychiatrists on the various steps that need to be followed for a commitment to be binding legally and that would guarantee a reasonable immunity from a malpractice suit. He did not, however, address himself in any way to the indications for initiating such a commitment but warned that, "A physician that cannot demonstrate to a judge that the patient is psychotic has a weak case."[12] A recent text by T.P. Detre and H.G. Jarecki offers no comments about involuntary commitment and, in fact, the words "commitment," "certification," or "involuntary hospitalization" do not even appear in the index.[13] What this review of major texts demonstrates is that there are no guidelines for psychiatrists when involuntary treatment is planned or when it should be considered a medical duty.

M.A. Peszke and R. Wintrob, in their study, found that there was a great looseness of thinking among psychiatrists about involuntary commitment. Many of the psychiatrists felt that this was a strictly medical issue and the majority were unaware of the background statutes which govern these procedures and their jurisdiction. Most, however, shared a medical concern that the indications for commitment were harm to self or others as a result of psychoses or inability to take care of self as a result of psychoses.[14]

The legal profession, concerned about looseness of definitions emanating from psychiatrists, concerned by the lack of treatment or inadequate treatment in many psychiatric institutions, has tended to argue that only the police power protection of the state in respect to the dangerous individual is the criterion for incarceration. Not all attorneys or not even all attorneys belonging to the Civil Liberties Union feel or agree with T.S. Szasz that mental illness is a myth.[15] However, they argue that the problems are too complicated to be left to physicians and that abuses can only be prevented by strict and constant scrutiny and the application of various adversary procedures transplanted from criminal law. Therefore, such concepts as probable cause and protection against self-incrimination are invoked to prevent the alleged "victim" from being hospitalized. Least restrictive alternatives are advanced and both the medical profession as well as society are needled to provide more comprehensive and better treatment opportunities for individuals.

In a symposium on ethics and mental health Morton Birnbaum coined the word "sanism" to describe the attitude of society in general toward the mentally ill.[16] He likens that feeling to other prejudices and makes a strong point in arguing that it is the inability or the lack of interest of many in our society, even established psychiatric professional groups, that has led to the current situation of neglect and of ideological acrimony. A physician and an attorney, Dr. Birnbuam has for the last ten years been closely associated with the right to treatment issue that saw its first successful action in the test case of *Wyatt* v. *Stickney* in Alabama.[q]

The case of *Wyatt* v. *Stickney*—the name of the plaintiff patient being Wyatt and the name of the commissioner of mental health in the state of Alabama being Dr. Stonewall B. Stickney (chief defendant and representative of the state facility)—has generated considerable satisfaction as well as concern in various circles. The suit was brought on behalf of Wyatt who argued that he had been unable to obtain reasonable treatment while committed. The judge ruled in favor of the plaintiff and came up with a very detailed set of recommendations based on American Psychiatric Association guidelines for standards. The fact of the matter is that the case, won by the plaintiff in court, has really not led to any significant improvements that can be documented in the general care of the mentally ill in that state or elsewhere. The case was appealed in 1974 and the original decision upheld. The significant thing is that Dr. Stickney stipulated to most of the criteria that were demanded by the plaintiff and that were within the guidelines of the Psychiatric Association's minimum criteria for Treatment. However, after this occurred,

---

[q]Awarded the Manfred Guttmacher prize in 1973 for contributions to legal psychiatry, he has written a number of outstanding articles in this area, among them: "The Right to Treatment—Some Comments on Implementation," in the *Duquesne Law Review,* 10:579-608, 1972. "Some Comments on the Right to Treatment," *Archives of General Psychiatry,* 13:34-45, 1965.

Dr. Stickney was dismissed by the Alabama Mental Health Board in September 1972, and was replaced by a nonmedical associate commissioner who has joined the state in appealing the case.[r]

Sick patients continue to be brought to psychiatrists, emergency rooms, and physicians, and no amount of legislation appears to stop them from experiencing the disabling anxieties of everyday life. The psychiatrists in private practice need not worry about this problem and, by and large, neither does the attorney, the legislator, or the Civil Liberties Union attorney. It is the emergency room staff, the welfare worker, the public health nurse, and the police officer who are confronted with these problems.[s] Changing the statutes does not make these people disappear, go away, or change their behavior. It would seem that as long as society turns to the physician, and nowadays specifically to the emergency room for help, then so should the physicians and the hospitals take a strong and emphatic stand in both developing criteria for emergency detention and making adequate provision for emergency psychiatric facilities. It seems perfectly reasonable for physicians to allow mental health specialists from the legal profession to advise and counsel the patients, but not to interfere at every step with the practice of medicine. The attorney always has recourse in the long tradition of Anglo-Saxon law to the habeas corpus proceeding.

Furthermore, peer reviews should be set up to help physicians take a second look at the practice of commitment as well as to help them develop the use of other agencies to strengthen the lifelines of their patients. This would help to implement the "least restrictive alternative" philosophy that is now being argued and advocated, one of the more constructive developments in the area. But continued enforced involuntary treatment has to be left to a

[r]Details of this are under 344 F Supp. 373,387 (M.D. Ala. 1972). The standards referred to were promulgated by the American Psychiatric Association, 1956 and revised in 1958, published by the Association under the tital "Standards for Hospitals and Clinics," Washington, D.C., 1958. A commentary on this was made by Dr. Solomon, who in his presidential address, remarked on the fact that in the majority of American state facilities, only fifteen states had more than fifty percent of the total number of physicians needed to staff the facilities according to the minimum standards suggested by the American Psychiatric Association, "American Psychiatric Association in Relation to American Psychiatry," *American Journal of Psychiatry*, 155:1, 1958. For a comprehensive discussion of the case, see Slovenko, R.: *Psychiatry and Law*, Boston, Little, Brown & Co., 1973 (particularly Chapter 14: "Rights of Committed Patients").

[s]In the majority of cases, it is the police officer who is stuck with trying to implement public safety and health while attempting to conform to a variety of statutory and accepted procedures. This was well commented upon by Mathews, A.R.: "Observations in Policy and Procedures for Emergency Detention of the Mentally Ill," *Journal of Criminal Law, Criminology and Political Science*, 61:283-95, 1970. In a similar vein, Dr. Zusman and Ms. Shaffer wrote about the inadequacy of trying to provide emergency treatment through a legal pathway. Zusman, Jack and Shaffer, S.: "Emergency Psychiatric Hospitalization via Court Order: A Critique," *American Journal of Psychiatry*, 130:132-36, 1973.

combined medical and judicial body or possibly, given the climate of the day, one that is strictly judicial.

The World Health Organization also addressed this point. While on initial reading it seems to be a rather platitudinous statement, in fact it is very perceptive and should be taken to heart by all involved. The problem lies in the fact that it can be read as condoning a religious-political approach to mental illness:

> What is required is to give these patients facilities for treatment and the possibility of guardianship and medical supervision in accordance with their medical needs and social inadequacy. The different methods of solving these problems are extremely complex since they must vary according to the social structure of each country. No one system can be applicable to several different countries and even in one and the same country the systems advocated by some will be repudiated by others. Any system which comes into conflict with legal or cultural conceptions is inapplicable. It would seem, therefore, that preference should be given above all to establishing laws strongly integrated into cultural traditions while at the same time leaving the way open for possible changes.[17]

Such mental health tribunals, however, should have more than the one alternative, which is currently the practice. I have written elsewhere that while medicine has many alternatives, the legal system has some options in criminal practice; yet, when it comes to the treatment of the mentally ill there is an all-or-nothing approach.[18] Patients are either committed or not, and there are no other options currently available.

Emergency detention appears to be strictly a medical matter. The issue of involuntary hospitalization following adjudication is one that will be determined by social values and legal concerns. Is this involuntary treatment for diagnosis or treatment? If for treatment, then what kind of treatment? How far and how heroic are the treatments that are justified and permissible? Is it reasonable to inject a patient with antipsychotic medication, or is it reasonable to shock a depressed patient to prevent suicide?

There is a serious misunderstanding among many nonmedical people as to the use and effect of phenothiazines which are the standard antipsychotic medications. It is quite surprising that while intelligent people comprehend the effectiveness of dilantin for the control of epilepsy, they refuse to accept the fact that phenothiazines play a similar role in the treatment of the psychotic. Over and over again one runs into a prejudice that these medicines are merely a "downer" to chemically restrain the mind (e.g., Cole, J. and Davis, J.: "Antipsychotic Drugs" in Bellak, L. and Leob, L.: *Schizophrenic Syndorme.* In this chapter literature pertaining to neuropharmacology is extensively reviewed, and the following facts of pertinence to this article are discussed and references given. From this body of medical literature it is shown that for schizophrenics, antipsychotic phenothiazines are significantly related to improvement, their withdrawal significantly associated with relapse and rehospitalization, and that these medicines are significantly better than sedatives or placebos and more useful than psychotherapeutic treatment without them.)

Just such a question was taken to the Supreme Court of the state of New York in New York County, and it was ruled that shock treatment could not necessarily be given to an involuntarily hospitalized patient if that patient refused to consent to its administration. This rather paradoxical finding in that a patient could refuse appropriate treatment for her or his illness and yet be involuntarily confined for his welfare can only be explained by the current climate of doubt as to the efficacy of electric-convulsive therapy and the general fear of manipulating the brain in any physical manner. The judge ruled that in view of the fact that there was some question as to the indication for this treatment, the patient should be given the benefit of the doubt and not subjected to this specific treatment.[t]

We might also ask if it is ethical and reasonable to put a patient in a behavior modification unit or perhaps to expose him to a psychosurgical procedure?[u] I am convinced that how society reconciles this concern about the right to treatment with the preservation of freedom will have to do with both the ethics and level of concern of the medical profession, and with the legal profession's own perceptions of this problem and its ideological commitments. These are bound by current mores, culture, and concerns, as well as by the interpretation of the credo behind this country's existence—the Constitution.

As psychiatry and the medical profession become better able to define specific forms of mental illness and thus guarantee therapeutic results, then social and ideological problems will be heightened and the issue of the therapeutic state will be a progressively growing dilemma. Success will lead inevitably to demands of society to control the deviant as well as to treat the ill; hence, the dangers emanating from this will heighten concern.

Having observed a number of different state procedures, I can think of no better approach at present than that of New York State. Involuntary treatment is legal if a physician certifies that the patient's mental condition is a threat to

---

[t]*New York Law Journal*, July, 1972.

[u]There is a progressive amount being written on the issue of behavior therapy and the two references listed are quite representative of the more enlightened concerns expressed in this area. Halleck, S.L.: "Legal and ethical aspects of behavior control," American *Journal of Psychiatry*, 131:381-85, 1974. As well as Wexler, D.B.: "Token and Taboo: Behavior Modification, Token Economies, and the Law," *California Law Review*, 61:81-109, 1973. Also reprinted in *Behaviorism* 1:1-24, 1973.

his welfare.[v] Yet, dangerousness may be invoked as a public health measure by a relative or a police officer and thus the patient is brought in for observation of his mental condition. This is more civilized, more appropriate to the needs of the mentally ill and of society in general that the Washington, D.C., statute which states that a person be hospitalized only if he is mentally ill and because of his illness is likely to injure himself or others if he is not immediately detained.

Washington, D.C., from having very loose and inadequate statutes for the protection of the civil rights of individuals as a result of congressional hearings in 1961, went to the other extreme and has what appears to be punitive commitment laws that must leave a great number of people in serious distress. The appropriate statute reads, Article 21-521:

> An accredited officer or agent of the Department of Public Health
> of the District of Columbia, or an officer authorized to make arrests
> in the District of Columbia, or a physician of the person in question,
> who has reason to believe that a person is mentally ill and because of
> his illness is likely to injure himself or others if he is not immediately
> detained may, without a warrant, take the person into custody,
> transport him to a public or private hospital, and make application
> for his admission thereto for purposes of emergency observation and
> diagnosis. The application shall reveal the circumstances under which
> the person was taken into custody and the reasons therefor.

The provision of attorneys to insist on these rights apparently has made a significant impact in the number of admissions to St. Elizabeth. However, this is not the case in the state of Connecticut where up until 1971 an emergency confinement could be expedited by a physician who had to state that he found the patient in immediate need of care and treatment for mental illness. In 1971, as a result of lobbying, this language was changed to, "I am of the opinion that the above named person is in immediate need of care and treatment in a hospital

---

[v]New York State Mental Hygiene Law, Amended 1973—Article 31 deals exclusively with hospitalization of the mentally ill and Article 31:35 with the appeal possibility for the patient or his relative. The statutory language for a two-physician certificate that seems to be the most reasonable and expeditious manner for admitting a sick patient reads that the undersigned physician certifies "that he finds that this individual has a mental illness which requires care and treatment as an inpatient for that individual's welfare and, furthermore, that there is such impairment of judgment that patient himself is unable to understand need for such care and treatment." The physician, furthermore, has to state that he has considered alternative forms of care and treatment, but that in his judgment, they are inadequate to provide for the needs of the patient or are not readily available. The patient's welfare is, furthermore, reasonably well protected by the New York Mental Health Information Service, which in two of the districts of New York State is staffed by attorneys and in two by social workers, a rather paradoxical situation. For an excellent review of the functioning of this agency, see Gupta, R.K.: "New York's Mental Health Information Service: An Experiment in Due Process," *Rutgers Law Review* 25:405–50, 1971.

for mental illness, because his mental condition presents a danger to himself or others." The issue of danger to himself or others has not been defined and it is difficult, at this point, to see any major difference in the practice.[w]

There is a paradox that makes no legal, logical, or ethical sense. If mental illness does not exist per se, and the commitment is activated by the "dangerous" criterion, then it is indeed preventive detention. If mental illness does exist, then it is cruel to deprive such a patient of treatment merely because he/she is not dangerous! Yet, the psychiatric specialty has been castigated bitterly for all its sins of commission and omission, the most recent attack being by Nader's group.[19]

The medical profession has to respond to these challenges not with a sense of bitterness, but with the honest and forthright approach of knowing its limitations as well as its capabilities. Physicians should not, under any circumstances, ignore the statutes written by jurisdiction, nor should they become advocates for the commitment of a patient. They should under no circumstance argue, but merely present the facts, and leave the conclusion to the tribunal or the probate judge. Psychiatrists should be responsive to the needs of their community but should not in any way allow themselves to become victims of the establishment by "fudging" the regulations to help the patient. At times, in Connecticut, I have observed physicians commit because the patient otherwise might go to jail, even though the grounds for commitment were not really fulfilled. The situation in the state of Connecticut where the expert panel advises the probate judge that the patient is "a fit subject for confinement" is archaic. Psychiatrists should not take such a position, but should leave it up to the tribunal and present the facts for that tribunal to adjudicate.

To conclude, physicians in their everyday practice are confronted by psychiatric emergencies that they are forced by reason of their mandate and by their traditional role to examine, diagnose, and, at times, treat. Emergency detention for psychiatric illness should be in essence no different from the protection of an accident victim. Detention should be subject to peer review, with input of consultants from other disciplines. The New York definition of welfare—an inability to understand the need to take care of oneself—seems reasonable and workable. Hospitalization is not, as critics would have it, a way to modify behavior, but merely to bring the patient back to his premorbid level of functioning. Such adjudication probably should be made by an independent tribunal that should be expert in the areas of both law and psychiatry; the English system appears an excellent model.[20] The facts should not be presented as conclusions. Such involuntary treatment should be continually

---

[w]A Canadian study showed that a statutory language change was not followed by any meaningful change in the practice of psychiatrists in the Province of Ontario. Page, S. and Yates, E.: "Civil Commitment and the Danger Mandate," *Canadian Psychiatric Association,* 18:267-71, 1973.

revised and progressively stricter criteria applied. That kind of tribunal should have the option of mandating outpatient treatment.

It does not appear unreasonable to consider the concept of incompetency as a major ground and criterion for involuntary hospitalization. If a patient is competent to exercise judgment about his life, then probably treatment should be urged but not enforced. At the same time, equating involuntary treatment with incompetency should mean that all reasonable treatments appropriate to the condition could and in fact *should* be applied. It seems at best illogical to state that a patient is so benighted as to need to be hospitalized and then to allow him a choice about treatment!

The medical profession should remember the prophetic words of de Tocqueville: "The government of democracy is favorable to the political power of lawyers; for when the wealthy, the noble, and the prince are excluded from the government, the lawyers take possession of it. . . . The courts of justice are the visible organs by which the legal profession is enabled to control the democracy." In a different setting, de Tocqueville states that the legal profession is the only defense against tyranny of the majority and that "if they prize freedom much, they generally value legality still more," and he advised the despotic prince to allow lawyers into the government.[21]

We as a profession are becoming a little like the man holding a tiger by the tail. It would be very useful if the responsibility in this area were evenly shared by the legal profession; in that event a more pragmatic attitude would develop quickly.

To conclude with Mill from *On Liberty:* "It is, perhaps, hardly necessary to say that this doctrine (i.e., individual liberty) is meant to apply only to human beings in the maturity of their faculties . . . but as soon as mankind have attained the capacity of being guided to their own improvement by conviction or persuasion (a period long since reached in all nations with whom we need here concern ourselves), compulsion, either in the direct form . . . is no longer justifiable . . . ."[22] There is no reason to think that Mill was writing about the mentally ill, but his willingness to admit exception certainly would apply to those whose level of functioning has reduced them to a helpless and incompetent state.

As a profession we do not wish to change people, only to revert them to that optimum state they had reached prior to illness. But to do it well we need the support and the understanding of the community.

Notes

1. Mill, J.S.: *On Liberty*, New York, Appleton-Century-Crofts, 1947, p. 9.
2. Sigerist, H.S.: "What Medicine has Contributed to the Progress of Civilization," *International Record of Medicine and GP Clinics*, 168: 383-91, 1955.
3. Overholser, W. and Weihofen, H.: "Commitment of the Mentally Ill," *American Journal of Psychiatry*, 102: 758-69, 1946.

4. The original of this can be found in Ray, I.: *Contributions to Mental Pathology*, Boston, Little, Brown & Co., 1973, chapter on "Confinement of the Insane."

5. Stevens, R. and Vermenlon, J.: *Foreign Trained Physicians in American Medicine,* Division of Manpower Intelligence, Bureau of Health Manpower Intelligence, N.I.H., 1972.

6. Group for Advancement of Psychiatry: Report #4, "Commitment Procedures," April 1948.

7. Brakel, S.J. and Rock, R.S.: *The Mentally Disabled and the Law*, rev. ed., Chicago: University of Chicago Press, 1971.

8. American Psychiatric Association, Position Statement on Involuntary Hospitalization, *Amer. J. Psychiatry,* 130: 3, 1970.

9. Beers, C.W.: *A Mind That Found Itself*, New York, Longmans, Green & Co., 1908.

10. Katz, J.: "Law and Psychiatry," in Redlich, F. and Friedman, D.X., *Theory and Practice of Psychiatry*, New York, Basic Books, 1966.

11. Freedman, L.Z.: "Forensic Psychiatry," in Freedman, A.M. and Kaplan, H.T., editors, *Comprehensive Textbook of Psychiatry*, Baltimore, Williams and Wilkins, 1967.

12. Davidson, H.A.: "The Commitment Procedures and Their Legal Implications," in Arieti, S., editor, *American Handbook of Psychiatry*, New York, Basic Books, 1959.

13. Detre, T.P. and Jarecki, H.G.: *Modern Psychiatric Treatment*, Philadelphia, Lippincott & Company, 1971.

14. Peszke, M.A. and Wintrob, R.: "Emergency Commitment—A Transcultural Study," *American Journal of Psychiatry*, 131: 36-40, 1974.

15. Szasz, T.S.: *Myth of Mental Illness,* New York, Hoeberger-Harber, 1961.

16. Birnbaum, M., "The Right to Treatment: Some Comments on its Development," in *Medical Moral & Legal Issues in Mental Health Care*, ed. Frank J. Ayd, Williams and Wilkins, 1974.

17. World Health Organization Technical Report #98, 1955, "Legislation Affecting Psychiatric Treatment," Geneva, July, 1955.

18. Peszke, M.A.: "Involuntary Treatment of the Mentally Ill: Law's All or Nothing Approach," *Connecticut Bar Journal, 46:*620-642, 1972.

19. Chu, F.D.: "The Nader Report: One Author's Perspectives," *American Journal of Psychiatry*, 131: 775-79, 1974.

20. Maclay, W.S.: "The New Mental Health Act in England and Wales," *American Journal of Psychiatry*, 116: 778-81, 1960; Wood, J.C.: "Mental Health Review Tribunals," *Medical Science and Law*, 7: 86-92, 1971.

21. de Tocqueville, A.: *Democracy in America*, Two volumes, New York, Alfred A. Knopf, 1963.

22. Mill, *On Liberty*, p. 10.

6 Psychiatric Hospitalization in New York: A Paradigmatic Approach
William A. Carnahan

The States have traditionally exercised broad power to commit persons found to be mentally ill. The substantive limitations on the exercise of this power and the procedures for invoking it vary drastically among the States. The particular fashion in which the power is exercised—for instance, through various forms of civil commitment, defective delinquency laws, sexual psychopath laws, commitment of persons acquitted by reason of insanity—reflects different combinations of distinct bases for commitment sought to be vindicated. The bases that have been articulated include dangerousness to self, dangerousness to others, and the need for care or treatment or training. Considering the number of persons affected, it is perhaps remarkable that the substantive constitutional limitations on this power have not been more frequently litigated.[1]

New York's recently recodified Mental Hygiene Law reflects current thinking on the subject of Justice Blackmun's opinion exerpted above. Its statutory scheme appears to obey emerging constitutional demands for functionally relevant admission standards, exploration of less drastic alternatives to psychiatric hospitalization, and rights to treatment. It will, no doubt, serve as both an anatomical and an analytical model for legislation in other states.

The main thematic issues that will be discussed here in relation to New York's Mental Hygiene Law include a definition of mental illness, admission standards, durational limitations, treatment, the Mental Health Information Service, counsel, and judicial review of psychiatric hospitalization.

Mental Illness

In psychiatry, diagnosis is used for informational purposes leading to prescriptions for various therapeutic interventions. For example, consider the following diagnosis of schizophrenia, paranoid type:

This type of schizophrenia is characterized primarily by the presence of persecutory or grandiose delusions, often associated with hallucinations. Excessive religiosity is sometimes seen. The patient's attitude is frequently hostile and aggressive, and his behavior tends

111

to be consistent with his delusions. In general the disorder does not
manifest the gross personality disorganization of the hebephrenic
and catatonic types, perhaps because the patient uses the mechanism
of projection, which ascribes to others characteristics he cannot
accept in himself. Three subtypes of the disorder may sometimes be
differentiated, depending on the predominant symptoms: hostile,
grandiose, and hallucinatory.[2]

Since this diagnosis is used primarily to trigger a therapeutic plan and is of
further value for statistical and epidemiological purposes, it is of little legal
concern whether it denotes a distinct clinical entity. In fact, it does not, as
the American Psychiatric Association's manual on mental disorders later
acknowledges.[a]

However, in psychiatric hospitalization proceedings, this diagnosis fairly
often leads to a prediction of dangerousness, and as a consequence, triggers
legally sanctioned social isolation. Since psychiatric diagnosis has not been
shown to be clinically or statistically reliable or valid as a behavior predicting
mechanism,[3] its use in such proceedings is questionable—if not pernicious.

In an effort to provide a functionally relevant connection between the
subject and the object of the diagnostic process, New York has defined mental
illness as "an affliction with a mental disease or a mental condition which is
manifested by a disorder or disturbance in behavior, feeling, thinking or judgment to such an extent that the person afflicted requires care and treatment."[4]
While clinical considerations are still relevant in shaping conceptual contours
of "mental disease or mental condition," this definition demands a bridge
between demonstrable mental pathology and proffered benefits of therapeutic
institutionalization. Where the institutionalization is of an emergency nature
or at the patient's option, inpatient status need only be appropriate.[5]   Where
legal compulsion is otherwise involved, inpatient status must be "essential."[6]

Admission Standards

Informal and Voluntary Admissions

Informal admissions may be characterized as superficially analagous to

---

[a]American Psychiatric Association, *Diagnostic and Statistical Manual of Mental
Disorders*, 34 (2 ed. 1968), XI. "Consider, for example, the mental disorder labeled
in this Manual as 'schizophrenia' which, in the first edition was labeled schizophrenic
reaction.' The change of label has not changed the nature of the disorder, nor will it
discourage continuing debate about its nature or causes. Even if it had tried, the Committee (on Nomenclature and Statistics of the American Psychiatric Association) could
not establish agreement about what this disorder is; it could only agree on what to call
it."

voluntary admissions into nonpsychiatric public or private hospitals. Formal admission procedures may be waived and the patient is free theoretically to leave at any time.[7]

Voluntary admissions are upon written application of a person over sixteen, or by the parent, legal guardian, or next of kin of a minor under sixteen.[8] Upon written notification by the patient of his desire to leave the hospital, he must be released within seventy-two hours, unless the hospital director moves for a judicial order of involuntary retention.[9]

The seeming virtues of both informal and voluntary admissions are somewhat blemished by the fact that at any time the patient may find himself a subject of a judicial involuntary retention hearing. In fact, a hospital might lose its operating certificate for failing to move for involuntary retention.[10] Incongruity creeps into the whole scheme by requiring of both informal and voluntary patients that they understand they are making application to a mental hospital and may be involuntarily retained,[11] yet, dispensing with any requirement of "legal capacity to contract."[12]

The fact that voluntary admissions may trigger involuntary retention has engendered controversy. Dr. Szasz would argue that due to the power of the state to compel retention, "(t)he distinction between voluntary and involuntary commitment is . . . not a significant one."[13]

However, Doctors McGarry and Greenblatt conclude:

> We believe that "conditional voluntary" mental hospital admission is a highly desirable alternative to involuntary commitment. It avoids the necessity of a court-mediated process with criminal overtones. Conditional voluntary status gives a much greater degree of dignity and autonomy to a patient than could possibly exist in a state that admits only on an involuntary basis. The conditional voluntary admission (rather than being a fraud) has proved in practice to be a reasonable contractual compromise in the best interests of both patients and the community. It has helped to destigmatize mental-hospital admission. It is hoped that informal or totally voluntary admission will be used increasingly, but there will probably continue to be a few mentally ill citizens who will require conditional voluntary admission and a few who will require involuntary admission.[14]

There exist no empirical studies concerning the use of voluntary admissions in New York. However, a recent Illinois study of voluntary commitment in that state has concluded:

> Both the medical and legal proponents of voluntary care share a conception of voluntary admission as an individual decision to

accept mental treatment, made entirely apart from involuntary commitment procedures, thereby avoiding the therapeutic and legal problems
of coercion. . . . The results of our study indicate that the foregoing
conception is wrong.

In a majority of cases voluntary admission is utilized to hospitalize
persons who are already in some form of official custody. Voluntary
admission avoids procedural complexity and the need for officials to
assume responsibility, both inherent drawbacks to compulsory commitment from the officials' point of view. Individuals are therefore induced
to voluntarily commit themselves with the threat of involuntary commitment as the principal means of persuasion, and with little concern for
the adequacy of the information on which the individual's decision is
based or whether it is "voluntary" at all. The foregoing situation raises
serious legal questions which have thus far gone largely undiscussed.[15]

Involuntary Admissions

Presentment of Patients

An individual may be involuntarily presented to an approved psychiatric
hospital in one of three ways:

1. *Peace Officers.* Should any police or peace officer determine that an
individual "appears to be mentally ill and is conducting himself in a manner
which is likely to result in serious harm to himself or others,"[b] that individual
may be taken into custody and removed to an approved psychiatric receiving
hospital, or temporarily detained "in another safe and comfortable place."[c]

2. *The Judiciary.* Should any court be informed by affidavit of anyone
that a person is "apparently" mentally ill and conducting himself in a manner
deemed to be either "disorderly conduct" or that is "likely to result in serious
harm to himself or others," the court shall issue a warrant directing the

---

[b]N.Y. Mental Hygiene Law 31.19 defines likelihood of serious harm to include:
"(1) Substantial risk of physical harm to himself as manifested by threats of or attempts
at suicide or serious bodily harm or other conduct demonstrating that he is dangerous
to himself or (2) A substantial risk of physical harm to other persons as manifested
by homicidal or other violent behavior by which others are placed in reasonable fear of
serious physical harm." This definition is based upon California and New York formu-
lations. See, Cal. Welf. & Inst'ns Code 5300 (West 1972); Mass. Gen. Laws Ann. Ch.
123 1.

[c]N.Y. Mental Hygiene Law 32.41 (McKinney Supp. 1974). However, penal facil-
ities may not be utilized. 1972 Op. Atty'y Gen. 18-19 (1972); Zusman, J. and Shafer,
S., *Emergency Psychiatric Hospitalization Via Court Order: A Critique,* AMER. J.
PSYCHIAT., 130 (1973), 1323.

presence of the person before the court.[d] Thereupon, if it appears that "such a person has or may have a mental illness that is likely to result in serious harm to himself or others, the court shall issue a civil order directing his removal . . ." to any approved psychiatric hospital for a determination by the hospital director regarding further retention.

3. *Director of Community Services or his Psychiatric Designees.* Upon notification by a parent, spouse, child, licensed physician, health officer, or peace officer that a "person has a mental illness for which immediate care and treatment in a hospital is appropriate and which is likely to result in serious harm to himself or others . . ." a director of community services or his psychiatric designee may direct the removal—with the aid of the police, of such person to an approved psychiatric hospital.[16]

Commitment of Patients

The director of an approved psychiatric hospital is vested with initial authority to involuntarily detain persons satisfying statutory standards for detention. Such authority may be exercised in emergency, short term, or extended commitment situations.

Emergency Commitment. Should a person be "alleged to have a mental illness for which immediate observation, care, and treatment in a hospital is appropriate and which is likely to result in serious harm to himself or others . . ." he may be detained for a period of up to fifteen days,[17] or if referred by a director of community services or his psychiatric designee, for a period of no more than seventy-two hours.[18]

Short Term Commitment. Upon application of certain designated persons together with certificates of two examining physicians, the director of an approved psychiatric hospital may detain any person "alleged to be mentally ill and in need of involuntary care and treatment . . ." for a period of up to sixty days.[19]

Extended Commitment. Upon judicial approval, commitment may be

---

[d]Id. at 31.43. Although the statute is silent as to the meaning of "disorderly conduct" sufficient to satisfy the affidavit requirements underlying judicial warrants, the provisions of the penal law provide guidance. N.Y. Penal Law 240.20 (McKinney 1967) provides: 240.20 *Disorderly Conduct.* A person is guilty of disorderly conduct when, with intent to cause public inconvenience, annoyance or alarm, or recklessly creating a risk thereof: (1) he engages in fighting or in violent, tumultuous or threatening behavior; or (2) he makes unreasonable noise; or (3) in a public place, he uses abusive or obscene language, or makes an obscene gesture; or (4) without lawful authority, he disturbs any lawful assembly or meeting of persons; or (5) he obstructs vehicular or pedestrian traffic; or (6) he congregates with other persons in a public place and refuses to comply with a lawful order of the police to disperse; or (7) he creates a hazardous or physically offensive condition by any act which serves no legitimate purpose.

extended in consecutive six-month, one-year, and thereafter two-year incre-
ments.[20] As earlier indicated, where inpatient status if other than emergency or
at the patient's option, such status must be deemed "essential" to the patient's
welfare.[e]

Durational Limitations

In an effort to end indeterminacy as the touchstone of psychiatric hospitalization, New York has chronologically circumscribed emergency, short term and
extended involuntary hospitalization. Moreover, both informal and voluntary
admissions require a yearly administrative audit by the Mental Health Information Service.[f]

Treatment

Regardless of the outcome of judicially elaborated concepts of a right to
treatment,[g] New York accords such a right legislatively. Specifically, there is a
right to "care and treatment that is suited to (one's) needs skillfully, safely and
humanely administered with full respect for . . . dignity and personal integrity."[h]

---

[e]Short-term and extended involuntary psychiatric hospitalization require that the
patient be "in need of involuntary care and treatment," which is defined as: "that a
person has a mental illness for which care and treatment as a patient in a hospital is
essential to such person's welfare and whose judgment is so impaired that he is unable
to understand the need for such care and treatment." N.Y. Mental Hygiene Law at 31.31

[f]N.Y. Mental Hygiene Law 31.25 (McKinney Supp. 1974). Such an audit is not
to be merely perfunctory, since: "If the mental health information service finds that
there is any ground to doubt the suitability of such patient to remain in a voluntary or
informal status or the willingness of the patient to so remain, it shall make an application
upon notice to the patient and the director of the hospital, for a court order to determining those questions. In any proceeding, the patient or someone on his behalf or the
Mental Health Information Service may request a hearing. If the Mental Health Information Service finds no ground to doubt the suitability or willingness of the patient to continue in a voluntary or informal status, it shall certify that no issue exists as to those
questions and the patient may be continued in the hospital in such status. A copy of
such certification shall be filed in the patient's record."

[g]See, for example, Donaldson v. O'Connor, 493 F. 2d 507, 520 (5th Cir. 1974):
"We hold that a person involuntarily civilly committed to a state mental hospital has a
constitutional right to receive such individual treatment as will give him a reasonable
opportunity to be cured or improve his condition."

[h]N.Y. Mental Hygiene Law 15.03 (McKinney Supp. 1974). To ensure such rights,
New York also requires: (1) careful and periodic reexamination of inpatients and evaluation of each patient; (2) periodic physical examination by a physician; (3) the order of
a staff member operating within the scope of a professional license for any treatment or

Of equal importance is the principle that treatment be rendered in a setting least disruptive to the patient's personal liberty. Formulated under labels such as "least restrictive alternatives,"[21] or "less drastic means,"[i] the principle sanctions institutionalization only as a last resort.[j] By Department of Mental Hygiene regulation, this principle is the law in New York State.[k]

Correlative to the right to treatment, is a right to decline treatment. By way of recognizing this latter right, New York requires consent for "surgery, shock treatment, major medical treatment in the nature of surgery, or the use of experimental drugs or procedures."[22]

Where the patient lacks capacity to consent, it is my successfully litigated view that absent either a medical emergency or an imminently life-threatening

---

therapy based on appropriate examination; (4) consent for surgery, shock treatment, major medical treatment in the nature of surgery, or the use of experimental drugs or procedures; (5) notation in the patient's clinical record of periodic examinations, individualized treatment programs, evaluations and reevaluations, orders for treatment, and specific therapies, signed by the personnel involved. [For a laundry list of items comprising a constitutional right to treatment, see, Wyatt v. Stickney, 344 F. Supp. 373, Appendix A, (M.D. Ala. 1972)].

[i]Cf. Shelton v. Tucker, 364 U.S. 479, 488, 81 S. Ct. 247, 252, 5 L. Ed. 2d 231, 237 (1960): "(E)ven though the government purpose be legitimate and substantial, that purpose cannot be pursued by means that broadly stifle fundamental personal liberties when the end can be more narrowly achieved. The breath of legislative abridgment must be viewed in the light of less drastic means for achieving the same basic purpose."

[j]In Lessard v. Schmidt, 349 F. Supp. 1078, 1095-1096, (E.D. Wisc. 1972), a three judge federal bench, in considering the Wisconsin civil commitment statute, observed: "Even if the standards for an adjudication of mental illness and potential dangerousness are satisfied, the court should order full-time involuntary hospitalization only as a last resort. . . . Perhaps the most basic and fundamental right is the right to be free from unwanted restraint. It seems clear then, that persons suffering from the condition of being mentally ill, but who are not alleged to have committed any crime, cannot be totally deprived of their liberty if there are less drastic means for achieving the same basic goal."

[k]14NYCRR 36.1 provides: Section 36.1 *Statement of philosophy.* "The long term rehabilitation of mentally disabled persons is promoted by maintenance of relationships with other persons and agencies in the community, avoidance of institutionalization, and minimization of disruption of life rhythms. The civil rights of mentally disabled persons require that such persons be treated and served in the least restrictive setting possible in which treatment or service goals can be met. Therefore, periods of inpatient service should be as short as possible in accordance with the individual patient's plan of care and treatment. This philosophy will, in many cases, require continued service to a patient on an outpatient basis at the conclusion of inpatient service." See also, N.Y. Mental Hygiene Law 31.27 (d) (McKinney Supp. 1974): 31.27 *Involuntary admission on medical certificate.* ". . . (d) Before an examining physician completes the certificate of examination of a person for involuntary care and treatment, he shall consider alternative forms of care and treatment that might be adequate to provide for the person's needs without requiring involuntary hospitalization. . . . "

situation, decisional authority must rest with a committee of the patient's person.[1]

The Mental Health Information Service

The Mental Health Information Service is a legislative response to a 1962 recommendation of the Special Committee to Study Commitment Procedures of the Association of the Bar of the City of New York.[m] Specifically, the service is charged with the following statutory responsibilities.

1. Study and review the admission and retention of all patients.

2. Inform patients and, in proper cases, others interested in patients' welfare concerning procedures for admission and retention and of a patient's rights to have judicial hearing and review, to be represented by legal counsel, and to seek independent medical opinion.

3. In any case before a court, assemble and provide the court with all relevant information as to the patient's case, his hospitalization, his right to discharge, if any, including information from which the court may determine the need, if any, for the appointment of counsel for the patient or the obtaining of additional psychiatric opinion.

4. Provide services and assistance to patients and their families and to the courts having duties to perform relating to the mentally disabled or the allegedly mentally disabled, who are admitted pursuant to articles thirty-one, thirty-three, and thirty-five of this chapter, as may be required by a judge or justice thereof and pursuant to the regulations of the presiding justice of the appellate division of each judicial department.[23]

Organizationally, each of the four judicial departments maintains its own staff under a departmental director appointed by the presiding justice of the

---

[1]Petition of the Director of the Edward J. Meyer Memorial Hospital Concerning Mary Fabian, 43 A.D.2d. 814, 350 N.Y.S. 2d 888 (4th Dep't. 1973); see also Winters v. Miller, 446 F.2d 65, 68-71 (2d Cir. 1971); Comment: Civil Commitment of the Mentally Ill: Theories and Procedures, HARV. L. REV. 79, 1288, 1296-97 (1966).

[m]See, New York City Bar Association and Cornell Law School, Mental Illness and Due Process—Report and Recommendations on Admissions to Mental Hospitals Under New York Law, 20-21 (1962). In commenting on the then existing situation, the committee observed: "Present judicial certification procedures, even when accompanied by a hearing, seldom sketch a full picture of the patient's background. The hearing may not even meet basic requirements of due process of law. Although the details of due process in a hearing involving mental illness are and probably should be different from the details of due process in trial of a criminal offense, certain fundamentals are not provided by the present kind of hearing. Ordinarily, no one represents the patient or outlines the possible alternatives to care in a state hospital. No one points out the factors and developments in his work or family life which may have created temporary emotional strain or which may now ease his return to normal life in the community. No one is charged with this responsibility."

respective appellate division.[24] Designed to promote regional flexibility, decentralization has produced differing staffing patterns and services throughout the state.[25] The first and second department is staffed primarily with lawyers. By choice, the service in the first department performs advocacy functions.[n] The third department is staffed primarily by—and the fourth department entirely by—professionals trained in social case work.[26]

Considering the presence of lawyers as a positive factor in affecting non-institutionalization outcomes, proposals are being advanced for a Mental Health Legal Assistance Panel.[27] These proposals envision:

> . . . a permanent panel of attorneys in each judicial department,
> trained in this area of law, who would be available to represent
> the patient. Indigent patients would receive free representation
> while nonindigent clients, if they so elect for MHLAP representa-
> tion, would reimburse the state on a fee schedule. The MHLAP
> could either be a permanent staff appointed by the State Admin-
> istrator or a contractually-based unit similar to the Law Guardians
> program of the Legal Aid Society. This tentative organization
> would serve to centralize the MHIS under the Administrative
> Board of the Judicial Conference and thus establish a truly state-
> wide agency serving those requiring its services and provide an
> effective accommodation for the expanded role of advocacy nec-
> essary for the effective safeguard of patients' rights.[28]

Unless and until patient advocacy becomes a function of institutional representation, patients' rights will continue to be protected by the fee-for-service legal profession.

Counsel

Reluctantly one must accept a recent characterization of the competence of the fee-for-service legal profession in areas of mental health law as "[a] desert in which untrained and unknowledgeable counsel appear . . . ."[29] Reasons for such parched performance are twofold. The area of the law is quite complex; the financial return is quite meager.

In an effort to irrigate the financial situation, New York provides compensation for court-appointed counsel, comparable to rates for representing indigent criminal defendants.[30] Statutory provisions also allow appointment of a psychiatrist to serve as an adjunct to a patient's appointed counsel.[31]

---

[n]See, for example, Kesselbrenner v. Anonymous, 33 N.Y.2d 161, 350 N.Y.S.2d 889 (1973).

Judicial Review

Emergency Commitment

As a practical matter, there is no review of emergency seventy-two-hour commitment period. The statute provides none, and while theoretically a writ of habeas corpus is available, the time necessary to secure both the writ, its return, and a hearing would exceed the length of commitment. Should, however, the person be detained into a fifteen-day period, he may demand a judicial hearing to determine whether "there is reasonable cause to believe the patient has a mental illness for which immediate inpatient care and treatment in a hospital is appropriate and which is likely to result in serious harm to himself or others."[32] An adjudication unfavorable to the person results in continuous detention to the end of the fifteen-day phase.

Short Term Commitment

During a sixty-day short term nonemergency commitment, a person involuntarily detained may demand a judicial hearing to determine whether by a preponderance of the evidence he is "mentally ill" and "in need of retention."[33] An adverse adjudication simply denies release to the patient for the balance of the sixty-day period.

Extended Commitment

The burden of initiating extended commitment is upon the hospital director. An application must be made within either fifteen days of an emergency commitment,[34] or within the sixty days of a short-term commitment, or if a short-term commitment has been judicially sanctioned, within thirty days of the court's order.[35]

Whether or not a judicial hearing is held, the court must be satisfied by a preponderance of the evidence that the person is mentally ill and "requires continued retention for care and treatment. . . ."[o] If the court so finds, a commitment

---

[o] N.Y. Mental Hygiene Law 31.33. (McKinney Supp. 1974). There is a growing demand for a standard of proof beyond a reasonable doubt in civil commitment proceedings. See, Lessard v. Schmidt, 349 F.Supp. 1078, 1094-1095 (F.D. Wisc. 1972); In Re Ballay, 482 F.2d 648, 662 (D.C. Cir. 1973); Note, *Developments in the Law—Civil Commitment of the Mentally Ill*, 87 HARV. L. REV., 1190, 1298-1303 (1974). New York has not responded to this emerging demand. See, People v. Fuller, 24 N.Y.2d 292, 304, 300 N.Y.S.2d 102, 108-109 (1969); Fhagen v. Miller, 65 Misc. 2d. 163,   , 317 N.Y.S.2d 128, 138 (Sup. Ct. N.Y. Co. 1970); modified on other grounds, 38 A.D.2d 926 321 N.Y.S.2d 61 (1st Dep't 1971); aff'd, 20 N.Y.2d 348, 328 N.Y.S.2d 393 (1972), cert. denied, 409 U.S. 845, 93 S. Ct. 47, 36 L. Ed. 2d 85 (1972).

order for a period not to exceed six months is authorized. Further, judicially santioned detention of one year and thereafter two-year periods is authorized.[36]

Should the patient or anyone on his behalf be dissatisfied with a judicial determination, a new hearing before a jury may be held to decide anew the questions of "mental illness and the need for retention of the patient."[37]

Habeas Corpus

Theoretically, the writ of habeas corpus is always available to challenge the legality of a patient's involuntary detention.[P] The disadvantage of the writ is that the evidentiary burden of persuasion on the issues shifts from the hospital to the patient. Thus, if the probabilities are balanced, the patient loses.

Conclusion

This chapter has attempted to illustrate legislative response to current legal issues affecting the psychiatrically hospitalized mentally ill. The response is one characterized by distrust of indeterminate involuntary hospitalization, hostility to merely custodial constraint, and insistence upon alternatives to institutionalization.

Whether legislative attempts to defend involuntary psychiatric hospitalization against judicial assaults will succeed remains to be seen. Voices confidently assert society's right to involuntarily hospitalize the mentally ill. Yet, one senses echoes of an incipient political ethos decrying psychiatric constraint as terminal to fundamental personal liberties.

Notes

1. Jackson v. Indiana, 406 U.S. 715, 736-37, 92 S. Ct. 1845, 1857-1858, 32 L. Ed. 2d 435, 450 (1972) (Blackmun J.) (footnotes omitted).
2. AMERICAN PSYCHIATRIC ASSOCIATION, DIAGNOSTIC AND STATISTICAL MANUAL OF MENTAL DISORDERS, 34 (2 ed. 1968).

[P]N.Y. Mental Hygiene Law 15.15 (McKinney Supp. 1974) provides in part: 15.15 *Habeas corpus.* "(a) A person retained by a facility, the department, or the narcotic addiction control commission or a relative or friend on his behalf is entitled to a writ of habeas corpus to question the cause and legality of detention upon proper application; (b) Upon the return of such a writ of habeas corpus the court shall examine the facts concerning the person's alleged mental disability and detention. The evidence shall include the clinical record of the patient and medical or other testimony as required by the court. The court may review the admission and retention of the person pursuant to the provisions of this chapter. The court shall discharge the person so retained if it finds that he is not mentally disabled or that he is not in need of further retention for in-patient care and treatment.

3. ZISKIN, J., COPING WITH PSYCHIATRIC AND PSYCHOLOGICAL TESTI-
   MONY, (1970), passim, Beverly Hills, California, Law & Psychology Press.
4. N.Y. Mental Hygiene Law 1.05 (17) (McKinney Supp. 1974).
5. Id. at 31.01.
6. Ibid.
7. N.Y. Mental Hygiene Law 31.15 (McKinney Supp. 1974).
8. Id. at 31.13 (a).
9. Id. at 31.13 (b).
10. Id. at 31.17 (b).
11. Id. at 31.17 (a).
12. Id. at 31.21 (b).
13. SZASZ, THOMAS. LAW LIBERTY AND PSYCHIATRY, Macmillan (1968),
    40.
14. McGarry, A.L., and Greenblatt, Milton, *Conditional Voluntary Mental-
    Hospital Admission*, 287 NEW ENG. J. OF MED. 279, 280 (1972).
15. Gilboy, J. and Schmidt, J., *'Voluntary' Hospitalization of the Mentally
    Ill*, 66 Nw. U.L.R. (1971) 429, 432.
16. N.Y. Mental Hygiene Law 31.45 (McKinney Supp. 1974).
17. Id. at 31.39.
18. Id. at 31.37 (a).
19. Id. at 31.27 and 31.31.
20. Id. at 31.33.
21. Lake v. Cameron, 364 F. 2d 657, 660 (D.C. Cir. 1966).
22. N.Y. Mental Hygiene Law, 15.03 (b) (4) (McKinney Supp. 1974).
23. Id. 29.09 (b) (McKinney Supp. 1974).
24. N.Y. State Assembly Ways and Means Committee, The Mental Health
    Information Service—A Program Review and Suggestions for Reform,
    3-4 (1973).
25. Id. at 9-10.
26. Ibid.
27. Id. at 15.
28. Ibid.
29. Shestack, Jerome J., Chairman, American Bar Association, Commission
    on the Mentally Disabled, The Mentally Disabled—A New American Bar
    Association Viewpoint, 5 (1974).
30. N.Y. Judiciary Law 35 (1) (a) (McKinney Supp. 1974).
31. Id. at 35 (3) (McKinney 1968).
32. N.Y. Mental Hygiene Law 31.39 (McKinney Supp. 1974).
33. Id. at 31.31.
34. Id. at 31.39.
35. Id. at 31.33.
36. Ibid.
37. Id. at 31.35.

7

Changing Roles and Structures of Mental Health Boards

Noel A. Mazade and John L. Sheets

The purpose of this chapter is to assess critically the status of various citizen boards in the governance and operation of mental health programs (including the state hospital and local community mental health centers). Rather than accepting the notion that such boards are required, this chapter will: (a) review the traditional roles these boards have played; (b) speculate upon the future organization and trends in mental health programming; and (c) offer several suggestions designed to utilize and structure citizen input more effectively.

There is little need to trace historically the advent of the community mental health (CMH) movement in this country and the prevailing ideology to increase the community's role in decision making. The first enabling federal legislation, most state statutes, and often local county regulations encourage the formation of various boards to monitor the planning and operation of a state's mental health program.

To this end, several functional types of boards are found in most states and include:

1. a state-level hospital board that often has ultimate responsibility for the state mental hospitals
2. a state-level mental health council that is responsible for CMH centers
3. county or multicounty boards that govern the development of local CMH centers, programs for alcoholics and drug users, and the mentally retarded
4. advisory boards, having no formal power, that assist the state hospital and/or the local CMH center by offering political support, raising funds, informing administration of pressing needs, and the like

It is not uncommon for state legislation to dictate the membership composition of these boards (particularly 1-3 above) and mandate their specific duties and responsibilities. In some states for example, the board must include a physician, minister, teacher, psychologist, minority group member, agency representatives, and local school superintendent. Such representation, it is assumed, will assure participation of all sectors of the community and, it is hoped, will help guarantee that programs are developed in relation to all community needs.

123

The legislatively defined functions of these boards generally encourage a myriad of duties. These include:

1. appointing and prescribing the duties of the local Mental Health Center director
2. raising funds for mental health and mental retardation programs
3. coordinating public and private mental health and mental retardation agencies
4. reviewing and evaluating services and facilities
5. submitting program plans and budgets to county commissioners, health planning agencies, and to the state department of mental health

Although many of the tasks inherent in these functions are carried out by the staff, the ultimate legal responsibility for their execution rests upon the board. Logically, one might assume that if the functions are within the legal authority and responsibility of the board, it is necessary that the board members have personal familiarity with the resources, skills, and tasks necessary to plan and maintain a high quality program. But in fact this is not always so.

To date, most states have had no difficulty structuring the various types of boards described above. This was easily accomplished since the state hospital and neighboring local CMH centers comprised distinct program entities, were geographically separated, and were administratively unique.

No doubt, the establishment of these independent boards perpetuates the dichotomy between the state mental hospital system and local community facilities. From a historical perspective, the integration of institutional and community systems may have been more easily facilitated had state and regional boards been created whose responsibility included developing policies and program plans for both sectors simultaneously.

In some communities, local CMH boards have begun to exert considerable influence in regard to establishing program emphases. They have become heavily involved in hiring professional staff, have created subcommittees to examine various aspects of the total program, and demand fiscal and programmatic accountability from administrative staff.

When viewed exclusively from the standpoint of community program development, one may conclude that the development of such boards has dramatically influenced the entire statewide mental health system. In the final analysis, this conclusion is inappropriately optimistic. As recipients of only 10 to 20 percent of all state mental health operating funds (the remainder earmarked for institutions), the supposed power-base represented by the statewide aggregate of boards may be decidedly minimal in terms of influencing state policy and subsequent resource allocation.

Some Research Findings

Traditionally, community participation has been practiced in community mental health centers in five major patterns. These have included participation through consumers, volunteers, indigenous staff personnel, organization, and interest group members, and through board membership.[1]

Mental health boards according to Holton, New, and Hessler[2] are primarily of three types: advisory, consumer control, and elitist.

The advisory model consists of a board composed of a majority of community residents or potential consumers, and functions as a "recommending liaison" between community residents and center staff regarding service needs and program responses.

The consumer control model consists of a cross section of catchment area residents and functions with various degrees of direct control over the operation of the mental health center.

The elitist model is comprised of community leaders and volunteers who provide sanction and support for the mental health program based on their political and power structure affiliations.

In a study reported in 1970, which was conducted in 27 OEO Neighborhood Health Centers, Sparer and associates concluded that the effectiveness of community boards was positively correlated with the degree to which they were well organized. It was pointed out that even if a group is formally limited to an advisory role, it can, by effectively organizing itself, develop active working relationships with center personnel, and thus position itself to exert considerable decision-making influence.[3]

During 1973-74, two independent studies of over 130 mental health boards in two states were conducted by the staff of the Community Psychiatry Division, Department of Psychiatry, University of North Carolina School of Medicine. Over 400 board members were included in these surveys that combined the use of questionnaires and interviews with CMH Center administrative staff, board chairmen, and board members-at-large.

The overall findings indicated that these boards were comprised of members who do not fully understand the nature of comprehensive mental health services nor their role in the development of those services. For example:

1. Almost one-third of the members felt that their boards had little or no knowledge of the needs of their service area population.
2. Over one-half felt that the staff of the mental health program had the most influence on board decisions v. the board members influencing one another.
3. Over 75 percent expressed inadequate knowledge in the following areas:
   a) program evaluation

b) the role of the board in relationship to the regional and state admin-
    istrative offices
c) program planning schemes and specific ideas to develop programs
    for the retarded and mentally ill
d) knowledge regarding the specific roles the board should be performing

Whether by intent or default, one may be compelled to conclude that these
particular boards closely paralleled the elitist model that Holton described as,
"Community leaders and resident volunteers who serve on boards largely for purposes of moneyraising, public relations, and imagebuilding. Most professional
decisions are left up to the staff, and the board is little concerned with representing the interest of clients or potential clients."[4]

Trends

In spite of its relative stability since its initiation in the late 1960s, the CMH
centers movement (and along with it, the state hospital) is undergoing change.
This change is in relationship to substantive alterations in the health care system
in general, resulting in specific trends that may appear within the next three years.
These trends include:

1. The nationwide trend to create "Departments of Human Resources" at
the state, regional, and county level: These superagencies seek to combine the
services of public health, mental health, social services, and vocational rehabilitation. At the fiscal and organizational level, the creation of such departments
has signaled the end of autonomy for mental health and has placed programs in
a competitive relationship with other public human services.

2. The increased use of extremely sophisticated management information
systems for program planning, monitoring, and evaluation.

3. A decline in federal government support for CMH programming and
special programs within state hospitals. The sizable reduction in available construction and staffing grants has already signaled the beginning of this trend.

4. The introduction of some form of national health insurance that will
provide third-party payments for specific psychiatric services.

5. Professional review of services by the utilization of provider-oriented
mechanisms such as the PSRO.

6. The development of regionalization in many human service programs.
Professional staff at the regional (multicounty) level will have responsibility
for initial program budget screening, setting and enforcing standards, program
evaluation, and the provision of technical assistance to local programs.

7. A greater emphasis on treatment programs that are highly "visible"
versus efforts to expand community education programs, consultation, and
the like. These latter programs are more difficult to evaluate and hence will

be reduced as agencies compete for scarce fiscal resources for services which are easily identified.

8. More program directors who are trained in administration. The non-administratively trained mental health professional (e.g., psychiatrist) will not be legislatively required to have ultimate authority and/or responsibility.

9. In conjunction with item no. 1 above, more efforts to understand and facilitate interorganizational linkage. Thus, consumers and providers must deal with a larger system of services and to manipulate such a system.

The development of such trends compels even the casual observer to question the viability of maintaining the system of mental health boards as it currently exists in most states. At best, the current composition, sophistication, and organization of such boards place them in a poor position to cope effectively with these trends.

The development of Departments of Human Resources is often accompanied by new state adminstrative policies and structures. More often than not, new priorities are established, leaving local programs in a dependent position both in terms of existing in an unpredictable, top-down administrative environment, and in relation to maintaining local program priorities that, when viewed by top-level state administrators, may appear to be less important.

The trend toward regionalization and the role of regional staff will gradually usurp the functions that have traditionally comprised the duties of the mental health board. This reality is most visible in relationship to functions such as budget review and program evaluation.

National health insurance and accompanying professional review mechanisms also incorporate traditional board activities. As services become more technical, the ability of the layman to make judgments of program efficiency and/or effectiveness diminishes.

Finally, whereas the board previously monitored and assisted the nonadministratively trained director, the arrival of generic administrators to operate the program substantially reduces the need for boards.

Suggestions for the Future

Utilizing a highly general framework, the planning and administration of a mental health program entails the successful performance of several key functions. These are assessing community needs; formulating program policies; developing specific program plans; maintaining and operating the program on a day-to-day basis; and evaluating programs.

In light of the tasks required to accomplish these functions, it would appear that the necessity to maintain a "board of directors" may be questionable. Such a viewpoint may be supported from several standpoints:

1. After six to ten years of existence, a substantial majority of boards are still ignorant and apathetic with regard to improving their knowledge in these key areas.
2. Professional staff at the mental health facility, utilizing appropriate consultation if required, should be quite capable of performing the program planning, operations, and evaluation functions.
3. The increased control by state governments of local mental health programs will gradually erode the degree of community "ownership," which may now exist, eventually leading to the bureaucratization of services. Rarely, if ever, do such state-operated programs include the provision for controlling boards.
4. Power in regard to priority-setting and the allocation of funds will rest with governmental entities such as county commissioners and state legislatures. This is in marked contrast to the early experience of the CMH movement in which localities designed, controlled, and operated their own program with federal funding.

It is not the intent of the authors to present the practice of organizing lay boards in a negative light, but rather to suggest that the purposes and mandates necessary in the early stages of the CMH centers movement may no longer be relevant. The political administrative realities of today may signal the need to critically examine the role of the board and to explore other methods of securing citizen input and support. In short, the question must be asked, "Boards for what?"

The following are several suggestions for increasing the scope of citizen input for program planning, operations, and evaluation:

1. Utilize participative techniques such as nominal group process[5] and key informants[6] to assess community needs and develop programs in relation to these needs. Such techniques are advantageous in that they insure participation by an unlimited number of persons, are heterogeneous in scope, have rotating membership, and are oriented more toward the accomplishment of specific clearly defined goals.

2. Make greater use of nonhierarchical temporary problem-solving groups that are time-limited, are comprised of individuals who have clear expertise in a given area (e.g. program evaluation) and who will be involved in the consequences of the decisions reached.[7]

3. Formalize the functions heretofore pejoratively ascribed to the "elitist board" described above and form specific ad hoc advisory and action groups to raise funds, develop public relations, lobby with state legislatures, and the like.

Summary

In response to developing trends in mental health care delivery, this chapter has sought to raise several issues related to the maintenance of permanent boards of directors. Given their lack of knowledge in critical areas, the high control exerted by program staff and state office administrators, and the characteristics of program tasks, the continued desirability of these boards is questionable. Citizen input in program planning, operations, and evaluation is nevertheless seen as a valuable adjunct to governmental authority. There is still a need for the layman's involvement in local mental health programs although the mechanisms suggested are of a more ad hoc variety, encompassing functions of a more promotional and advisory nature.

Notes

1. Kaplan, S.R. and Roman, M., *The Organization and Delivery of Mental Health Services in the Ghetto*, New York: Praeger Publishers, 1973.
2. Holton, W.E., New, P.K., and Hessler, R.M., "Citizen Participation and Conflict," *Administration in Mental Health,* National Institute of Mental Health, Fall, 1973.
3. Kaplan and Roman, *Organization and Delivery.*
4. Holton, et al., "Citizen Participation," p. 99.
5. Van de Ven, A. and Delbecq, A., "The Nominal Group as a Research Instrument for Exploratory Health Studies," *American Journal of Public Health,* March, 1972, pp. 337-42.
6. Hollister, W.G., et al., *Experiences in Rural Mental Health: Developing Citizen Participation.* Book III in a series in Rural Mental Health, Community Psychiatry Division, UNC School of Medicine, Chapel Hill, North Carolina 27514.
7. Thayer, F., "Temporary Organizations and Interdepartmental Committees: A Note on the 'New Administration,' " (paper) Graduate School of Public and International Affairs, University of Pittsburgh, 1971.

8

Citizens and Consumers Look at
Their State Mental Hospitals
Irving Blumberg

The precipitous and continuing decline in the resident patient population of state hospitals literally compels a basic reassessment of the
total mental health delivery system within which these costly, generally
isolated, and essentially custodial institutions have played so dominant a
role. To some, the progressive dissolution of these massive facilities,
warehousing from two to nine thousand human beings, inspires hope for
a better future for the oncoming waves of the mentally disordered. To
others, the same phenomenon presages the death knell of the orderly, dis-
ciplined, authoritative, and serene lives they have for so long been accustomed to enjoying.

For the most part, those engaged in both debating and deciding the
issue have been mental hospital administrators and commissioners, system
theoreticians, heads of university departments of psychiatry, and others
presumed to be knowledgeable in the field of human welfare engineering
The input from citizens generally, and from consumers of mental health
services specifically, has, until fairly recently, been negligible at best.
This writer respectfully submits that the future we should be talking
about is not the future of state mental hospitals—a time and use-limited
artifact of society—but the present and future of human beings in
distress.

The real questions bear on what is needed and what is best for defined
groups of human beings who have special problems in living, in each community. Who will work with and serve them, where, and how? Why is
there such a major preoccupation with the fate of state mental hospitals
when, in fact, they constitute only one in a proliferating number of other
subsystems of mental health care? A look at the annual budgets of many
state governments showing enormously disproportionate sums allotted
for the continued sustenance of these facilities provides a big part of the
answer.

To cite an example, New York State appropriated for its Department
of Mental Hygiene almost a billion dollars for fiscal 1974-75. A significant portion of this came from patient resources, federal funds, and other
third-party sources. Whenever the status quo is imperiled, and in this the
future status and role of mental hospitals are no exceptions, passions
become heated, rhetoric becomes more florid, vested interests take up
arms, and partisans in the ideological scrimmage become increasingly

131

polarized. What major points of view have emerged in the escalating debate, and where do citizens and consumers fit into the picture?[a]

Opposing Points of View

On the left, there are those who see no future whatever for the more than 300 archaic state mental hospitals that have dotted the country for the past hundred years. They are seen as hopelessly countertherapeutic, and the "dissolutionists" strive only to hasten the day when they are merely unpleasant memories in the historic march to a new era of community-based and community-operated services. Efforts by hospital administrators to eliminate the most noxious aspects of institutionalization or to transform the hospitals into "therapeutic communities" are viewed as ineffectual and diversionary, as tactics designed primarily to still criticism and perpetuate the status quo. Interestingly enough, the advocates of these doctrines contain a curious mix of preeminent leaders in the field of psychiatry, including a past president of the American Psychiatric Association, the younger and more radical breed of mental health workers, and a sizable segment of sophisticated consumers and concerned citizens.

On the right there is the vast army of "protectionists" who see, or profess to see, dire economic and professional disaster if the demands of the "radicals" are met. Not surprisingly, a preponderant number of traditional hospital administrators, their second and third echelon staffs, and the bulk of professional and nonprofessional personnel ministering to the needs of patients can be found in the ranks of the militant antidissolutionists.

These stand-patters are facile in supplying profound theoretical arguments justifying the continued need for state operated institutions. Reluctantly, and only under considerable pressure, will they sanction even the mildest accommodation to the winds of institutional reform. They hope that by acceding to minor reforms whose net effect is to provide a cosmetic facade to the instituions that they operate, they can achieve a legitimacy for them before the demolition process sets into an irreversible pattern.

The center group takes into account the realities of the political, economic,

---

[a]For the purpose of this chapter, "consumers" of mental health services include patients (inpatients or outpatients); residents (of facilities for the retarded); persons in foster or group homes, hostels, etc.; former patients and prospective patients. "Concerned citizens" would include parents, relatives, or friends of consumers; hospital volunteers; interested professionals; citizen groups such as Mental Health and Mental Retardation Associations (even though some of these nonprofit agencies operate services for categories of individuals); parent federations and coalitions. "State Mental Hospitals" may be defined as facilities operated or services rendered directly by state governments whether such facilities are designated as hospitals, schools for the retarded, developmental or psychiatric centers, or otherwise.

and psychological constraints involved in making any basic alteration in an encrusted bureaucracy. They aim to achieve simultaneously two major goals: (1) to reduce both the number and size of state operated mental hospitals to an irreducible minimum; (2) to capacitate public and private local agencies to assume an increasing share of responsibility for the care, treatment, and rehabilitation of their disabled populations.

This is no easy task. Pursuing the first goal implies a redirection, reorganization, and redeployment of physical and human resources. It means "humanizing" the operation of the hospitals and making them less restrictive; offering more intensive treatment; developing outreach programs into the community; fostering outpatient, partial hospitalization and rehabilitative services; decentralizing staffs and administration, and encouraging unified services planning with local governments and voluntary agencies. It is no secret that state legislatures are signally unenthusiastic about approving radical changes in their administrative structures, unless they perceive a clear and imminent fiscal gain by so doing. The exceptions are few and far between.

With respect to the second goal—community support—governors and legislatures move ponderously and only by small incremental steps to rectify the present disproportionate balance between the large sums annually appropriated for traditional state institutional services as contrasted to the meagre resources allocated for community-operated programs. State and local governments currently are caught in the vise of a raging inflation as well as high taxpayer resistance to increased levies. At such a time, it takes a feat of legerdemain to squeeze out of tax-conscious legislators funds required both to humanize existing state mental hospitals and simultaneously expand community based alternatives.

Yet, this is the formidable task facing concerned citizens, voluntary agencies, consumers, and dedicated professionals; which brings us to the point—what, in this complex and challenging dilemma should be the role of consumers and concerned citizens? How can they make their views known and accepted by those who have the power to decide policy? What should be their stance in relation to "establishment" forces—the government, administrators, the professionals, and others? Should it be one of exposure and confrontation, or of cooperation on agreed objectives, or perhaps a pragmatic mix of the two? What strengths do they bring to bear and what weaknesses do they labor under in seeking to advance their interests, as they see them?

On one fact there should be little dispute—that is that mental hospital patients have the highest stake in the proximate and ultimate outcome of decisions affecting their future and their very lives. They are inevitably destined to be the chief beneficiaries of any purposeful reorganization of the mental health delivery system.

A Look at the Future—for Patients and Hospitals

State hospitals have become more ecumenical in that they have been accepting, in addition to those with psychiatric, neurologic, and developmental impairments, sizeable populations with primary or mixed diagnoses of alcoholism or drug abuse. They have also resorted to housing in a single institutional framework individuals with a variety of disabilities and special treatment and rehabilitative needs. The needs of persons requiring special preventive treatment, rehabilitative, and other life support services argues for the development in each community, however defined, of a comprehensive, coordinated, integrated, available, and accessible network of services and programs whose basic and ultimate goal should be to capacitate the individual to function at maximum effectiveness in as normal and nonrestrictive an environment as possible, considering the individual's impairments and capabilities.

Some of the implications of this view have been recently spelled out by knowledgeable and forward-looking practitioners and administrators. Dr. Nicholas Stratas, chairman of a subcommittee of the NIMH Federal-State-Local Relations Committee has stated that "state mental hospitals as isolated delivery systems be phased out as soon as possible. They should continue in existence only as part of a unified and purposeful system of delivery of mental health services."[1]

Dr. Jack Zusman, formerly director of the Division of Community Psychiatry at SUNY/Buffalo, predicted the time will come when the state "will no longer provide direct mental health services, since state hospitals will become the property of and be administered by local communities."[2]

The inutility of the overwhelming number of present state mental institutions has been clearly depicted by Dr. Milton Greenblatt, former commissioner of the Massachusetts Department of Mental Hygiene, who stated the alternative as "*phase out* before we go *bankrupt*" (italics are Dr. Greenblatt's).[3] While Dr. Werner M. Mendel, another critic, asserts, "The hospital as a form of treatment for the severely ill psychotic patient is always costly and inefficient, frequently anti-therapeutic, and never the treatment of choice."[4]

This writer agrees with the substance of the above comments. Only experience and experimentation will reveal to what extent and for what populations state mental hospitals can perform *any* useful service. Even if it were conceded that specialized facilities may be required to house and treat the violently aggressive psychotic, the alcoholic, the drug abuser, "chronic" schizophrenics, etc., it does not necessarily follow that such facilities need to be state operated. Why cannot city, county, regional, or area authorities incorporate virtually any facility or service within its administrative structure, subject only to minimum standards, monitoring, priorities, evaluation, quality controls and plans determined by state mental health authorities in conjunction with local government, citizen, consumer groups, and voluntary agencies' input and involvement?

This should leave state mental health authorities free of operational responsibilities, except for extremely restricted functions. They could then engage in
major research, education, and training activities, both on a statewide basis
and in support of local initiatives. It would make it possible for the state
authority to encourage, on a broader basis than heretofore, pilot and demonstration projects, and to provide assurance, through fiscal, technical, and other
forms of support, that no area within a state would be lacking in essential
services required by its residents—at least, insofar as a state's resources can permit.

Goals of Consumers and Concerned Citizens

These goals may be briefly summarized, as follows:

1. to assure that their views are heard, respected, and acted upon
2. to assure, so long as state mental hospitals are in the picture, that they
    provide human care, treatment, and rehabilitation to patients, under con-
    ditions of dignity and privacy
3. to assure a reordering, restructuring, and reorientation of the mental health
    and other related delivery systems, to meet the life serving needs of the
    population
4. to assure that communities will be furnished with the necessary resources
    to provide adequate aftercare, residential, transitional, treatment, and
    rehabilitative services to those who could benefit from such services
5. to play an effective role in helping to bring these changes about

With respect to the second goal enunciated above—conditions in the state
hospitals—the first concern of consumers and concerned citizens relates to pre-
serving the human, the civil, and the constitutional rights of the patient. These
rights range all the way from the right to oppose improper, illegal, or innappro-
priate admission or retention; to appeal; to habeas corpus; to decent food,
clothing, and amenities; to recreation, education, and training; to privacy and
confidentiality; to access within and without the institution; to payment for
work; to humane and considerate treatment by staff; to medical care; to involvement in decisions affecting his (her) treatment, transfer or living conditions; to
heat and air conditioning; to clean, private toilets and showers; to privacy and
freedom of correspondence; to self-organization; to vote; to consent to or
deny consent to treatment under specified conditions all the way to proper
discharge and aftercare; to employment without discrimination; to drive a car
or fish.

While the "right to treatment" has been enunciated in a number of recent
court cases, the complementary right to habilitation and rehabilitation has not

been so clearly spelled out. A recent article from the publication "Silent Majority," by the President's Committee on Mental Retardation, describes it in the following terms: "The legal right to habilitation has evolved from the recent applications of established constitutional concepts. It grew from an analogy to the right to treatment of the mentally ill."[5]

Dr. Andrew S. Adams, United States commissioner of rehabilitation, recently delineated the freedoms he believed all mentally and physically handicapped persons should enjoy as members of a community. He issued a proclamation, subsequently reprinted in the *Congressional Record,* which listed the following rights: "the right to employment; the right to education; the right to housing; the right to transportation; the right to use public accommodations; the right to recreation; the right to health care; and the right to access to cast an election ballot."[6]

Consumers—The "Establishment" and Change

With reference to the third and fourth goals referred to earlier—the reorganization of the mental health delivery system and the strengthening of community based services—the principal concerns of citizens and consumers are to accelerate the pace of change and to guarantee their full involvement as co-agents, together with legislators and administrators, in plans to implement the necessary changes. As indicated earlier in this chapter, the resistance to change is enormous and comes from a formidable array of opponents as well as bureaucratic inertia. Poor preparation and planning, as well as failure to establish a balanced and unified system of services during the process of transition from state-operated to locally operated services, accounts for some measure of failure in such states as California and elsewhere.

Dr. Greenblatt, in the above cited article, lists some of the forces opposing or retarding the phasing out of mental hospitals. He includes:

1. opposition of legislative bodies
2. resistance of hospital personnel
3. anxieties of patients and families who fear the effects of dislocation, or the return of unwanted family members
4. resistance from labor, concerned with security or relocation problems
5. opposition from communities, both with regard to patients who are unceremoniously "dumped" on their community doorsteps or the intrusion of facilities providing services to any group of "deviant" or problem individuals. (A number of communities have already reacted by passing zoning laws restricting the uses of land and property to avoid what they conceive to be blots on their fair community.)

In some states, it should be noted, opposition to reductions in capital expenditures for new mental hospital construction stems from the close political alignment between the executive branch of government and the construction unions and construction industry. A more insidious form of opposition toward change finds its source in the unreadiness, particularly on the part of many psychiatrists and hospital administrators, to grapple with the practical problems involved in rehabilitating and reintegrating human beings into community life. Such mundane problems as vocational rehabilitation, housing, leases, welfare, jobs, transportation, etc. appear alien to the experience, training, competences, and traditions in which too many professionals have been nurtured. There is a reluctance by psychiatrists, for example, to abandon the role of the leader or to accept the notion that a shop foreman, a vocational specialist, a housing expert or a special educator may have an equal or, in some instances, greater impact in restoring an impaired human being to a state of social usefulness than he or she may have.

Consumers and concerned citizens clearly have their work cut out for them. They must be determined enough to assert countervailing power to the bureaucrats and the "edifice complex" proponents. They must be patient enough to help allay the legitimate concerns of patients and families. They must be adroit enough to be able to offer the hand of friendship and cooperation to dedicated professionals, without being smothered by their "expertise" or self-assurance. They must be skilled enough to educate their neighbors in the communities—that is, "we"—our fathers, mothers, sisters, and aunts—not "they" who need and deserve support when vulnerable human beings are returned to community life. Above all, they must be organized and strong enough to make it clear that, while cooperation is their first desire, confrontation may have to be exercised. Acknowledging the predilection of the media to play up harrowing stories of injustice and dramatic scenes of confrontation, who can say with certainty, that had there not been an element of confrontation, the "Willowbrook" story (see Chapter 4) would never have reached the public eye.

Those who look beyond the present confines of the community mental health movement to an even broader vista, now speak of a more generic human services ideology.

Dr. Frank Baker, in an unusually perceptive article, had this to say in analyzing the future human services ideology:

> Although the human services ideological structure is still undergoing refinement and development, five general themes can be identified as characterizing this belief system.
>
> These themes are: systematic integration of services; comprehensiveness and accessibility; client troubles defined as problems in

living; general characteristics of helping activities; and accountability
of service providers to clients.[7]

He elaborates on each of these with singular acuity and provides a useful
antidote to those who hug the so-called medical model too closely to their
chests. While this approach gives no comfort to those who simplistically assert
that the solution to what they define as the "myth of mental illness" is the
political liberation of a distressed human being, or that psychiatry per se is
irrelevant, he does reflect the growing awareness that the social and personal
functioning of an individual, including the clinically impaired, is potently
influenced by the social and economic environment.

The Strengths and Weaknesses of
Consumer Roles

Dr. Greenblatt has recognized the potential of the citizen movement to
reshape the present delivery system when he declared, in the article mentioned
earlier that, "this massive citizen army will prevail, we hope, in the fight for
the mentally ill and retarded and they will close many more hospitals, if indeed,
that is what they think is proper in the long run."[8] Referring to the role of
consumers in the initiation of community mental health centers that, notwithstanding some of their faults, are seen by many as a basic community alternative to mental hospitals, Dr. Lucy Ozarin of the National Institute of Mental
Health noted that "active involvement of consumers in a center program has
led in some places to the formation of mental health corporations."[9]
    While some federal legislation or regulations provide for specific represen-
tation of consumers or concerned citizens on various councils or advisory
boards, and this is paralleled at state and local levels, it is fair to say that
increasingly the consumers have become disenchanted with symbolic roles.
They are demanding—and getting—a larger share in the planning process,
and in the deliberations on policy and fiscal issues. Although not neglecting
such roles as they can perform usefully on advisory bodies, consumers and
citizen groups are moving more aggressively and independently in the area of
influencing public policy and public legislatures, and, as will be noted by
other writers in this volume, addressing their grievances to the courts—not
without significant results.
    Community mental health boards, boards of visitors to institutions, and
similar bodies, generally appointed by governors or mayors to serve as representatives of the public interest, often fail to keep pace with changing needs.
Their preference for nonactivist roles has prompted parents, who, as one of
them put it, has "the monkey on my back," to place reliance on their own
organized strength to safeguard the welfare of their loved ones. To an even

greater degree, and in a variety of ways, consumers, especially in poverty areas, are moving from consumer and citizen involvement and participation to demand for effective consumer control. This demand may be less clearly articulated at present with regard to the state mental hospital than, let us say, with community services such as local hospitals and community mental health centers. However, the trend is unmistakable and, with regard to the poor and minority segments of the population, is not likely to be denied for long.

As the president of the Federation of Parents Organizations for New York State Mental Institutions stated in a recent address to the Annual Conference of the National Association of State Mental Health Program Directors:

> We want the old approaches, which have debilitated and dehumanized people, discarded. We want vibrant new methods and programs instituted. And most important of all, we want accountability for all of your actions. Self-accountability is self-defeating and leads to a bureaucracy that stifles growth, ideas, needed change, and the hopes of those within the system who have the desire and motivation to move forward.[10]

Perhaps the major impact that citizen groups and consumers have had in the redirection of mental health and mental retardation services and in meeting the service needs of the mentally disabled has been in influencing public policy, as expressed in legislation and budgetary appropriations. This influence is being exerted at all levels of government—federal, state, and local. It is reflected in the enactment of and amendments to such basic legislation as the Community Mental Health Centers Acts, the Developmental Disabilities Act, the Vocational Rehabilitation Act, the Comprehensive Mental Health Planning Act, the provisions and appropriations for Special Educational Services for the Handicapped, the Health Maintenance Organization legislation, and others.

The battle for improvements, expansions, and funding of programs embodied in these measures, together with counterpart legislation at state levels, will impact directly and indirectly on the future role of state mental hospitals. What ultimate effect subsequent enactment of a National Health Insurance Bill will have on the present mental health delivery system remains to be seen.

In discharging their responsibilities to their constituencies, the major national and state citizen organizations have performed two indispensible functions: (1) They have served as interpreters to the public and to the legislators who determine policy of the needs of the mentally disabled; and (2) they pioneered in providing services to categories of human beings for whom no public programs were initially available.

In this latter function, they still continue to provide services that in many instances serve as benchmarks of excellence to which counterpart public services might well aspire.

Candor, however, compels the observations that many of these citizen groups and voluntary agencies have, to some degree, limited the impact of their total potential by failing to arrive at a consensus on commonly agreed-upon priorities. Narrowly conceived concerns, overcategorization according to diagnostic labels, a competitive rather than cooperative approach, have in too many instances made the efforts of citizen groups vulnerable to the "divide and conquer" tactics of these legislative economizers whose astigmatic views on governmental priorities place human services at the bottom of the totem pole.

To the extent that parent and citizen groups surmount these separatist tendencies and develop effective coalitions based on minimum, high-priority common programs, to that extent they can more fully discharge their role as ombudsmen for their respective constituences. They will then be in a better position to fulfill the role suggested by Dr. Saul Feldman of the National Institute of Mental Health, when he asserted: "Finally 'consumerism' is affecting health services, with 'citizen participation,' 'community control,' and 'relevance' becoming part of our common jargon. The goal, of course, is to ensure that mental health services will be responsive to consumers rather than to providers."[11]

The New York State Experience

The following comments on New York State are offered not because the state's experience is either typical or exceptional, but because the writer has a closer familiarity with the New York scene. A brief historical review would be in order as background for the comments to follow.

In 1954 the state legislature enacted the Community Mental Health Services Act, the first of its kind in the nation. This act provided the programmatic framework for the development of community-based and -operated mental health services, with shared fiscal support emanating from the state. In 1964 the state legislature enacted an amendment to the Mental Hygiene Law, which established a Mental Health Information Service. This service is designed to assist the state's appellate courts in a process designed to prevent improper commitment or retention of state mental hospital patients. The same year also saw amendments authorizing the state to assist local agencies in funding construction costs of mental health facilities.

In 1965 a voluminous report was submitted to the governor by a broadly representative group of citizens and professionals comprising the New York State Planning Committee on Mental Disorders. The report analyzed and made recommendations for the whole spectrum of needs of the state's population in the areas of mental health, mental retardation, alcoholism, and drug abuse. It analyzed the programs and activities of the State Department of Mental Hygiene, as well as of the local community services. Among other recommendations, it called for the state hospital system to limit the size of mental institutions to a maximum of 1,000 patients. Early in the same year, Governor Rockefeller had announced the launching of a massive five-year construction program to provide facilities to carry out modern concepts of care and treatment for the mentally ill and mentally retarded as developed in 1962 in the state's Master Plan for Mental Health. The total cost of this program would be in the magnitude of $500 to $600 million.

The Mental Health Section of the 1965 New York State Planning Committee listed its planning goals as follows:

1. sharing of staff between State and local facilities and services
2. a shift in the locus of service from a few remote state-operated institutions to the localities in which people live
3. the full conversion of the state hospitals to active treatment centers, reduced in size and located in the centers of the population they serve, close to major medical or university centers wherever possible, and adequately staffed to provide a therapeutic program for all patients, with emphasis on rehabilitation and return to community
4. a corresponding shift of primary responsibility for providing continuity of patient services to local government, with continued state fiscal responsibility
5. clearer definition of roles between state and local governments and between "mental health" agencies and other service agencies in health, education, welfare, employment, law enforcement, and corrections.[12]

In 1966 the Department of Mental Hygiene prepared for its own guidance a Proposed Reorganization Plan in which it reviewed its programmatic objectives and noted the need for further redirection of its institutional systems and operations. While many of the objectives were thoroughly laudable, apparently the department had not yet forsaken its commitments to construction of new facilities since it included a specific recommendation for "a vast construction program encompassing at once radically new concepts in program, design, size and location."

In 1972 the legislature enacted a long overdue Recodification of the Mental Hygiene Law, which, *inter alia,* further strengthened and expanded the civil rights of state institutional patients and included the mentally retarded and alcoholics among those to whom the Mental Health Information Service could provide assistance. The same year, 1972, saw the release of a significant document relating to the objectives and organization of mental health services in the state.[13] The document, using Long Island institutions as a geographical base of analysis, set forth a detailed critique of some of the weaknesses of the existing mental health delivery system and offered a number of alternative approaches to restructuring the components of the system within the communities involved.

Interestingly, the document quotes another statement by Dr. W.M. Mendel regarding state hospitals:

> I propose that mental illness is never well treated in a psychiatric hospital, that taking the patient into a psychiatric hospital further complicates the disorganization resulting from the mental illness and in no way propels him to resume his life in the community.[14]

In 1972 also, as a result of exposure by the media of conditions in some of the wards of the Willowbrook State School for the Retarded, the then Secretary of Health, Education, and Welfare, Eliot Richardson, issued a report of a Special Federal Team that cited among major needs the need to develop more community based services and to increase consumer-parent participation.[15]

In 1973 and 1974 the Department of Mental Hygiene began the process of decentralization by setting up a number of regional offices throughout the state to bring the process of administration closer to the "grass roots." The year 1973 also saw the enactment of the Unification of Services Law, which sought to accomplish two principal objectives:

1. the development of a system of joint planning of services for each community between the State Department and City or County Mental Health, Mental Retardation and Alcoholism Boards, the voluntary agencies, and citizen-consumers
2. the establishment of a more rational system of shared funding between state and local services to remove incentives tending to inappropriately shunt disabled individuals into state institutions.

A second important internal document of the Department, entitled *Toward a Balanced, Community Based Mental Health Service System,* sets forth the goals and planning tools required to further align mental health services with rapidly changing needs in the state. Its principal thrust was to delineate basic directions and options for reorganizing and redeploying the state's and the community's total resources in a manner designed to achieve maximum benefit to populations at risk. Considerable emphasis was placed on transitional services and rehabilitative programs. Presumably, over a period of time, a smoothly integrated state-local system would evolve with more and more emphasis on the community role in the total process.

New York State and Citizen-
Community Involvement

The New York State Department of Mental Hygiene early in 1972 organized a Task Force on Greater Community Involvement and Consumer Participation in Department of Mental Hygiene Programs. Represented on the task force were spokesmen for citizens, consumers, and voluntary agency groups as well as representatives of the department. The final report submitted to the commissioner in December 1972 contained, to the writer's knowledge, the most detailed series of recommendations pertaining to the rights of patients and residents made thus far to any mental health official. Also outlined in considerable detail were the policies and procedures that would enable concerned consumer and citizen groups to become involved in virtually all matters pertaining to the welfare of institutionalized patients. Many of the recommendations of the task force were subsequently incorporated into the department's official regulations.

A special office was created in the department to implement the department's policies in the aforementioned areas, and an advisory council to the office was set up.

In 1973 the commissioner established a citizen, consumer, multistate agency, Task Force for the Development of Community Residential and Rehabilitative Programs, which will be issuing its final report to the Commissioner in 1975. The above historical recital of the evolvement of mental health services in New York State would suggest that progress, on a modest incremental basis, is being made. What is essentially at issue, in this writer's view, is the pace and vigor of the change and the depth of commitment to a substantive and rapid restructuring of the delivery system. There is no need to rehash the obstacles and restraints, both internal and external, which tend to slow the process of change. The difficulties are real enough.

The present (1974-75) disproportion between state funding for state-operated services (approximately $753 million) and state assistance to community-operated services (approximately $70 million—for a total *local* expenditure of $200 million) obviously needs to be put in balance if the "balanced system of services" is to become a reality. It is hoped that 1975 will be the year when the present imbalance will begin to be significantly rectified. The likelihood of this coming to pass will depend in no small measure, on the extent to which concerned citizens, consumers, and dedicated professionals can fashion a grand alliance.

Notes

1. National Institute of Mental Health. Report of the Sub-committee on the Future Role of the State Hospitals, Federal-State-Local Relations Committee, NIMH. Washington: GPO, 1973.

2. Zusman, Jack, M.D. "The University, the Community and the State—
   Partners in Community Mental Health," (mimeo) Division of Community
   Psychiatry, State University of N.Y., Buffalo, N.Y. 1973.
3. Greenblatt, Milton, M.D. "Historical Forces Affecting the Closing of
   Mental Hospitals," in *Where Is My Home?* Proceedings of a Conference
   on the Closing of State Mental Hospitals, Menlo Park, Calif., Stanford
   Research Institute, 1974, p. 8.
4. Mendel, W.M., "Dismantling the Mental Hospital," in ibid., p. 18.
5. Department of Health, Education and Welfare, *Silent Majority*, Publication No. (OHD) 74-21002, p. 9.
6. *Congressional Record*, June 10, 1974. E-3689.
7. Baker, Frank, M.D. "From Community Mental Health to Human Services
   Ideology," *American Journal of Public Health* 64 (1974): 576-81.
8. Greenblatt, Milton, M.D., "Historical Forces."
9. Ozarin, Lucy D., M.D. "General Hospitals Support Centers," *Hospitals,
   Journal of the American Hospitals Association* 48:10, 51-55.
10. Schneier, Max. Remarks at the Annual Conference of the National Asso-
    ciation of State Mental Health Program Directors, Washington, D.C.
    January, 1974.
11. Feldman, Saul, M.D. "Problems and Perspectives: Administration in
    Mental Health," *Mental Health Digest* 5:4 (1973): 12-15.
12. Master Plan, New York State Planning Committee on Mental Disorders,
    N.Y.S. Department of Mental Hygiene, vol. 1, 1965, p. 20.
13. Urbahn, Max O., Associates, Inc. *This is a Lily Pad: The Responsive Men-
    tal Health Service System*: A Study of Mental Health Services in Nassau
    and Suffolk Counties for the New York State Department of Mental
    Hygiene, February, 1972, 47 pp.
14. Mendel, W.M., "On the Abolition of the Psychiatric Hospital," *in Com-
    prehensive Mental Health: The Challenge of Evaluation*, ed. by Roberts,
    L.M., Greenfield, N.S., and Miller, M.H. University of Wisconsin Press,
    1968, pp. 237-48.
15. Department of Health, Education and Welfare, Report of the Secretary's
    Special Federal Team: "The New York State Mental Retardation Pro-
    gram," Washington, D.C., 1972, p. 6.

Part III
New Treatment Modalities

Introduction to Part III

As the responsibilities of state hospitals and the nature of the populations they are serving have changed, the types of services provided have had to change accordingly. New knowledge of effective treatments has had a significant impact on the shape of state hospital services. Indeed, there are many who believe that the success of drug therapies—specifically the phenothiazines—has been one of the major triumphs of psychiatry during the twentieth century, and the principal reason why it is now possible even to consider closing state hospitals. Other major successes have been in sociotherapies—attempts to use the twenty-four-hour-day hospital environment to shape and support patient behavior—and in the behavior therapies—use of learning principles discovered from animal study to control the frequency of appearance of desirable or undesirable behavior in patients.

In Chapter 9, Dr. John Cumming, who spent a number of years as the deputy commissioner in the New York State Department of Mental Hygiene with primary responsibility for administration of the state hospitals, discusses the problem of chronic patients. Over the years of the development of community mental health centers and the acute treatment units in state hospitals, it has become clear that some patients simply are not suitable for short-term treatment. These individuals do not recover rapidly, if they recover at all. As the number of these individuals in the caseload of an acute treatment-oriented facility increases over the years, there is the "silting up" described by a number of authors. It is conceivable that after some period, all of the treatment places in an acute unit will be occupied by these chronic patients who are not able to make appropriate use of the facility and who will then block the access of those who can use the facility. The resulting temptation for the facility administrator is somehow to rid himself of these patients even if it means turning them out without anyone to care for them. Dr. Cumming discusses strategies of dealing with these patients.

In Chapter 10, Dr. Robert Liberman and his co-authors discuss current use of behavior therapies in a number of state hospital settings. In the past two years or so, a variety of uses of the principles of learning developed by Skinner and co-workers have been widely applied in state hospitals. Although evaluations of the effectiveness of these approaches have begun to be reported, behavior therapy is far from having been demonstrated as effective. Yet, there is much to suggest that it is a valuable addition to the armamentarium of the state hospital psychiatrist and worthy of careful study. Dr. Liberman

147

has been involved in state hospital use of behavior therapy for a number of years and was able through his knowledge of the national scene to recruit several co-authors to describe their work.

In Chapter 11, Dr. Leonard Gottesman deals with one of the great unsolved problems of the state hospitals—the rapidly enlarging geriatric population. These individuals, who in many ways are unsuitable for state hospital care but yet have no other place to go, are among the group mentioned above as "silting up" the hospitals. State hospital clinicians and administrators are not accustomed to dealing with this population. In fact, in New York State not too long ago, they responded to the issue by refusing to admit many individuals over age sixty-five who were referred to the hospitals. Dr. Gottesman, on the basis of his experience in working with geriatric programs, presents a number of interesting, innovative ideas that can serve either to help get state hospitals out of the geriatric service business, or to help the hospitals do a better job of serving their older patients.

In Chapters 12 and 13, one of the major forms of sociotherapy used in helping patients to adjust outside of the hospital are described and analyzed. Mrs. Mildred Cannon, a member of the staff of Biometry Division of the National Institute of Mental Health, uses national data to provide a picture of current operation in halfway houses for various types of populations. Halfway houses provide supervised group living for individuals not in need of the close supervision and medical treatment of the mental hospital but who are not ready for independent community living. For several years Mrs. Cannon has been following the development of halfway houses through data gathered in the repeated surveys that the National Institute of Mental Health has conducted of the rapidly increasing number of halfway houses throughout the nation.

Mr. Charles Orndoff, director of an agency devoted to providing a full spectrum of transitional housing to discharged patients, describes how he has carried out his work. Starting in Buffalo, New York, with only partial interest in the community and no facilities at all, he has managed to build up an agency with several hundred spaces for residents, carrying out an intensive rehabilitation program in combination with offering housing at various support levels.

9

Who Will Care for the Chronically Disabled?
John Cumming

Who will care for the chronically disabled? If this question were not asked so persistently, it could be dismissed with a facetious or a cynical comment. Historically, the chronically ill have never been cared for properly, so why would anyone expect that care for them would begin at this somewhat inauspicious time of minimal public funding. A slightly less cynical response might result from examining those agencies that have traditionally supplied what care has been made available—jails, poor houses, and large mental hospitals. Good conservative principles then predict that these agencies will continue to provide this care, such as it is. Indeed, those who operate the large mental hospitals sometimes legitimately ask who will care for the chronically disabled when they are confronted with plans for community services that they suspect will deplete their resources without taking responsibility for this group who use the greatest part of their budgets.

Perhaps the real title should be, "who will care for the chronically disabled; because *we* are not going to"—disclaimers that appear to be made chiefly by politicians and operators of community mental health centers at this particular time.

Over the last twenty years, beliefs about both the nature of psychiatric illness and our legal structures have changed. These changes have caused mental hospitals to examine their practices and their patient groups and to restate their policies. It is no longer considered good practice to retain in institutions patients whose illnesses are stable and who are not dangerous to themselves or others. Furthermore, hospitals have stopped receiving without question every patient who is sent to them, and have abrogated their function of removing from society large numbers of persons who are poor, elderly, physically ill, eccentric, incompetent, or some combination of these.

Because the hospital is not accepting or retaining this latter group does not mean that these patients do not need assistance. But their presence in the community places new demands on the fiscal and human resources, a matter of some concern to the local politican and the operators of community treatment services.[1] Whether their objections can be wholly justified, however, is open to question.

Political and Community Objections

A majority of the chronically disabled who are discharged from the hospital will need welfare services for a time. But it should be remembered that most of them were on welfare before they first went to the hospital.[2] Furthermore,

149

those who are refused admission to hospitals also include a high proportion of welfare recipients. Thus, the welfare rolls are increased by the new policies.

However, if all mental hospitals were closed entirely, the numbers of new welfare clients would be extremely small relative to the total welfare load. Further, if release of these chronic patients is indeed increasing welfare costs, the amount of increase is offset by a corresponding reduction in hospital costs resulting on the whole in a saving to the average taxpayer. Yet, the local politician often tries to make good political capital with his constituents by decrying mental hospital "dumping" of chronic patients onto welfare rolls. The local citizens thus addressed are known to be already apprehensive about having more mental patients in their midst, and to this apprehension the politican adds his false concern over taxation.[3] It is not surprising that there is public resistance to the care of chronic disabled patients in the community; politicians may take much of the credit.

The complaints of community mental health centers about the discharge of chronic patients from mental hospitals probably relates to the way in which most of these services have developed—with an acute inpatient service as their core. In such organizations it is traditionally assumed that if patients do not respond to treatment within a certain time period, they should be transferred to a mental hospital. Most patients who are considered for transfer are not hard to reintegrate into the community, given a supporting structure, but where this structure is lacking, there is no alternative to the mental hospital. The fact that supportive, rehabilitative structures have not more often been developed in communities has to be an indictment of the psychiatric profession. Either they are ignorant of how to develop and use community services for the chronically disabled or they are not interested in so doing.

Both the people centrally concerned with treatment, (i.e., psychiatrists), and people centrally concerned with fiscal support for treatment, (i.e., politicians), have too often turned their backs on the chronically disabled. The question remains, who should assume the burden of their care?

The chronically disabled can best be cared for in the community by the same therapists and within the same system that provides initial treatment for the acute episode of illness. Justification for this belief can be found by examining who are the chronically disabled; what are their numbers; whether or not it is feasible to treat them in the community; and whether such treatment is humane, effective, and fiscally sound.

Definition of the Population

It is quite plain that the majority of those known as the chronically disabled, or the chronic patient, are chronic schizophrenics. Schizophrenia is the most common diagnosis of the longterm patient in the mental hospital. A.M. Kraft[4] in his study of the development of a chronic population in a new, modern, psychiatric hospital reports that 94 percent of this chronic group was labelled as schizophrenic. While some schizophrenic patients may fail to respond to treatment because of an inappropriate treatment method, some authors feel that there is reasonable evidence of discrimination at admission of a "sicker" subgroup of schizophrenics.[5] Even disregarding those criteria that seem tautological, for example, early onset and numbers of previous admissions, it seems reasonable to discriminate at least statistically a subgroup of schizophrenics less likely to respond to the usual therapies on the basis of a mental status examination alone.[6]

Nor is this group who suffer from persistent illness an inconsequential one. In describing a cohort of patients admitted for services with a two-and-a-half year period at risk, Kraft found that 81 of 590, or 14 percent had been receiving service continuously for two years. What is perhaps more important, only four of these, or less than 1 percent, had been inpatients over the whole period. However, Strauss and Carpenter,[7] in recent careful perspective studies, found that the only variables that predicted the level of social functioning of schizophrenics after hospitalization, for example, satisfactory work or interpersonal relationships, were the previous levels of these same variables. The weak correlation of these variables to schizophrenic symptoms leads to speculation that competence may somehow be orthoganal to the presence or absence of symptoms.[8] Whether symptoms or performance are used, however, there does appear to be a basis for deciding who among schizophrenics will need long-term care. Thus, while we perhaps must resign ourselves to providing long-term attention to a considerable number of patients, this is not synonymous with expecting a large number of chronically hospitalized patients.

Pasamanick[9] has perhaps more clearly than anyone else demonstrated the feasibility of treating and maintaining an unselected group of schizophrenic patients in the community. He demonstrated that after an initial period, in which the therapeutic team was presumably learning its new role, only eight percent of the patients selected as needing hospitalization actually required inpatient care. The use of drugs played a major role in the prevention of hospitalization, although the presence of the public health nurses who "visited the patients' homes, delivered medications, gathered research data systematically by interviewing significant others, and gave family members practical assistance and support" also contributed significantly to the encouraging treatment results. After two and one half years the project was abandoned and the patients were returned to the routine care of the state system. A follow-up five years later indicated that under state system care, all groups of patients had deteriorated and about three out of five had been hospitalized.

Pasamanick views "schizophrenia [as] a chronic disorder primarily genetic or congenital in nature, with precipitants not basically psycho-social in origin, but rather an organic process with still undetermined precipitants resulting in exacerbations and remissions or acutely unacceptable symptoms." This inability to find precipitating stress, also detected by Beck[10] and others, may result because they have not followed the kind of interesting lead that Brown[11] and his co-workers explored. These workers suggest that the crucial event for relapse is one that upsets relationships with significant others and it is this altered relationship that is the direct cause of the acute episode. To hold to a basic genetic or congenital causation does not mean that social events are without influence.

Treatment Alternatives

An important paper providing a possible basic link between biological and neurophysiological studies on one hand and those dealing with social variables on the other was recently published by Claridge.[12] Beginning with a review of the neuropsychological findings related to schizophrenia, Claridge quotes Kerry's well-known observation that the only consistent findings in such studies seem to be that schizophrenics show a greater variance on neurophysiological variables than is found in normal subjects.[13] He goes on to postulate that the basic schizophrenic difficulty may be found not in the variation of a single factor but in a disturbed relationship between two or more factors. Elaborating on this hypothesis he presents evidence that the relationship between arousal and attention is indeed anomalous in schizophrenics. In normal people the relationship is reciprocal: as arousal increases, the field of attention is simultaneously narrowed in a way that suggests an automatic control system, or governor. In the schizophrenic the relationship appears to be direct; that is, high levels of arousal are accompanied by an opening of the field of attention and a flood of stimuli, while at a low arousal level there is a stimulus lack and the individual becomes relatively inaccessible. There is, of course, a middle ground of moderate arousal levels where the relationship between these factors is very much the same in the schizophrenic and the normal.

These findings are suggestive. They suggest a rationale for the effectiveness of drug therapy in controlling acute symptoms, they also suggest that it might not require too much work to develop a method of titrating an individual's drug requirement. The necessity for this will be considered later. Perhaps more importantly, Claridge's findings provide a more rational basis upon which to plan a therapeutic environment for the schizophrenic patient.

Brown, Wing, and Birley[14] have done more than any other group to describe the sorts of environments in which schizophrenics are likely to develop acute symptoms. While originally entirely pragmatic, they have lately developed a general theory of environmental influences on the schizophrenic. In doing so,

they have drawn upon previous work on arousal by Venables and Wing.[15] As
these workers reformulated their concepts in preparation for a replication of
their earlier work on the influence of various types of family settings on
schizophrenics they have, from one point of view, provided a test of the validity
of Claridge's basic neuropsychological constructs, and these constructs seem to
be supported by the results.

Brown and Wing confirmed the relationship, found in their earlier work,
between a high degree of expressed emotion among family members and the
likelihood of relapse. The emotional behavior observed in the Brown study
was almost always criticism and hostility expressed toward the patient. These
expressions of negative emotions had often been preceded, during the previous
three weeks, by a significant change in the patient's social environment, accompanied by a raised level of tension in the home. The onset of florid symptoms
and relapse was likely to follow such a change. These authors conclude that
the "optimal social environment, for those who remain handicapped . . . [is] a
structured and neutrally stimulating one with little necessity for complex
decision making." They also find that the key moment for the use of drugs
in the regimen of care was during these periods of interpersonal strife.

We[16] as well as others have postulated that the chronic patient is protected
from the development of acute episodes by the acquisition of skills that enable
him to deal more competently with ordinary environmental problems. A crisis
that has been met once and overcome is less critical when it reappears. Further,
if a patient so shows himself competent in playing the reciprocal roles expected
of him relative to those he lives and works with, we can expect that the "high
expressed emotion" situations will be less frequent. While we know that those
who relapse seem to be less competent than those who do not, we have had
little good work to enable us to predict stability on the basis of competence.

A specific exception to this general lack of evidence on the usefulness
of competence comes from the recent work of Lamb and Goertzel.[17] At the
termination of hospitalization they randomly assigned patients either to a
traditional boarding home situation, which they called a "low expectation
situation" or to a system of halfway house, sheltered workshop, and independent apartment house living, which they termed a "high expectation situation." As might be expected, those who were assigned to the high expectation situation had more flareups of acute symptoms and were rehospitalized
more frequently than were the group assigned to traditional boarding homes.
Nevertheless, at any follow-up period, those subjected to high expectations
were more often to be found in the community and were functioning on more
socially acceptable levels.

All in all, these recent studies give considerable hope that chronic psychiatric patients can be managed in the community with less danger of deterioration, with more humanity, and at probably no greater costs than result from
traditional methods of care.

Summary

The elements needed in a system to care for the chronically disabled are the following:

1. *Housing.* On the one hand, when programs of placement have been sponsored by large hospitals they often have been based on the boarding home; yet, recent studies of these[18] have discovered them to be "new back wards." On the other hand, when the problem of housing is left to local welfare departments, patients are often segregated into welfare hotels, the target of a similar phrase "from the back wards to the back alleys." (See notes 1 and 3). Neither one of these alternatives is good enough. Housing must be of good quality, provide privacy and be integrated into the monitoring and care services of the community mental health system.

2. *Someone who is responsible for the patient's welfare.* A chronically impaired person needs long-term help, and a basic mental health worker who plays the role of advisor, helper, advocate, friend, and therapist is the cornerstone of the system of services that must be provided. This worker sets up the "high expectations" that are needed. He uses his influence to get the patient to take his drugs; he helps the patient to maintain his position in the world of work; he is available in moments of stress.

3. *The proper use of psychotrophic drugs.* While the effectiveness of drugs in the control of symptoms is unquestioned, their greatest disadvantage is that patients do not take them. There has been little experimentation on methods for increasing complaince with prescribed drug regimens. Evidence exists that mildly ill acute patients recover more quickly on placebos than on drugs;[19] that drugs are most important in specific social situations;[20] that taking a placebo regularly protects against relapse;[21] and that not all patients who stop taking drugs inevitably relapse. More needs to be known about drugs and their proper use and dosage. Greater sophistication in drug use, would achieve greater acceptance of drugs by patients.

4. *The opportunity to work, as a support to the patient's own self-image, to increase his competence, to lessen the time he may have to spend in high expressed emotion situations with kin, and for monetary rewards.* A high percentage of schizophrenics do, of course, work. In a follow-up of a comprehensive sample of those so diagnosed, R.J. Turner[22] reported that 75 percent were employed. This is not an argument, however, against the need to provide rehabilitation and sheltered work for those who are temporarily or permanently unable to compete in the open market.

5. *Addressing the problem that Grad and Sainsbury[23] have referred to us the "burden on the community."* The chronically ill person does indeed place a burden on families and friends. The fact that these families and friends are willing to assume this burden should not blind us to their need for help and support in discharging this duty. Presumably such support would do much to

obviate the effect of events that otherwise create an emotional climate that is the prelude to relapse.

At the present time, the concept of community care for the seriously mentally ill is under critical scrutiny, and with considerable justification. The populations and budgets of mental hospital systems have been reduced and the funds from new sources spent for community services to a different population, seriously jeopardizing resources needed to finance a broad spectrum of community services. While there are few examples of how an adequately financed mental hospital could deal with the problem of the chronically impaired, there are also few examples of an adequately organized system of community care for the chronically ill. Considering the spiralling costs of hospital care, it would not seem wise to abandon efforts to create an alternative community system. Further, there is no reason to suspect that abandonment of a community approach will result in increased funding for hospitals. There is enough money now. The imperative remains to devise ways of using it effectively.

Notes

1. The City of New York Commission on State-City Relations, "A Shuffle to Despair," June, 1972, mimeo.
2. Cumming, J.H., "The Inadequacy Syndrome," *Psychiat. Quarterly*, 37:4 (1963): 723-33.
3. Aviram, Ari and Segal, S.P., "Exclusion of the Mentally Ill," *Archives of General Psychiatry* 29 (July, 1973): 126-31.
4. Kraft, A.M., Binner, P.R., and Dickey, B.A., "The Chronic Patient," in *Community Mental Health*, ed. R. H. Williams and L. Ozarin, San Francisco: Jossey-Bass, 1968.
5. Evan, J.R., Rodnick, E.H., Goldstein, M.J., and Judd, L.L., "Premorbid Adjustment, Phenothiazine Treatment and Remission in Acute Schizophrenics," *Archives of General Psychiat.* 27 (1972): 486-90.
6. Kraft, "The Chronic Patient."
7. Strauss, J.S. and Carpenter, W.T., "The Prediction of Outcome in Schizophrenia, Characteristics of Outcome," *Archives of General Psychiat.* 27 (1972): 739-46; ____, "The Prediction of Outcome in Schizophrenia, II, The Relationships Between Predictor and Outcome Variables," American Psychiatric Association Annual Meeting, Honolulu, May, 1973, mimeo.
8. Turner, R.J. and Cumming, J.H., "Theoretical Malaise and Community Mental Health," in *Emergent Approaches to Mental Health Problems*, ed. E.L. Cowen, E.A. Gardner, and M. Zax. New York, Appleton-Century-Crofts, 1967.
9. Pasamanick, B., Scarpitti, F. and Dinitz, S., *Schizophrenia in the Community:*

An Experimental Study in the Prevention of Hospitalization, New York: Appleton-Century-Crofts, 1967; Davis, A.E., Dinitz, S., and Pasamanick, B., "The Prevention of Hospitalization in Schizophrenia," *Amer. J. of Ortho-psychiat.* 42 (1972): 375-88.

10. Beck, J.C. and Worthen, K., "Precipitating Stress, Crisis Theory and Hospitalization in Schizophrenia," *Archives of General Psychiatry* 26 (1972): 123-29.

11. Brown, G.W. and Birley, J.L.T., "Crisis and Life Changes and the Onset of Schizophrenia," *J. of Health and Social Behavior* 9 (1968): 203-14.

12. Claridge, G., "The Schizophrenias as Nervous Types," *Brit. J. of Psychiat.* 121 (1972): 1-17.

13. Ketty, S.S., "Recent Biochemical Theories of Schizophrenia," in *The Aetiology of Schizophrenia*, ed. D.D. Jackson, New York: Basic Books, 1960.

14. Brown, G.W., Birley, J.T., and Wing, J.K., "Influence of Family Life on the Course of Schizophrenic Disorders: A Replication," *Brit. J. of Psychiat.* 121 (1972): 241-58.

15. Venables, P.H. and Wing, J.K., "Level of Arousal and the Subclassification of Schizophrenia," *Archives of General Psychiatry* 7 (1962): 114-19.

16. Cumming, J.H. and Cumming, E., *Ego and Milieu*, New York: Atherton Press, 1962.

17. Lamb, H.R. and Goertzel, V., "Discharged Mental Patients: Are They Really in the Community?" *Archives of General Psychiatry* 24 (1971): 29-34.

18. Murphy, H.B.M., Penee, B., and Luchens, D., *Foster Homes: The New Back Wards?* Canada's Mental Health Supplement #71, September-October, 1972.

19. Evan, et al., "Premorbid Adjustment."

20. Brown, Birley and Wing, "Influence of Family Life."

21. Hogarty, G.E. and Goldberg, S.C., "Drug and Sociotherapy in the Aftercare of Schizophrenic Patients," *Archives of General Psychiatry* 28 (1973): 54-64.

22. Turner, R.J., *The Implications of Psychiatric Disorder for Employment*, Department of Sociology, University of Western Ontario, 1973, mimeo.

23. Grad, J. and Sainsbury, P., "The Effects that Patients have on Their Families in a Community Care and a Control Psychiatric Service: A Two-Year Follow-up," *Brit. J. of Psychiat.* 114 (1968): 265-68.

10

Behavior Therapy in State Hospitals

Robert P. Liberman, Thomas S. Ball,
Lois Sibbach, William DiScipio,
Irvin P.R. Guyett, Peter A. Magaro,
and *Charles Wallace*

Behavior therapy, as an applied science, builds upon principles of learning and behavior change derived from research in psychology and psychiatry for the alleviation of human suffering, the enhancement of human functioning, and the fulfillment of the learning potential of individuals. Behavior therapy is not a mere collection of techniques. Behavior therapies develop and adapt a wide variety of techniques that can be demonstrated empirically to be effective in clinical situations. Techniques, therapeutic methods, and interventions are simply by-products of the creative use of social learning and operant conditioning principles and the adherence to empirical evaluation and experimentation. Behavior therapy improves the quality of personal and social life only through the bringing about of favorable changes in the patient's environment. For behavior therapy to succeed, it is mandatory that the milieu be enriched with greater social stimulation, more consistent and positive staff-patient interaction, and a wider array of rewards, reinforcers, and privileges. As such, behavior therapy or behavior modification could be more aptly renamed "environmental modification."

The clinical strategy of behavior therapists requires answers to the following questions obtained through specific tasks:

1. What behavior is maladaptive or problematic? *Task*: To specify concretely the observable behavior that should be increased or decreased, thus clarifyin the therapeutic goals.
2. How often does the behavior occur? *Task*: To measure or record the frequency or intensity of the undesirable and desirable behavior, a procedure necessary for following therapeutic progress.
3. What environmental and interpersonal contingencies currently support the problem behavior and reduce the likelihood of more adaptive responses? *Task*: To specify the functional relation between behavior and those events and reactions that determine the frequency of the behavior. A retrospective analysis uncovers the conditioning history of the patient.

The views expressed in this chapter are those of the authors only and should not be construed as official policy of the institutions or agencies for whom they work.

Dr. Robert P. Liberman had responsibility for the overall organization of this chapter and for inviting contributions from the additional co-authors. The introduction and conclusion sections were written by Dr. Liberman.

157

4. Which interpersonal transactions, particularly between therapist and patient(s), or other interventions can alter the problem behavior in a more adaptive direction? *Task*: To develop therapeutic tactics and strategy—using modelling, reinforcement, instructions, punishment, and counter-conditioning—that will modify behavior effectively.

The Therapeutic Community

The therapeutic community incorporates principles of learning in its approach. With the change of the norms and culture of a ward, contingencies of reinforcement are clearly altered. Patients are given feedback as responsible humans rather than as custodial cases. Opportunities to behave in more adaptive directions are increased with the emphasis on democratic, group decision making; freedom of movement; more informal patient status; the blurring of the lines between patient and staff; and increased social interaction in group activities. There is a great emphasis on group pressure and expectancy directed toward more normal functioning.

However, the contingencies that are set up under the therapeutic community are often haphazard, not monitored in any consistent way, and at times can work at cross purposes to each other. For example, because the goals of the therapeutic community are not concretely specified, emotional expressiveness tends to be reinforced regardless of the effect it has on rehabilitation or on the other patients. Thus, some patients get rewarded for unconstructive griping, expression of hostility, and acting-out behavior, which makes it that much more difficult to rehabilitate them for discharge into the community. The greatest weaknesses of milieu therapy have been the failure to focus systematically on instrumental role training, the elimination of bizarre behavior, and the provision of community support and after-care. We simply cannot expect patients who have been hospitalized for many years to be able to stay out in the community without very special preparations and continued support even after receiving the most favorable milieu therapy.

Description and elaboration of the principles of learning and conditioning upon which behavioral methods are based is beyond the scope of this chapter; hence, you are referred to any one of the many available and informative texts on behavior therapy and behavior modification.[1] Clinicians in psychiatry, psychology, social work, and allied disciplines are beginning to reap the benefits of the empiricism generated by behavior therapists. From studies of the effects of behavior therapy with a diversity of clinical problems, data are accumulating that reveal the type of therapeutic interventions that have discernible and significant impact on the problem behaviors of specific groupings of patients.

Much of the initial work in behavior therapy during the 1950s and early 1960s was carried out in state hospitals and veterans' hospitals, some distance

from the academic mainstream of clinical psychiatry and psychology. Conducting therapy with "hopeless" patients on the back wards, the pioneers in behavior
therapy met less resistance and competition from traditionally trained professionals. Similarly, the nursing-level staff in large, custodial institutions were
relatively deprived of professional stimulation and supervision and lacked
training in the conduct of any form of active treatment for patients. Those
nursing personnel who sustained therapeutic idealism in the face of institutionalized inertia were responsive and enlivened by the young psychologists
and psychiatrists who came onto their units to demonstrate new treatment
methods with the chronic mental patient.

The basic principles and the methods of behavior therapy were concrete,
practical, and easy to understand—these methods were sometimes referred to
as the systematic and consistent application of common sense. By 1965 a new
optimism began sweeping large mental institutions as the first reports were
published of the success of behavior therapy with mute and withdrawn psychotics, autistic children, anorectics, apathetic, and bizarre schizophrenics, and
retardates.[2] By 1963 Ayllon and Azrin[3] had established the first "token
economy," the application of reinforcement principles to an entire ward of
patients.

The Token Economy

A systematic approach with chronic patients, the token economy uses
clear specification of treatment goals and contingencies of reinforcement. The
goal of the token economy is to prevent or reverse the "social breakdown syndrome" from enveloping the chronic psychotic in a custodial milieu. Instead
of receiving food, bed, privileges, and small luxuries like cigarettes free of
charge, patients must work and perform at a higher level of functioning in
order to earn tokens, which then can be exchanged for the good things of
life. Each patient's goals are calibrated periodically allowing success to occur
easily and frequently in small steps of therapeutic progress.

The aim of a token economy is to induce more socially appropriate
behavior in patients, on a ward-wide basis, through the use of tokens. The
tokens serve as common currency for a wide variety of back-up reinforcers,
which then can be chosen on an individual basis by the patients. The token
economy also enables the staff to reinforce more adaptive behavior immediately by rewarding the patient with a token, rather than having him wait
to receive some desired item or privilege at a later time. It is well known in
both laboratory and clinical studies that immediate reinforcement is much
more effective in the teaching of new behaviors than is delayed reinforcement. The dispensing of tokens also cues staff members to give frequent
praise and recognition to the patients. Ultimately, this more natural "social

reinforcement" will supplant the tokens as the motivational support for the patient's behavior.

The emphasis in the token economies, then, is to make patients' responses have clear-cut, consistent consequences. Presenting a shaved face in the morning, grooming oneself carefully, participating in the ward clean-up, and working on a hospital job all have the consequences of being reinforced with tokens and approval. On the other hand, failure to engage in socially appropriate behavior leads to absence of reinforcement (extinction of maladaptive behavior), or occasionally to punishment (i.e., fines) where tokens are taken away from the patient.

In the token economy the patient's behavior does mean something and patients are required to take responsibility for their behavior. No patient in the token economy starves or goes without a bed, however. If not enough tokens are earned during the day, the patient subsists in a "welfare state." He may eat his meals on a steel tray rather than using more pleasant dinnerware; he may do without cigarettes and T.V., and he may sleep on a hard cot rather than a comfortable bed. Thus, tokens are immediate rewards that can be used to improve behavior much as money does in the natural economy. The ethical problems of using contingencies of reinforcement with dependent, institutionalized patients are being confronted and resolved by concerned professionals in law and psychology.[4]

What have been the results of behavior modification experiments in the token economy. Ayllon and Azrin illustrated the effect that tokens have on work performance in ward and hospital jobs at Anna State Hospital in Illinois.[5] When tokens are provided to patients contingent upon their work efforts, the patients show high levels of activity. When tokens are withdrawn or given free without any need to work, patients' participation rapidly declines. It is clear from the data, that the tokens are crucial in maintaining high levels of performance. Findings from studies such as these, using patients as their own controls, have been replicated many times in different hosptials.[6]

Since the original aims of managers of token economies were to minimize and counteract the apathy and regression of the social breakdown syndrome, most of the documented effectiveness of the token economy has been with work activities and self-care behaviors. In recent years, however, investigators have reported beneficial effects of token economies on more functional and complex behaviors. Decreases in aggressive and destructive behaviors, delusional speech and hallucinations,[7] and increases in self-esteem[8] have been reported. There is evidence that bizarre behaviors can be decreased through "functional displacement" as tokens reinforce more adaptive behaviors.[9]

Some of the most disastrous effects of long-term institutionalization of mental patients are the destruction of interpersonal responses and withdrawal from social interaction. The "good" patient in a custodial setting is a quiet, unobtrusive one. Enhancing the social repertoires of such patients is critical for their being capable of leaving the hospital, for adjusting to and remaining in the community. Competence in carrying on conversations is instrumental in developing relationships, asking for directions, obtaining necessities, and, in general, navigating the social pathways that are required for a successful adaptation to community life.

One study involved four chronic schizophrenic women, hospitalized over fifteen years each, whose social conversation was reliably and quantitatively recorded during fifty-minute group sessions.[10] Contingent token reinforcement increased conversational participation by four to five times over the baseline and noncontingent reinforcement phases (see Figure 10-1). Other reports of significant improvements in social behavior of schizophrenics have been made in hospitals and community mental health centers using behavioral procedures.[11]

Using more conventional measures of effectiveness, managers of token economy programs have reported considerable success in releasing long-stay patients, increasing durations of community living, and decreasing rehospitalization or the "revolving door syndrome." Recently, studies have been published

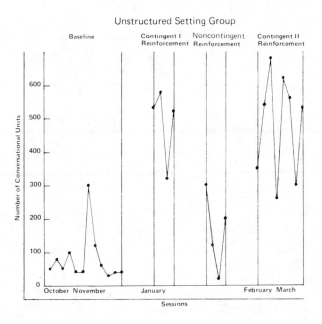

Figure 10-1. Conversation Among Group Members Under Baseline, Contingent, and Noncontingent Reinforcement Conditions. (Reprinted from Liberman, R.P. "Reinforcement of Social Interaction in a Group of Chronic Schizophrenics." Chapter in *Advances in Behavior Therapy,* vol. 3, R. Rubin, C. Franks, H. Fensterhein, and L. Ullmann (eds.). New York: Academic Press, pp. 151-60.

showing the comparatively greater effectiveness of behavior therapy v. milieu
or custodial treatment with chronic mental patients.[12] Paralleling the reports
of the effectiveness of behavior therapy, the number of institutions using
behavior therapy has quickly increased. By the end of 1969 there were twenty-
seven ongoing token economy programs with veterans administration (V.A.)
hospitals alone, and the V.A. had issued a policy statement supporting and
encouraging the implementation of token economies. In Figure 10-2 the
exponential rise in published reports on token economies referenced in *Psychological Abstracts and Index Medicus* is shown. Unfortunately, there remains
a paucity of information in the literature concerning the practical problems
and solutions in developing and sustaining a successful behavior therapy
program.

Many behavioral programs, heralded in journal reports, have folded hardly
before the ink is dry on the journal page. New programs are set up with their
administrative and clinical leaders making the same fatal mistakes or omissions
that have led to the collapse of similar programs in other institutions. Some
token economies are "token" efforts with little additional enrichment of the

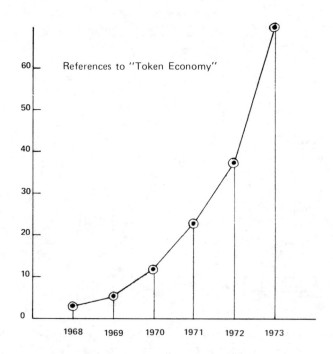

Figure 10-2. Number of Bibliographic References to "Token Economy" in
Psychological Abstracts and Index Medicus, 1968-73.

milieu other than the haphazard and inconsistent dispensing of mental coins or coupons. The basic principles of learning and conditioning that form the strategy for behavioral programs are not sufficient for operational success. Administrative, organizational, and group process variables are the real determinants of an effective behavior therapy program.

To avoid perpetuating an unsophisticated and naive "advertising" of behavior therapy, the senior author (Robert P. Liberman) conceived this chapter as an opportunity to bring together some practical and sobering viewpoints on behavior therapy in state hospitals. Ten psychologists who had developed token economy and behavioral programs in state or veteran's hospitals were invited to contribute brief narratives that would address the following questions:

1. How did you train your staff in behavioral interventions and maintain their performance over time?
2. Which results and outcomes were most significant in terms of impact on patients? Which patients (types defined behaviorally) did best in the program? Which did worst? How did you deal with unresponsive patients?
3. How long has your program continued? If it has terminated, why? If ongoing, how much dissemination and penetration has occurred into other parts of the hospital or the state system?
4. How much generalization across settings, responses, and time (durability of improvements) has been observed? What procedures do you employ to facilitate generalization and which seem practical and effective?
5. What administrative issues facilitated or impeded the development and progress of your program?

While each of the invited contributors had published accounts of their programs in books and journals, the senior author encouraged them to use the forum of this chapter to present previously unreported results, retrospective reflections, and speculative interpretations of their experiences, both positive and negative. Five individuals agreed to contribute and their narratives, edited by the senior author, follow in alphabetical order. Their contributions should not be viewed as inclusive of the experiences of all program managers, but they are broadly representative. It is hoped that the candid descriptions of their experiences will be instructive to current and future program managers and informative to administrators and policy makers upon whose actions the success of behavior therapy in state hospitals depends.

Pacific State Hospital
Pomona, California

Thomas S. Ball and
Lois Sibbach

Pacific State Hospital, located thirty miles east of Los Angeles, is one of four hospitals solely for the mentally retarded in the state of California. The establishment of a token economy program was inspired by a successful demonstration of the token economy with the mentally ill conducted by Drs. Hal Schaefer and Pat Martin at nearby Patton State Hospital.[13] In 1966, when the hospital's Treatment Program Planning Committee was approached, it was already aware of the undisputed success at Pacific State Hospital of a self-help skill program based on operant conditioning. Token economy is but another application of operant technology. But this time it was proposed to take over an entire ward of adolescent and young adult female retardates with a tightly controlled program. Following the Patton model, patients would have to earn tokens to pay for all aspects of their daily living, including food. We also proposed the control of parental visits.

Such features aroused great resistance, primarily from the social work department, but from other departments as well. The proposals "rocked the boat" insofar as the definition and delineation of professional roles were concerned. They also challenged some notions of professional intervention with parents. It was predicted that control of parental visits would break the tenuous bond that existed between many parents and their institutionalized children, that it would encourage parents to rationalize a complete break in the relationship. The proposal also placed the prospective psychologist-director of the program in a unique position. In our institution a psychologist had never had major administrative responsibility for an entire ward program.

Although emphasizing from the outset the primacy of medical authority in ward problems of a medical nature, the psychologist insisted on policy control of the behavioral aspects of the program. After a series of meetings, the Treatment Program Committee approved the token economy, a result of the strong support of the hospital administration, especially the superintendent, Dr. Vernon Bugh.

One thing learned from those meetings was the need to value informed, intelligent, articulate opposition. Such opposition forces one to evaluate one's own assumptions, sharpen one's own thinking, and to develop a position statement. For example, largely in response to the perceptive objections raised by our chief social worker, a position statement was formulated and circulated to key hospital staff on the rationale, value, and ethical safeguards of the token economy program. The fact that the program was actually launched in January

1967, an uncertain and difficult time for the California State Department of
Mental Hygiene, was due to the vigorous support received from Dr. Bugh and
Mrs. Mary Roberts, superintendent of Nursing Services. We requested our own
ward, time to select and train our own staff prior to the arrival of patients, and
control over the selection of patients. And we were doing this with no outside
funding. The result was a strain on already limited resources, but key administrative people felt that we had something of value and were willing to back
us up.

Because of the special nature of the program, written parental approval
was required before patients could be transferred to the token economy ward.
Parents were approached with a "contract" that they could either accept or
reject. In group meetings with parents all aspects of the program were explained
in detail. Considerable opposition was anticipated but much to our surprise
over 90 percent of the parents attending gave written approval for their daughters
or charges to be admitted to the program. Many parents have shown unusual
cooperation and some have been willing to carry the program, including the use
of tokens, into the home.

Training

The nursing level staff were selected for their noninstitutional attitudes,
initiative, and enthusiasm for learning new methods. The initial training of the
token economy staff was conducted by Dr. Ball, program director, three psychologists selected by him to be ward consultants, the ward physician, and the social
worker. Orientation to behavior modification and the use of tokens as condi-
tioned reinforcers was implemented through lectures, films, selected reading, and
discussion sessions. All formal training was done during the week prior to the
admission of residents to the token economy.

Nursing-level staff are involved in contributing ideas for the treatment programs, thereby assuming a certain amount of responsibility and obtaining credit
for their efforts. Supervisors view the nurses and psychiatric technicians as
intelligent, creative, skillful individuals who should be helped to develop to their
maximum potential. Supervisory personnel know first-hand the problems
encountered by the nurses and technicians, as they work directly with them,
sharing in maintaining the consistency of the program. This close working
relationship reinforces a cohesive team. The entire team, from project director
to technician, works at all levels of responsibility, always keeping in mind that
top priority must be given to staffing the immediate therapeutic environment
with the resident and her treatment program. Giving nursing-level personnel
specific training skills, opportunities for designing individual treatment programs,
and involving them in the decision-making process have contributed to the
development of a highly motivated team.

Significance of Results

The token economy has been an ongoing program since January 1967. Begun as a six-month demonstration project, the program was extended to a year, then a second year. In June 1969 the program was doubled in size, with an increase in resident population from twenty to forty-five residents and a concomitant increase in staff and physical area. Patients admitted to the token economy program have multiple behavioral problems that can be categorized into the following dimensions:

Immature and dependent behaviors: pouting, clinging, baby talk, whining, giggling, crying, requiring assistance in eating, grooming, and toileting.

Asocial behavior: withdrawn, shy, little or no conversation, isolated, avoiding social or recreation contact.

Antisocial behavior: negativistic, noncompliant, stealing, tantrums, verbal abusiveness.

Aggressive behavior: self-destructive, physically assaultive to staff and patients.

Twenty-three residents did poorly in the token economy and were transferred to other units at the hospital. Of these, four were so profoundly retarded that they could not grasp the contingencies of reinforcement operative within the token economy, in spite of lengthy pairing of primary reinforcers with the tokens. Thirteen residents exhibited frequent aggression, against self or others, that could not be controlled by the positive contingencies of the token economy. Two patients repeatedly ran away from the unit, which is an unlocked, open program.

The most recent data available on the effectiveness of treatment in the token economy reveal that sixty residents have been placed in community programs since 1967. Fifty-two of them (87%) have maintained a successful and uninterrupted community adjustment averaging 92.44 months. Their average stay on the token economy ward was twenty months.

Maximum effort is made to provide as "normal" a living environment as possible for residents. Treatment not only extinguishes maladaptive behaviors but also develops skills that will enhance a successful return to community living as productive family members. Formal schooling, speech therapy, sensory motor training, homemaking, grooming, and training in self-help skills are integral parts of daily programming. Whenever possible, residents are involved in community-learning experiences that best suit their individual needs.

One of the most important and practical learning environments for residents was a two bedroom home located on hospital grounds and used to prepare patients for community living. No other single aspect of the program had given staff the insight into the degree of institutionalization possessed by a significant number of residents. An often cited example is the resident who could operate a commercial dishwasher most efficiently on the ward but was at a complete loss when asked to wash dishes manually in the kitchen at the home.

The token economy's policy has always been to work closely with parents and potential foster parents to aid the transition to community living. "Transitional placements," or gradually lengthened visits, are recommended in some instances with consultation and follow-up available whenever needed. "Booster" sessions, or returns for short periods for evaluation have been arranged when problems arose. Treatment programs and schedules of activities for daily living have been written as guidelines to be followed by parents or foster parents.

A critical factor in a resident's successful adjustment to community living has been the involvement of those in the "placement business," the state-funded regional centers for the developmentally disabled that designate where a resident will live. There has been a direct relationship between the attention and consideration given to the selection of a "proper" placement and success in remaining in that placement.

Dissemination

While the token economy aroused much controversy during its first eighteen months of operation because of its novel approach, behavior modification and token economy programs are currently operating on a majority of wards at Pacific State Hospital. Every state hospital in California now utilizes the token economy as a customary method, especially with retardates. Personnel from other California state hospitals who have wished to begin token economy programs have been trained at the Pacific token economy, some groups staying as long as six weeks. Psychologists, students, psychiatrists, and individuals from related disciplines have visited the program from Germany, Ireland, Spain, Japan, Mexico, Canada, and many parts of the United States. Psychiatric technician trainees, employed after graduation by the state hospitals of California, spend from six weeks to two months assigned to the Pacific token economy, receiving both formal lectures and direct clinical experience.

As a result of the Pacific State Hospital self-help skill and token economy programs, and similar projects at Patton State Hospital, the California Department of Mental Hygiene's Bureau of Training obtained a federal grant to fund the training of nursing-level staff in behavior therapy on a statewide basis. The training was carried out on a demonstration ward at Pacific State Hospital with sixty profoundly retarded boys under the direction of Dr. Thomas Ball. During 1969-70, rotating groups of nurses, supervisory personnel, and psychiatric technicians lived on the grounds of Pacific State Hospital while undergoing the three-week, intensive-training practicum. Each trainee was assigned to a resident and conducted twenty-minute therapy sessions twice daily under the supervision of a teaching assistant. The trainees were taught how to use shaping (reinforcing successive approximations to the desired behavior) in helping residents acquire improved self-help skills. A key element in the training sessions was the modelling done by Larry Payne, the teaching assistant, who demonstrated a warm and genuine concern for the patients as he deftly carried out the conditioning procedures.

Daily critiques, sessions in which all trainees were present, were led by the teaching assistant. Since each trainee observed the performance of every other trainee, many viewpoints were expressed in the ensuing discussions. Frequently, during the discussion period, trainees would express their opposition to or skepticism about operant conditioning. Debate would proceed openly and freely. Most of the skepticism related to the fact that operant conditioning concerns itself primarily with behavior that can be seen, heard, or felt. Most trainees sought to explain behavior in terms of an inferred inner state rather than in terms of environmental factors. Opposition was often strongest among those employees who had been in state service the longest. Often opposition was expressed on the grounds that operant conditioning procedures seem extremely rigid. Beyond this, many trainees believed that the mentally retarded should *not* be held responsible for their actions and, therefore, teaching them through rewards is inhumane. This was countered effectively with the point that allowing these individuals to continue living on a regressed level is the more inhumane alternative and that we were merely providing them with the tools for dealing appropriately with their environment.

What really convinced the trainee of the effectiveness of operant conditioning was his ability to see for himself how he could change behavior. When the trainee discovered that through his actions he could teach the child a certain skill, he then became convinced of the effectiveness of the approach.

Facilitating the training project, from inception to completion, was a reorganization of treatment services for the retarded within state facilities. Thus, while the inpatient population comprising the mentally ill was steadily declining, demand for services for the mentally retarded remained at a high level. As a result, retardation programs were being established at facilities previously devoted entirely to the care of the mentally ill. It was clear that traditional methods for training the mentally ill were not suitable for this population, most of which is severely or profoundly retarded. Concern for the development of adequate programming was generated, not only at the headquarters level of the Department of Mental Hygiene, and the administrative level of individual facilities, but also in the California Council for Retarded Children, an organization with considerable political influence in the state of California. Because of the need to train personnel from the Department of Mental Hygiene (DMH) in the newer methods, the DMH Bureau of Training actively entered the picture. This set of circumstances provided an optimal context within which to establish programs. We found that the support was there and we did not hesitate to draw upon it.

From the outset it was evident that technical training in the application of operant conditioning methodology had to be combined with a strategy for ensuring programmatic implementation. Experience has demonstrated that without such safeguards, excellent demonstration projects may have absolutely no generalized influence on overall hospital programming.[14] To deal with this problem, the notion of the "administrative umbrella" was developed; that is, we asked each facility seeking training at Pacific State Hospital to send, in addition to psychiatric technicians (aides), administrative staff in certain key administrative roles. For example, the mental retardation (MR) program at Napa State Hospital began with a single ward that would come to function as a demonstration and training unit, the "hub" of an administrative-therapeutic "wheel" from which other programs would radiate. It was critically important that we train and obtain the commitment of all of those involved in the administrative hierarchy influencing practical policies and decisions regarding this single ward.

We sought to erect an administrative umbrella with no "holes." It was not sufficient to have the support of the ward charge and the supervisor if middle management within nursing services was not similarly committed. For example, given conditions of staff shortages, a nursing supervisor can readily "float" a PT from a demonstration ward to help cover an understaffed ward. Because the need of the second ward may well be a valid one, it is difficult to challenge the legitimacy of the request and the decision to transfer a staff member temporarily to meet the immediate need. What is required, however, is a long-term point of view. Up to a certain point sacrifices must be made to achieve long-term objectives. Middle management must, of course, sense the continued support of top management in order to carry out decisions that prove unpopular in the immediate situation. In the case of most facilities, we did succeed in obtaining key administrative personnel from every level of the decision-making hierarchy.

Training Programs of Other Hospitals

All hospitals that have sent trainees to the Pacific project have established their own training programs in operant conditioning. These programs have been conducted by graduates of the Pacific program. The programs provide training for ward personnel in both classroom and ward settings. As of 1970 approximately 15 percent of the employees assigned to the mental retardation programs at the state hospitals were receiving training at any one time. This was to continue until all were trained. In-service training in operant conditioning was provided new employees also. Over 500 employees have received training in behavior therapy. More than 2,100 patients have been affected by such efforts; that is, this is the number of patients on wards with behavior modification programs. The number of community placements made possible by these programs exceeds 100. This has been possible primarily because of the elimination of inappropriate behaviors and by the establishment of behavior necessary for patient self-care (dressing, feeding, and toileting).[15]

Bronx State Hospital
New York, New York
William J. DiScipio

Training in behavior modification at Bronx State Hospital grew from a small core group of six psychologists whose major theoretical and clinical skills were strongly based in behaviorism. Where these psychologists held administrative roles, behavioral programs were applied to the services under their auspices. Many of these psychologists were approached for informal consultation by a wide range of hospital staff interested in seeking advice and information about the efficacy of behavioral methods.

Beginning in 1969 behavioral programs flourished under the direction of these behavioral psychologists who functioned as mavericks within the hospital system. The extent and effectiveness of their programs were largely dependent upon their individual competence and the positions they held in the supervisory hierarchy of clinical services. In a hospital of 1,500 employees and 900 beds, six psychologists applied their skills to slightly more than 1,000 patients over a period of five years. Patients were treated in one of three distinct types of programs designed and run by the behavioral psychologists.[16]

1. A hospital-wide clinic was established for the purpose of providing a source of behavioral expertise for referrals from any of the hospital's units or services.
2. As new and special problems arose for the hospital staff (for example, retarded-psychotic patients and chronic patients), behavioral psychologists were called upon to develop treatment programs.
3. Several psychologists periodically designed and conducted special research projects in behavior modification on the regular, rapid-turnover wards.

In only two programs were efforts made to maintain the performance of staff in behavioral methodology over an extended period. In one case, the psychologist trained his staff in the method and theory of the "therapeutic community" in addition to behavior modification and the token economy. Decisions concerning patient treatment and ward policy were team decisions involving both staff and patient members.[17] This structure has maintained a stable and continuous token economy over the course of three years, in spite of numerous staff changes and the departure of the psychologist-administrator in 1974. The second program designed to maintain staff performance over time was part of a research project involving a token system that provided trading stamps for staff as well as patients.[18] While temporarily effective, this approach did not sustain itself beyond the conclusion of the research study.

Behavioral treatment generally had a therapeutic impact on patients only as long as the program was applied actively, systematically, and consistently. For example, short-term interventions that occurred during research projects were effective only while response contingencies were under programmed control. Severely psychotic patients responded well only when the staff was fully prepared to follow through with the contingencies, such as not permitting the patient into the dining room without a token. Less severe patients did not improve if their therapists did not themselves "buy" the behavioral model of treatment. Those nursing level staff who participated in behavioral treatment programs passively and inconsistently were ineffective in their work with patients.

Experiences at Bronx State Hospital have demonstrated that to sustain significant treatment effects a service or unit must define itself as one in which behavior modification is the predominant treatment modality. The scientific rigor upon which behavior modification is based necessitates built-in evaluation of program efficacy and a style of professional thinking that rules out the possibility of classifying behavior modification as an "adjunct therapy." This is not to suggest that behavior modification cannot be fostered by and integrated with certain treatment philosophies that involve the active process of open and meaningful communication. The "therapeutic community" and "family therapy" provide a useful sociopsychological frame of reference within which the techniques of behavior modification might be applied.

The generalization of patient improvement produced by behavioral methods depends upon the ability of the change agent to reach others in the social network surrounding the individual patient. If that network is a custodial staff in a state hospital, the entire treatment team must employ consistent contingencies or reinforcement in an enriched environment. In the case of after-care for the rehabilitated patient, community agencies and family members must be worked with conjointly in order to develop and coordinate sources of reinforcement for adaptive and functional behavior.

Dixmont State Hospital
Dixmont, Pennsylvania
Irvin P.R. Guyett

Hindsight provides a comfortable if not nostalgic position for abstracting about this particular token economy and about psychiatric institutions generally. Among these abstractions is a recognition of three major factors that operated upon the development and eventual termination of this token economy program for chronic schizophrenics at Dixmont State Hospital. First, the federal funding for the program (known as the HIP Cottage) was six months old when the author came to the unit at the institution. It was another six months before the physical facilities and staffing requirements could be completed. A decision not to continue funding the program when federal monies would end was made after the unit had been operating only eighteen months. This decision was partly a spin-off of a larger political-policy debate on institutional appropriations in the state and partly due to the low discharge rate from the unit at the end of the first year's operation—two patients. The program closed after twenty-two months of operation in April 1970. It seems reasonable to say that the unit started with a two-year time deficit.

The second factor to bear in mind in reviewing this program is that the author was concerned with going beyond a simple demonstration that reinforcement procedures have relevance for treating deviant behavior. It was recognized and repeatedly found in the HIP Cottage program that using narrowly defined, specific behaviors as the exclusive means for obtaining major primary rewards was extremely effective in "shifting" patients' performance. However, it was also recognized that most of the long-term, schizophrenic patients had multiple problems, often of a complex nature, with the controlling stimuli being extra-institutional. It was suspected that generalization effects would be modest under the narrower conceptions of simple target responses. Therefore, the HIP Cottage program was designed to develop broader behavioral "styles" or "competence strategies" by reinforcing what have been called "response sets," or behavioral strategies. This approach utilized cognitive, social learning theories in addition to the narrower Skinnerian model generally employed. Operationally, this often meant a focus on the informational and feedback value of reinforcement in addition to its more restrictive hedonic/physiological aspects. The goal of the program was the development of personal and interpersonal competence defined behaviorally along dimensions of self-care, work, socialization, and constructive spontaneity.

The third factor consistently influencing the development and operation of the HIP Cottage program was the plan to construct a system that maximized technical sophistication but minimized the necessity for decision-making expertise. It was felt that the system should be capable of handling the variety and intensity of clinical problems normally present in a state hospital setting.

Training

Training of aide and nursing staff was a continuous process carried on by the unit's very competent head nurse. Two regular weekly meetings covered basic principles and implementation of procedures. Staff performance was socially reinforced by peers and supervisors and by permitting staff to attend out-of-city training seminars and to select special duties, such as off-grounds treatment activities. A formal procedure was set up to reinforce with "time off" those staff members who came to work on time and did not take sick leave except with a written medical excuse.

During the last six months of the program, both patient and staff "specialists" were trained. Specialists among the staff were responsible for developing extra skills for certain treatment areas; for example, self-care, analysis of data (night shift), clubs, dining room, and work supervision. Staff members increasingly assumed roles as teachers. Correspondingly, patients were given roles that demanded greater autonomy and mutual support. It was intended that patients should eventually learn to operate the HIP Cottage and most of its routine treatment programs. Patients were expected to learn new roles by being placed in positions that required them to model more competent functioning for the benefit of less adequately functioning individuals. For example, a patient became a foreman to teach and supervise other patient-residents during daily two-hour assignments. Patients served as "orientors" or "counselors" to new residents, visitors, or for residents having special problems where peer-tutoring seemed more appropriate than staff directiveness. Patient and staff roles began to merge or at least overlap. To the extent that this was occurring, maintenance of "therapeutic" interventions by residents was monitored formally and reinforced extensively.

Significance of Results

Although the constantly evolving nature of the program made most prepost measures ambiguous, several ways of demonstrating change were developed.

Every resident showed substantial gain in at least one specific behavioral area, for example, anorexia with weight loss, wearing strange clothes, verbal abuse, fighting, odd mannerisms, sloppy eating, not bathing, and mutism. Yet, some behavior problems remained extremely resistive to change and seemed to require more intensive, one-to-one training than either personnel time or skill permitted. The specialty programs and having patients assume a greater share of the responsibility for running the unit were strategies to deal with these problems that were not sufficiently tested before the program folded. Using broader categories of behavior, results indicated that the token economy led to large scale improvements in socialization, self-care, and constructive spontaneity.

At the end of the first fourteen months of operation, the program director reviewed his notes, data, and impressions, and made subjective, "clinical" judgments on changes in residents during this period. Self-care and work were the major areas where change occurred. While substantial gains were seen, there was a sufficient amount of improvement to warrant discharge for only two patients. An elaborate but reliable system was developed for rating nursing note entries of specific behavior. A person who was totally unfamiliar with the residents rated all the nursing note entries for residents. The ratings reflected small but reliable shifts in positive directions. Low-functioning residents progressed more slowly and did not attain the same final level of performance as did higher functioning residents. The Psychotic Reaction Profile, a ward rating procedure based on general observations, was completed quarterly by staff members for each resident. Small reductions were noted in "agitated depression" and "withdrawal" but "thinking disorganization" and "paranoid belligerence" were slightly increased. These changes were not statistically significant.

Dissemination

Few of the methods used on the HIP Cottage were incorporated into the rest of the institution. Only one psychiatrist ever spent any time on the unit solely to provide medication. Several "token" programs were eventually initiated by isolated personnel on a very modest one to two hours per week basis. How much penetration the HIP Cottage has had into the state system is a difficult question, but it would not be easy to find any direct influence. Thus, the impact of the Dixmont token economy on other colleagues and hospitals has been marginal, except in adding another "voice" to the growing swell of interest in behavior therapy.

Dissemination of behavioral procedures within the institution was impaired by the administrative isolation of the token economy. As a traditionally custodial institution, the staff at Dixmont State Hospital viewed the token economy as a threat to the status quo. The HIP Cottage was barely tolerated as an innovative "thorn" in the side of the hospital. Receptivity to the token economy improved during the last four months of the program when the rest of the institution's staff had begun to believe that the program was there to stay. In addition, the HIP Cottage staff had begun to generate and reinforce systematically collaborative, amicable relationships with other administrative and clinical personnel.

One of the most positive attributes of the program was the degree of autonomy allowed the program director. In comparison with many other token economy programs around the country, it appeared that this autonomy was substantial. All treatment decisions, except medication and discharge orders, were made by the program director. Also of considerable value was the fact that the program director had sole responsibility for hiring and firing all staff members.

There are probably only two conditions under which the former program director would attempt to lead such a program again, as superintendent or as an independent contractor. Either option provides the most necessary ingredient for success and impact—ability to cope with an entrenched system. Procedurally, the other desirable change to make is to emphasize training for self-responsibility of patient from the beginning. This could be done by greater staff development, better use of automated equipment, and more active involvement with the community.

**Bangor State Hospital and Mental
Health Institute
Bangor, Maine**

Peter A. Magaro

In the process of designing research and treatment procedures, deriving grant support, gaining hospital support for program initiation, and finally directing token economy programs at two state hospitals, it has seemed that possibly the most important consideration in determining program outcome is the social-political milieu of the institution. Reports of procedure and specific results of the token economies themselves have been covered elsewhere.[19] The present discussion, therefore, will be an attempt to consider the seldom measured facilitative and inhibitive effects of the institutional mentality upon a token economy. Hopefully, such a discussion will be instructive concerning the limitation upon the results that could be obtained from a token economy when it is embedded within a total institution maintaining the status quo.

It seems that a large number of token economy programs of the 1960s were undertaken within the context of a custodial institution. Our token economy program was initiated in a relatively humane, custodial institution that had all the traditional indicators of maximum patient-management and little active treatment of patients. For example, prior to the program, there was only one psychiatrist, and no Ph.D.-level psychologists for some 1,400 patients. The superintendent was a physician with a background in tuberculosis and most staff maintained a pride in the custodial procedures, especially the tender-loving and total care of the patient.

The introduction of a token economy into a state hospital is an action of institutional change. Possibly one of the greatest benefits of the token program is that it forced many institutions to offer alternatives to custodial care. Although token economies usually required the additional payment of a relatively inexpensive consulting psychologist, additional aide staff, and some funds for reinforcers, this was relatively cheap and usually could be handled within existing resources. The principles of behavior modification are also relatively understandable to traditional hospital staff. You rewarded appropriate behavior and punished inappropriate behavior. That sounded familiar and the fine points of procedure could be seen as questions of technology that would be left to the behavioral engineer. Also, by the late 1960s, the token economy as a hospital treatment modality was becoming respectable and even a bit avant-garde. If one wanted to initiate institutional change in moving from a custodial to a treatment model, the token economy was the method of choice.

With institutional change as a goal involving the demonstration that patients

176

can be considered individuals capable of being responsible for themselves, staff and patient selection for the token economy followed specific patterns. The patients selected were mainly long-term residents, in some cases having a reputation for being unmanageable. Difficult patients were accepted to allay fears of the hospital staff. Even though behavior modification techniques were understandable, they were still relatively novel and in some ways a radical form of treatment. The possibility of harmful consequences to the patient would not be as great a matter of concern when applied to accepted treatment "failures." If acute patients were to be used, there would be too great a concern that the treatment would prove harmful to the individual. Using treatment failures minimized this fear and facilitated the acceptance of the program. Another more political reason for choosing such patients was that the probability of the "Pinel Principle" working on at least a few was relatively high. That is, simply removing the patients from isolation or from an attitude of being chronic should result in some improvements, and discharges would be considered as dramatic successes. Treatment successes would increase the acceptance of the token economy and the validity of the custodial approach could be questioned.

Staff Training

Staff were selected mainly in terms of youth and their lack of institutionalization. Since an active interpersonal interaction between patient and staff was desired, staff were selected to be outgoing and not needing roles as nurses or aides to shield them from personal interactions. The staff, therefore, was enthusiastic, and a real pleasure to socialize and work with. There was the usual training involving the showing of films on behavior modification plus a course of instruction on elementary learning principles. The most meaningful instruction, however, was the daily staff meetings that devised individual behavioral programs and reviewed individual patient progress on specific behavioral programs. These meetings increased staff morale and taught behavior modification procedures as tailored and applicable to individual patients. Possibly the most efficient method in teaching a behavior modification approach was supplementing the regular staff at the beginning of the program during the summer with psychology graduate students. The students were familiar with behavioral techniques, at least academically, and taught the rest of the staff by demonstrating the procedures. It was found that by the end of the first six months, the program was fully entrenched to the point where the patients could be rewarded for assuming the major program duties. For instance, maintaining the "store" where goods can be exchanged for tokens takes a great deal of staff time, therefore decreasing the time working with patients. This task was quickly assigned to a patient at a respectable token income and was handled efficiently. In terms of staff training, therefore, my experience has been that the best preparation for the permanent aides is an initial infusion of students who can demonstrate behavioral modification techniques. The work situation becomes immersed in behavioral language so that the token economy becomes a living, personal system involving the application of procedures with patients seen as individuals.

The results were somewhat predictable. Besides the measurable patient change,[20] the immeasurable results were probably more striking. Staff enthusiasm led them to devote more than the required forty hours of work per week. Patients were taken throughout the hospital and the community as part of their involvement in the staff's normal activities. The expected "Pinel effects" did occur. A woman hospitalized for thirteen years, who believed that she was a queen and wore her crown as ultimate proof, decided that even though she was a queen she did not need to tell anyone and removed the crown when entering the community. She was discharged within three months of the start of the program. The disappointments were those patients who were capable of functioning within the community but who refused to leave no matter what we did, including packing their bag and ushering them to the door. Empirical support[21] was found for the observations that some patients were capable of learning the tasks required in the token economy easily while others had difficulty learning even the most simple tasks. Those who performed well, were discharged into the community, and then returned, did so not from a lack of generalization of appropriate responses, but from a lack of supportive opportunities and reinforcers for functional behaviors. For example, discharged ex-patients would have been able to work or interact socially, but there was no job available or not one with whom to interact. The lack of financial possibilities and appropriate social living facilities made the hospital appear as an attractive domicile that had more benefits than the community.[22]

Dissemination

The program ran approximately a year at which time it was terminated. Remembering our goal of modifying the structure of the institution, we attempted to modify the authoritarian pattern of control over patients. Helping patients learn autonomy and self-control required increased ward staff responsibility and freedom. This led to the program being terminated. The director of nursing was threatened by our desire to remove our nursing staff from the control of ward supervisors. The "Big Nurse" stereotype did exist and required the nursing supervisor to evaluate nursing personnel. Our program, which evaluated the aide staff on program proficiency, used different criteria for staff evaluation. We attempted to remove the aide from a double standard imposed by the new program requirements and older nursing staff requirements. Aide standards in the custodial model specified medical duties v. interpersonal contact, nursing charts v. behavioral charts, uniforms v. street clothes, and starting a shift at eight rather than seven A.M.

The second set of administrative procedures that created conflict was the degree of freedom permitted patients. Regulations separated male from female patients on the grounds. We attempted to increase patient responsibility and learning of interpersonal relations with males and this directly conflicted with various regulations sequestering females from the "dirty old male" schizophrenic. The token economy contradicted another unwritten regulation by permitting a patient to create a "scene" in the community that could be defined as being noticed. The community traditionally was protected from patients by the hospital while the token economy encouraged patients to interact within the town as part of the reward system.

The program itself was terminated but the token economy procedure lives on in full force. The hospital has now adopted behavioral procedures but in name only. Four Ph.D. psychologists with some background in behavior modification have been given program leadership, including a new superintendent who is a psychologist. The name of the state hospital has been changed to "Mental Health Institute." However, changes in staff and printed philosophy have not produced institutional change. In fact, the switch from a custodial to a behavior modification institution has been minimal in its impact on patients. Patients are now subject to a new order that is as rigid as the old. The population has decreased dramatically, mainly by transferring patients to nursing homes where the older custodial systems are still in effect but on a smaller scale.

Behavior modification can be a warm interpersonal relationship between two people engaged in learning through helpful techniques or it can mean that one person controls another in order to provide a position of power and financial benefits to those managing the institution. The state hospital as the residence through time of the underprivileged in the society should not be concerned with which procedure is used as much as how it is applied. Without a prescriptive approach to treatment[23] that applies specific treatments to definable groups, all patients are going to be forced into a system in which much of the energy is devoted to keeping the system running smoothly rather than directing efforts to the specific behavioral problems of individuals.

Camarillo State Hospital
Camarillo, California
Charles Wallace

The Clinical Research Unit (CRU), located at Camarillo State Hospital and part of the Camarillo-Neuropsychiatric Institute Research Program, has provided intensive behavior modification to a variety of clinical disorders since November 1970. The CRU is relatively small, with a patient census of twelve and a staff complement of fourteen nurses and psychiatric technicians, a research psychiatrist, a clinical psychologist, a social worker, and a research assistant.

The flow chart in Figure 10-3 describes the administrative operations of the CRU. Patients are referred to the CRU both from other units within the hospital and directly from agencies in the community. Each referral is screened by a nursing staff member who interviews the patient and discusses with the referring personnel such topics as the patient's behavioral excesses and deficits and their frequency, possible reinforcers, and the ineffectiveness of past treatment modalities. The referral is discussed at a twice-weekly staff meeting, and the decision to accept or reject a referral is a cooperative decision made by all members of the treatment team.

A basic element in the CRU's treatment milieu is an individualized token economy that is used both for the completion of essential unit tasks and for the attainment of specific, therapeutic goals for each patient. In addition to receiving tokens for getting up in the morning at the appropriate time, for grooming, and for room cleaning, patients are assigned various tasks according to their current level of functioning. These tasks are written on a standard data sheet that provides spaces for the indication of completion or noncompletion of tasks. All token economy programs are changed every two weeks in conjunction with the patient who is given a copy of his or her program.

Apart from the token economy, individualized programs are developed that specify interventions for from one to three target behaviors for which the patient was referred to the CRU. To evaluate the effectiveness of these programs, a data collector and collation system has been developed, which includes several steps:

1. The frequency of the target behavior is determined by a variety of recording techniques ranging from continuous recordings, event recording during sessions, interval recording, and time sampling.
2. Data collection sheets are devised for each specific program.
3. Memos detailing each program are dittoed and distributed to all staff members' mailboxes, which are located in the nursing office.

Clinical Research Unit
Camarillo-Neuropsychiatric Instit. Research Program
ADMINISTRATIVE PROCEDURES

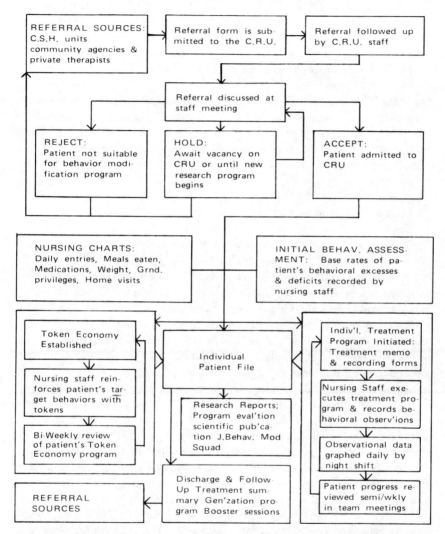

Figure 10-3. Flow chart of administrative and clinical operations on the Clinical Research Unit at Camarillo State Hospital, Camarillo, CA. (Reprinted from Liberman, R.P., Wallace, C., Teigen, J., and Davis, J. Interventions with psychotic behaviors, Chapter 9 in *Innovative Treatment Methods in Psychopathology,* K. Calhoun, H. Adams, and M. Mitchell, (eds.). New York: John Wiley & Sons, 1974, pp 323-412).

4. A clipboard is kept in the nurses office for each patient, which contains
    that day's data collection sheet and all program memos that pertain to
    that particular patient.
5. Each day's data sheets are removed from their clipboards by the night
    shift (12 midnight to 8 A.M. shift) and results graphed separately for each
    patient. New data sheets are then placed on the clipboards.
6. The data thus graphed provide day-by-day information to revise the
    individualized programs when necessary.

In the three and one-half years of it's operation, the CRU has developed
methods to (1) maintain appropriate staff behavior, (2) generalize appropriate
patient behaviors to the eventual facility to which the patient is transferred,
and (3) interface with the other sections of the hospital in as harmonious and
helpful a manner as possible.

Staff Behavior and Recording Systems

The shaping and maintenance of appropriate staff behavior is the key to the
CRU's research and clinical productivity. Basically, staff behavior is controlled
by five systems that specify the behaviors staff are to emit in order to modify
certain patient behaviors. The five systems deal with patients' appropriate completion of unit chores, (token economy) appropriate mealtime behaviors, appropriate showering and grooming, reduction of assaultive or destructive behavior,
and improvement in individually targeted behavioral excesses or deficits. Each
of these five systems has a similar means of data collection, and these data collection devices specifically cue appropriate staff behavior.

The system that deals with individually targeted behaviors of patients is
the unit's most important and complex system. Placed in the nursing station are
clipboards for each patient. Each clipboard contains: (a) a data sheet, individualized for recording of that patient's targeted behaviors; and (b) a dittoed memo
detailing the interventions and observations that constitute that patient's program. Each patient's data sheets are formulated so that they cue staff to perform
correctly the programmed observations and/or interventions. At any time, the
nursing staff may be called upon to use a wide array of procedures to observe
and/or consequate from twenty to forty individually targeted behaviors. These
daily procedures may include thirty-six randomly spaced, one-minute observations; six fifteen-minute conversations; four sessions of twenty-five questions
per session; thirty minutes of assertion training followed by on-the-spot training
as necessary; event recording of defined behaviors; and nine randomly spaced,
one-minute observations. Given such variety in procedures, the clipboard-memo-
data sheet system becomes critical in maintaining appropriate staff behavior and,
in particular, staff-patient interaction.

To maintain the cueing function of the data sheets, several steps are taken by the professional staff. All programs are previewed at biweekly team meetings, the appropriate observation and consequation procedures are modelled by the program writer, and continuing feedback is given about staff performance.

In contrast, the token economy is a system in which there has been a deliberate attempt to program a high degree of standardization. The goal of the economy is to use unit maintenance "jobs" to teach those behaviors that the staff of after-care facilities indicate are quite desirable. These include making beds, sweeping floors, and cleaning tables. The number and sequence of unit jobs depend only upon the scheduling of the units' major daily events such as mealtimes and bedtime. Since these events are the same from day to day, a consistent daily schedule has been established which encompasses 102 jobs grouped according to twenty-three major "routines" such as cleaning the dining room after lunch, cleaning the T.V. room in the evening. The jobs vary considerably in complexity so that patients of differing levels of functioning can participate in the economy. Jobs are assigned for two-week periods, and staff are informed of the assignments by means of a "job board" that is placed in the nursing station and that displays the name of each job, the criteria for appropriate completion, the sequence of all 102 jobs, and the names of the patients to whom the jobs have been assigned. A data sheet is used for the two-week period that essentially duplicates the job board and that asks staff to rate patient performance based on the number of prompts necessary for correct completion.

Since the appropriate supervision of a job requires several behaviors on the part of the supervising staff member, the token economy data sheet tends to be less efficient in controlling staff behavior than the data sheets of the individual treatment system. These latter data sheets prescribe only one or two behaviors necessary for observing and consequating targeted patient behaviors. For the token economy, appropriate supervision behaviors are maintained by a combination of modelling by the professional staff and continuing feedback.

An experiment performed on the CRU indicates that the unit is productive principally because the nursing staff authority figure models the appropriate staff behavior.[24] In that experiment, staff attendance at a scheduled recreational activity for patients increased only when attendance was modelled by either the professional staff or by the nursing authority figure, with greater attendance associated with the latter. Neither instructions to interact nor the removal of competing activities had any effect. This was in spite of the fact that instructions were given in the dittoed memo format with which all staff members were quite familiar.

Staff training consists primarily of familiarizing the nurses and technicians with the required behavioral observations and interventions using on-the-job instructions and modelling. Since consistency in the application of contingencies is a sine qua non of behavior modification approaches, communication among all members of the treatment team is vital. Twice weekly meetings are held in which patients' progress, program changes, referrals, and unit problems are discussed. These meetings are scheduled so that all three shifts attend at least one meeting per week. The program memos discussed above serve a vital communication function as does a written link between shifts, the Communication Book. Training sessions in the techniques necessary to conduct the individualized programs are scheduled whenever a new program is to be implemented. Although scheduled training meetings are held, the emphasis is placed on the day-to-day maintenance of treatment procedures by the staff through modelling and reinforcement by the professional supervisors. Thus, the use of the record systems makes the CRU flexible enough for modifying a wide variety of behavioral disorders and yet allows for the precise specification of staff behavior necessary to conduct well-controlled, clinically oriented research projects.

Generalization of Patient Behavior

The generalization of changes in patients' behavior has not been systematized to the same extent as the control of staff behavior. It is often difficult to predict the exact facility to which a patient will be transferred, and contingent control over that facility's staff cannot be exerted. Nevertheless, several variables anecdotally seem to be important in generalizing patient behavior successfully.

If the patient is to be transferred to a facility that is in close proximity to the CRU, contact between the CRU and the facility takes place from several weeks to several months prior to the projected transfer date. Generalization procedures are the responsibility of the CRU's social worker, and he uses this initial contact to establish a positive relationship with the staff of the aftercare facility and to determine what type of program is feasible for the facility. It seems important during this and subsequent contacts to avoid any appearance that an outside agency (the CRU) is telling the staff of the new facility how to treat a patient, particularly since that staff oftentimes did not request that they receive the patient. It seems important to also reassure the staff that the CRU will be available at any time and at their request to further assist them in working with the patient.

Once a feasible treatment program has been developed, the patient's CRU treatment program is then gradually changed so that it is soon the same as the one to be implemented in the aftercare setting. If the patient's behavior remains appropriate, an effort is then made to establish stimulus control of the behavior by the new facility through a series of visits that increase in duration and decrease in the supervision provided by the CRU nursing staff. If the behavior remains appropriate, the patient is transferred. The CRU continues to follow up the generalization program with a decreasing frequency of visits, giving social reinforcement to the aftercare staff for continuing with the program.

Furthermore, the CRU makes a deliberate attempt to develop behaviors in patients that will have a high probability of being rewarded in the "natural" environment and in a manner that will make them more resistant to extinction. Thus, a great deal of effort is spent in assertion training sessions to shape appropriate interpersonal behaviors, particularly for patients who may eventually be able to live on their own. Programs are systematically changed to variable schedules of reinforcement, and social reinforcement is systematically introduced while more tangible reinforcers and specific prompts are faded.

In spite of these planned activities, certain programs are implemented successfully while others are not even attempted by the after-care facility. Anecdotally, it would seem that an extremely important variable in the process, much as on the CRU, is the modelling of the program by the facility's authority figure. If sanction is not given and modelling not performed, the probability of successful generalization seems significantly reduced.

If a patient is transferred to a facility that is distant from the CRU, then the primary means of attempting to shape the facility's program is through telephone contact and a written treatment summary that details the CRU's programs and that suggests a program suitable for potential implementation.

Dissemination

Although the traditional means of disseminating information from research projects is used (e.g., journals), such information rarely, if ever, has an impact on the hospital staff. Hence, the CRU uses several other techniques for being active in the hospital. Training programs are conducted for interested professional and nursing staff as requested by the hospital administrators. Consultations are performed with other hospital units so that a patient's behavior can be modified without the necessity of admission to the CRU. Tours are conducted, and treatment summaries of all CRU patients are routinely distributed to the hospital administrators and all interested parties.

In spite of this, the CRU often hears the contention that it is an elitist organization that exists solely as a reinforcer for the researchers. This suggests that the publication of the CRU's involvement with the rest of the hospital has to become more systematic. Publicity and professional information methods are currently being formulated.

Conclusion

The narrative description of behavior therapy programs in five state hospitals underscores the importance of the administrative skills of the program directors in maintaining and sustaining an innovative form of treatment. The longevity of each token economy appears to be related directly to the positive relationships established between the program director and other elements in the hospital's power hierarchy. While behavior analysis and therapy are being applied with increasing clinical effectiveness to psychotic patients, the limiting factors in the enduring success of a treatment program lie in the resistance of institutions to change, both at administrative and service levels.

The sine qua non of any behavior modification program is an alliance between the research or professional staff and the clinical or paraprofessional personnel. Since the actual work with patients—the reinforcement of target behaviors—is done primarily by the nursing staff, the staff's training, consistency, and cooperation are of first-order importance. A challenge to behavior modifiers concerned with innovation and diffusion of new methods is the training of administrative and staff personnel at all levels in the rationale, utility, and methods of the social learning approach to mental patients. It is fallacious to assume that mental health workers will change their habitual ways of managing patients quickly or easily. Just as the "social breakdown syndrome" is resistant to change in patients, the methods used by staff members to induce this syndrome are also resistant to change.

The innovator must bring to bear principles of reinforcement for modifying staff behavior as well as patients' behavior. The staff must receive careful training and incentives or reinforcers in using new methods. Time off for attending training sessions, bonuses and certificates for fulfilling training courses, and, most importantly, the constant attention and encouragement by a dedicated project director are all examples of needed incentives. Thus, the principles of behavior that are applied to patients must also be taken into consideration when retraining of staff is undertaken. Similar attention must be given to the administrative hierarchies in the hospital. Vertical staffing patterns and authoritarian superintendents who receive status for managing large hospitals are inimical to a behavior modification approach. Administrators must be persuaded that the behavioral change of patients is more important to them than a high patient census or neat rows of beds that are well made. Vested interests, institutionalized staff members, and the persistence of past behavior (traditions) must all be contended with if basic behavioral principles are to have a chance to succeed.

186

Critical areas for improving the durability of treatment effects are after-care environments that prompt and reinforce maladaptive behavior, and insufficient and poorly planned efforts by clinicians to anticipate and program for generalization. Thus, a challenge to behavior modifers will be to harness the variety of contingencies from different directions that concurrently have an impact on the patient's behaviors. Of necessity, this systems approach requires more skills than straightforward application of behavior therapy. Sophistication in community organization and mechanisms for interagency communication and planning must be developed. It should also be clear to behavior modifiers, whether they be psychologists, psychiatrists, social workers, or paraprofessionals, that the learning model is not the only relevant theory in understanding and treating behavioral disorders. As long as there are individuals with major behavioral deficits and excesses, whether in large state mental hospitals or in small community boarding homes, we must devote our energies and creativity to developing therapeutic interventions that will assist these individuals to learn functional and happier roles in society.

Notes

1. Liberman, Robert P. (1972), *A Guide to Behavioral Analysis and Therapy*, New York: Pergamon Press; Bandura, Albert (1969), *Principles of Behavior Modification*, New York: Holt, Rinehart & Winston; Yates, Aubrey (1970), *Behavior Therapy*, New York, Wiley & Sons; Rimm, David C. and Masters, John C. (1974), *Behavior Therapy: Techniques and Empirical Findings*, New York: Academic Press.
2. Ullmann, Leonard and Krasner, Leonard (1965), *Case Studies in Behavior Modification*, New York: Holt, Rinehart and Winston.
3. Ayllon, Teodoro and Azrin, Nathan (1968), *The Token Economy,* New York: Appleton-Century-Crofts.
4. Wexler, David B. (1973), "Token and Taboo: Behavior Modification, Token Economies, and the Law," *California Law Review* 61: 81-109; Davison, Gerald and Stuart, Richard B. (1974), Behavior Modification and Civil Liberties. Paper presented to The Annual Meeting of the American Civil Liberties Union, Madison, Wisc., June 16, 1974.
5. Ayllon, Teodoro and Azrin, Nathan H. (1965), "The Measurement and Reinforcement of Behavior of Psychotics," *Journal of Experimental Analysis of Behavior* 8: 357-83.
6. Liberman, Robert P. (1972), "Behavioral Modification for Schizophrenia: A Review," *Schizophrenia Bulletin (NIMH)* 6: 37-48; Kazdin, Alan E. and Bootzin, R.R. (1972), "The Token Economy: An Evaluative Review," *Journal of Applied Behavior Analysis* 5: 343-72.
7. ibid; Richardson, Roger A., Karkalas, Yani, and Lal, Harbanas (1972),

"Application of Operant Procedures in Treatment of Hallucinations in Chronic Psychotics," pp. 147-50 in *Advances in Behavior Therapy*, vol. 3., R.D. Rubin, H. Fensterheim, J.D. Henderson, and L.P. Ullmann (eds.), New York: Academic Press; Liberman, R.P., Patterson, R., Teigen, J., and Baker, V. (1973), "Reducing Delusional Speech in Chronic, Paranoid Schizophrenics," *Journal of Applied Behavior Analysis* 6: 57-64; Wincze, J.P., Leitenberg, H., and Agras, H.S. (1972), "The Effects of Token Reinforcement and Feedback on the Delusional Verbal Behavior of Chronic Paranoid Schizophrenics," *Journal of Applied Behavior Analysis* 5: 247-62; Patterson, Roger and Teigen, James (1973), "Conditioning and Posthospital Generalization of Nondelusional Responses in a Chronic Psychotic Patient," *Journal of Applied Behavior Analysis* 6: 65-70; Liberman, R.P., Wallace, C.J., Teigen, J., and Davis, J. (1974), "Interventions with Psychotic Behaviors," Chapter 9 in *Innovative Treatment Methods in Psychopathology*, K.S. Calhoun, H.E. Adams, and K.M. Mitchell (eds.), New York: Academic Press, in press.

8. DiScipio, W.J., and Trudeau, P.F. (1972), "Symptom Changes and Self-esteem as Correlates of Possitive Conditioning of Grooming in Hospitalized Psychotics," *Journal of Abnormal Psychology* 80: 244-48.

9. O'Brien, F. and Azrin, H.H. (1972), "Symptom Reduction by Functional Displacement in a Token Economy: A Case Study," *Journal of Behavior Therapy and Experimental Psychiatry* 3: 205-207.

10. Liberman, Robert P. (1972), "Reinforcing Social Interaction in a Group of Chronic Schizophrenics," Chapter in *Advances in Behavior Therapy*, vol. 3, R. Rubin, C. Franks, H. Fensterheim, and L. Ullmann (eds.), New York: Academic Press, pp. 151-60.

11. O'Brien, F., Azrin, N.H., and Henson, K. (1969), "Increased Communications of Chronic Mental Patients by Reinforcement and by Response Priming," *Journal of Applied Behavior Analysis* 2: 23-30; Bennett, P.S., and Maley, R.F. (1973), "Modification of Interactive Behaviors in Chronic Mental Patients," *Journal of Applied Behavior Analysis* 6: 126-35; Horn, J. and Black, W.A.M. (1974), "The Effect of Token Reinforcement on Verbal Participation in a Social Activity with Long Stay Psychiatric Patients," *Australian and New Zealand Journal of Psychiatry*, in press; Fichter, Manfred M., Wallace, Charles J., Liberman, Robert P., and Davis, John (1974), "Increasing Social Behaviors in a Chronic Psychotic Using the Premack Principle: Experimental Analysis and Generalization," *Journal of Applied Behavior Analysis*, in press; Liberman, Robert P., King, Larry W., and DeRisi, William (1972), "Building a Behavioral Bridge to Span Continuity of Care," *Exchange* 1: 22-27; King, Larry W., Liberman, Robert P., and Roberts, Johnie (1974), "Evaluation of Personal Effectiveness (Assertion) Training in Group Therapy," *International Journal of Group Psychotherapy*, in press.

12. Liberman, "Behavioral Modification for Schizophrenia"; Liberman, Robert

P. (1974), "Behavior Therapy for Schizophrenia," Chapter in *Treatment of Schizophrenia*, L.J. West and D. Flinn (eds.), New York: Grune and Stratton; Kazdin, "The Token Economy"; Kazdin, Alan, E. (1974), "New Developments in Token Economy Research," in *Progress in Behavior Modification*, vol. 1, M. Hersen, R. Eisler, and P. Miller (eds.), New York: Academic Press.

13. Schaefer, H.H. and Martin, P. (1969), *Behavioral Therapy*, New York: McGraw-Hill.

14. Ball, T.S. (1969), "Introduction and Overview," in T.S. Ball (ed.), "The Establishment and Administration of Operant Conditioning Programs in a State Hospital for the Retarded," *California Mental Health Research Symposium*, no. 4., pp. 1-12.

15. Ball, T.S. (1971), "A Statewide Operant Conditioning Training Program for MR Hospital Employees: The Practical Results," *California Mental Health Research Digest* 9: 10-20.

16. DiScipio, W.J. (ed), (1974), *The Behavioral Treatment of Psychotic Illness*, New York: Behavioral Publications.

17. Glickman, H. (1974), "Can a Token Economy Find Happiness in a Therapeutic Community?" in DiScipio, W.J. (Ed.), *The Behavioral Treatment of Psychotic Illness*, New York: Behavioral Publications, 1974.

18. Hollander, M.A. and Plutchik, R. (1972), "A Reinforcement Program for Psychiatric Attendants," *Journal of Behavior Therapy and Experimental Psychiatry* 3: 297-300.

19. Gripp, R.F. and Magaro, P.A. (1971), "A Token Economy Program Evaluation with Untreated Control Work Comparisons," *Behavior Research and Therapy* 9: 137-49; Allen, D.J. and Magaro, P.A. (1971), "Measures of Change in Token-economy Programs," *Behavior Research and Therapy* 9: 311-18.

20. Gripp and Magaro, "A Token Economy Program Evaluation."

21. Allen and Magaro, "Measures of Change in Token-economy Programs."

22. Braginsky, B.M., Grosse, M., and Ring, K. (1966), "Controlling Outcomes Through Impression-Management: An Experimental Study of the Manipulative Tactics of Mental Patients," *Journal of Consulting Psychology* 30: 295-300.

23. Magaro, P.A. (1969), "A Prescriptive Treatment Model Based upon Social Class and Premorbid Adjustment," *Psychotherapy: Theory, Research and Practice* 6: 57-70; Magaro, P.A. and Staples, S.B. (1972), "Schizophrenic Patients as Therapists: An Expansion of the Prescriptive Treatment System Based Upon Premorbid Adjustment Social Class, and A-B Status," *Psychotherapy: Theory, Research and Practice* 9: 352-58.

24. Wallace, C., Davis, J., Liberman, R.P., and Baker, B. (1973), "Modeling and Staff Behavior," *Journal of Consulting and Clinical Psychology* 41: 422-25.

11

The Mental Hospital's Role in Developing Programs for Geriatric Residents

Leonard E. Gottesman

As the care of the geriatric patient moves more and more into the community there are three roles for the mental hospital. First, employees can teach nursing homes what has been learned in mental hospitals about good geriatric inpatient care; second, the twenty-four hour mental hospital can be modified to offer partial hospitalization; and third, the resources of the mental hospital can be used to offer services to elderly persons in their own homes.

Trends in Use of Services

In the last two decades, mental hospital census for patients of all ages has been reduced nationally by 40 percent from a resident population of 512,501 in 1950 to 275,995 in 1972. The trend has been even more marked among the aged. For example, in 1950 the *resident* patient rate in state and county mental hospitals for women aged sixty-five years and over was more than one per 100 elderly women in the population; by 1971 it was less than half as high. Admission rates have dropped even more sharply. In 1962, 163.7 out of every 100,000 people aged sixty-five and over were admitted to a mental hospital; by 1972 the rate had declined more than half to 69.2 per 100,000. As projected by Earl S. Pollack and Carl A. Taube in Chapter 2 of this volume, resident rates for the aged in mental hospitals are likely to go down another 56 percent by 1975.

For most other ages, decreasing use of mental hospitals has meant increased use of community facilities like the general hospital psychiatric service, outpatient clinics, and community health centers. For all ages, mental hospitals decreased in a decade from 28.9 percent of all patient care episodes to 18.5 percent. Among the aged, in spite of a marked decrease in numbers in residence or admitted, state mental hospitals still account for 51 percent of all patient-care episodes. In essence, this means that alternative mental health resources have not been used for the aged. Instead, the elderly have gone to nursing homes. From 1964 to 1969 (as Pollack and Taube point out) elderly residents of nursing homes increased by 153 percent from 214,000 to 542,000 persons, or possibly even higher.[1] This use of nursing homes as an alternative to the mental hospital is still a growing trend.

In spite of the development in the last twenty years of several promising psychosocial treatment programs for mental hospital residents,[2] the decreased use of mental hospitals did not result from the success of these programs. In fact, just as these programs were beginning to influence mental hospital treatment, three other developments occurred. First, psychotropic drugs were introduced to control extreme behavior. Second, the federal government decided to reimburse the care of the mentally ill in nursing homes; and third, state legislatures began to use federal rather than state resources for care of the elderly mentally ill by insisting that elderly patients be moved out of state mental hospitals.

There is evidence that elderly persons in these new settings are no better off than when mental hospitals were the main resource for their treatment. Time-sampled observations of elderly mental hospital patients in 1966 found that most of them received little except drug treatment and that they spent almost all of their time sitting idly in their wards.[3] In 1972 a study of a representative group of nursing homes in a large metropolitan area revealed a similar picture. Contracts between residents and staff for nursing, personal, or psychosocial care occurred during 9.6 percent of more than 27,000 observations of 1,144 residents.[4] Among the residents, 27 percent were almost never observed receiving personal care; 53 percent received little or no psychosocial care; and 77 percent were never observed receiving nursing care from a staff member. Finally, most resident/staff contacts observed were with nurses aides.

The vivid implication of these results is not only that resident care has not improved as a result of its shift from mental hospitals to nursing homes, but also that we may have lost the ground gained by successful mental hospital treatments. Rather than being closer to treatment, elderly nursing home residents are farther away from planned psychosocial treatment, from medical directors, psychologists, social workers, and all other professionals. In nursing homes, unlike mental hospitals, nurses and nurses aides seldom have other professionals to back them up.

Nursing homes do have some advantages, however. Most are smaller than 100 beds and therefore could institute planned programs with considerably less effort than is needed in the 1,000-bed or larger state hospitals. Most nursing homes are urban and close to families, churches, stores, and other noninstitutional resources. Finally, family members view nursing homes with less fear than they do mental hospitals.

As the resource of the mental hospital becomes less available, the group of disturbed older people living in the community becomes larger. Signs of the need for services in this group have only now begun to be seen in the concern for a growing group of elderly Skid-Row residents, for elderly boarding home residents, and for the needful elderly person who lives alone. Some estimates put this group of needful persons between 5 percent and 10 percent of the total elderly population. There are now few services available for this high-risk population in spite of the fact that they account for nearly one quarter of all mental hospital admissions. They constitute fewer than 10 percent of mental health center episodes, and are often excluded completely.[5]

In-Service Mental Hospital Programs

Mental hospitals may be in an ideal position to meet some needs of many inpatient and community-living elderly persons. Using mental hospitals as their laboratory, Bruno Bettelheim, Maxwell Jones, G.W. Fairweather, and many who followed them documented that it is possible to overcome the problems caused in an institution by the caste-like relationship among staff members and residents. They have shown that when these relationships are reorganized to become more equalitarian and goal-oriented, marked improvement in morale and diminution of symptoms occur.[6] This insight should be reflected in all continuing mental hospital programs and should be immediately transferred to all nursing homes.

In spite of the shifting of emphasis from mental hospitals to nursing homes, the isolated disabled elderly person continues to be a likely candidate for institutional care. Lacking family resources to provide the services, relationships, and protection he needs, a congregate communal life may often be the most sensible substitute for family. Although nursing home admission comes as a result of need for care, it is seldom, in fact, a transient service. Instead, the average nursing home stay is two years and is usually terminated by the death of the resident. If we acknowledge that both the staff and the residents of nursing homes and mental hospitals are members of a community it becomes very important to apply the insights that help make the community more satisfying.

A more satisfying community may also be a therapeutic community. Since between 50 percent and 80 percent of nursing home residents and all mental hospital residents have a mental disorder that disturbs their interpersonal relationships, the work of establishing a community in the institution is a direct therapy for this disability. There is now evidence that, when the techniques of therapeutic communities are applied, measurable improvements in residents' ability to relate normally to others are predictable.[7]

Gottesman, Coons and Donahue[8] have reported increased normal behavior among geriatric mental patients when they were provided opportunities and faced with expectations for normal behavior. The research showed that the patients' many hours of staring into space were not necessarily a manifestation of mental disturbance or of medication overdosage. For example, when they began working in a state mental hospital, they found 90 percent of its patients not using either knives or forks at meals. Simply providing these utensils improved both behavior and attitudes! Less obvious marked behavioral improvements were brought about by structuring opportunities and expectations for heterosexual roles, consumer roles, work, friendship, and self-management. The major interventions used were the creation of a sheltered workshop, the introduction of money and a ward store, and frequent instrumental contacts with the nonhospital community. The result was more active residents, more social interaction, and more ego skills among those treated.

Theories of Treatment

Changed social relationships and increased opportunities are two of four interacting elements in a model for psychosocial therapy.[9] The theory states that any behavior is the result of interaction among (1) the capacity of the actor; (2) his or her own attitudes and wishes; (3) the opportunities and expectations of society; and (4) the most significant people in his or her life. Capacity, attitudes, society, and significant others are all variable. Planning and influencing changes in the variables is the process of psychosocial therapy.

Several examples illustrate the relevance of this theory to the role of the mental hospital in treating the elderly. Basic is the assumption that both direct and indirect influences effect each element. Eyesight, for example, may worsen organically, but may be improved by a mechanical aid—glasses. Anxiety, which may be caused by intrapsychological conflict, may be alleviated by interpersonal therapy or by drugs. Severe visual deficit can be a major cause of depression. Conversely depression can impair vision.

The mental hospital and nursing home are both total life systems in which interaction among the four behavioral elements can be planned and controlled. Often, when only one element is changed, total system impact follows. This was apparent in the milieu treatment study described above. Increased opportunity for normal behavior brought about not only improved overt behavior, but also improved attitudes and apparent changes in capacity.

Spectacular behavioral changes in residents can result from changed institutional expectations, because in spite of multiple disabilities very few residents are required to operate at the limit of their capacities. In fact, most institutions intending to protect their residents overprotect them. In relation to aging residents, institutions usually overrespond to both the limitations of age and of mental disorder. Very few life tasks require sustained high-level performance. Even with substantial visual loss, dressing, eating, and most kinds of work can be done well. Likewise, even pathology like delusions or hallucinations may permit a person to carry on most activities.

The principles of milieu therapy come from the observation that too much and too little demand both have negative effects. When capacity is greater than opportunity not only behavioral decline, but depression and loss of capacity may also result. If demands are at or above capacity for long periods, behavioral decline characteristic of stress occurs. When opportunity and expectation exceed current behavior, but not capacity, the behavior ego growth will occur.

Teaching Principles of Treatment

Mental hospitals should be leaders in teaching others the principles and practice of therapeutic intervention with the geriatric patient. Unfortunately, they themselves had only begun institution appropriate programs when mass transfers

of geriatric patients out of state hospitals began. Certainly, if the political decision to close all state hospitals—or at least to remove all geriatric patients from
them—is carried out, then the state hospital may maximize its therapeutic role
by assisting in preparing patients for their move to another facility. There is
compelling evidence that without an opportunity to discuss their forthcoming
move and perhaps visit the place where they will live, death rates among geriatric
patients will double.[10] The greatest increase in death rates will be among those
who are most physically frail and senile. The mental hospital staff—recalling
that it has more professional expertise than most receiving facilities—can spear-
head both the insistence that patients be prepared for moves and the actual
preparation process.

Once the residents have entered a nursing home, another therapeutic program—Reality Orientation—can be used. This program, developed in a mental
hospital by J.C. Folsom,[11] sharpens the capacity of the resident by marking
the environment clearly. It emphasizes architectural features (like doors) and
personal possessions by use of colors and good lighting. It enhances orientation
by use of clocks with large numerals, calendars, and frequent personal reminders
by significant staff. In addition, noticing time, place, and person cues is made
a focus of staff expectation, taught, and rewarded. The technique is precisely
what is needed by many organically impaired residents.

Most behavior modification techniques in use today were developed in
mental hospitals.[12] There is considerable evidence that they lead to improved
overt functioning. One of their more salient features is that they clearly differentiate among behavioral expectations and provide opportunities for the
behaviors that are expected to occur.

New Nursing Home Programs

Nursing homes themselves have also begun developing programs for their
residents, more than half of whom are mentally infirm. For example, in a new
building at the Philadelphia Geriatric Center (PGC), Dr. M. Powell Lawton is
attempting to use architectural details to enhance capacities of mentally
impaired residents. Doors, clocks, light switches, etc. are all being marked
boldly. In addition, rugs used as wall hangings will provide color, texture, and
sound control. The interior design places resident rooms around a large activity
area, implicitly communicating to both staff and residents that they are part of
each other's lives.

Another program developed at PGC is "individualized treatment."[13] It uses
a multidisciplinary team to analyze each resident's needs in order to prescribe
specific areas where improvement can be expected. By so doing, the program
not only establishes the assumption that improvement can occur, but shows
both residents and staff what to do and where to expect change. One year after

applying the individualized treatment, objective tests and independent ratings by judges not informed of the treatment priorities confirmed that residents actually improved in the expected ways.

A feature of each of the programs described here is that in formulating and operating their plans, they bring together staff members of differing disciplines and status. This approach, first developed in mental hospitals, is now used in some nursing homes. At the Philadelphia Geriatric Center this cooperation is formalized through the development of an interdisciplinary team approach that operates at two levels of care. The first—called the Unit IDT (interdisciplinary team)—is composed of medicine, nursing, social service, and others operating at the unit level. It takes responsibility for the individualized treatment of each unit resident. In regular weekly meetings the UIDT develops a treatment plan and monitors it. The IDT Coordinating Committee is composed of department heads, who in monthly meetings both sanction and support by examples the cooperation among disciplines that is central to effective long-term treatment. The IDT-CC also plans overall policy, reviews unit performance, and considers differential programming for each unit.

Community Treatment

Today, geriatric care, like the care of other patients, is moving out of the institution. For younger patients, the most prominent push today is toward the day hospital, from which geriatric patients in the United States generally have been excluded. In part, this exclusion can be attributed to the traditional reluctance to include the geriatric patient in programs of any kind. But since geriatric patients respond well to other innovations in long-term institutional care, less restrictive treatment is likely to be just as appropriate for them as for younger people. The literature from geriatric day programs attempted until now to suggest special needs for transportation, easy availability of medical care, rest periods, nutritional supplementation, and help with housing during nondaycare hours. During the day geriatric patients play many normal roles successfully. There is also marked reduction in both institutional change and dollar costs. For example, The American Psychiatric Association reports that the total annual cost of operating Council House in Pittsburgh for 1,200 clients is less than the twenty-four-hour costs of caring for thirty-two patients over a comparable period. Even a more conservative estimate puts day care at half of the twenty-four-hour cost.[14]

A final program is now on the horizon—the use of the institution as a community resource to prevent institutionalization. Institutional facilities contain a wide variety of experts who can use their skills to coordinate and deliver service, which helps to keep people in their homes. No doubt, physicians, psychologists, nurses, and social workers can offer needed services. But since personal care makes up a large part of the need of nursing home candidates, maintenance men can also help to keep their private homes livable; institutional kitchens can provide them home and congregate meals; the institution's buses can provide transportation; workshops can provide work. Since administrative frameworks already exist, the service givers may be able to do extra duty without substantial additional cost. A kitchen preparing 300 meals can as easily prepare 325. The Philadelphia Geriatric Center, with support from AoA (Administration on Aging), is now evaluating whether these services can be provided to community residents without first admitting them.

All these programs, born out of mental hospitals, provide solid bases on which we can plan programs for the elderly. Both institutional services and community services are needed by them today, and more will be needed tomorrow as the population increases. Mental hospitals will continue to play a direct care role. Nursing homes and other institutions that have emerged in the last decade must become the beneficiaries of the programs which have been developed in the mental hospital.

Notes

1. Gottesman, L.E. and Hutchinson, E., "Characteristics of Institutionalized Elderly," in Brody, E.M., *A Handbook on Social Work with the Aged*, NIMH, 1973.
2. Gottesman, L.E., Quarterman, C.E., and Cohn, G.M., "Psychosocial Treatment of the Aged," in C. Eisendorfer and M.P. Lawton (eds.), *The Psychology of Adult Development and Aging*, Washington, D.C.: American Psychological Association, 1973.
3. Gottesman, L.E., Coons, D., and Donahue, W., Milieu Therapy and Long-Term Geriatric Patients. Final report to Gerontology Branch Division of Chronic Diseases Public Health Service, DHEW, 250 pp., 1966.
4. Gottesman, L.E., "Milieu Treatment of the Aged in Institutions," *The Gerontologist* 13 (1973), 1: 23-26.
5. Kramer, M., Taube, C.A., and Redick, R.W., "Patterns of Use of Psychiatric Facilities by the Aged: Past, Present, Future," in C. Eisendorfer and M.P. Lawton (eds.), *The Psychology of Adult Development and Aging*, Washington, D.C.: American Psychological Association, 1973.
6. Gottesman, Quarterman, and Cohn, "Psychosocial Treatment of the Aged."
7. Fairweather, G.W., *Social Psychology in Treating Mental Illness. An Experimental Approach,* New York: Wiley, 1964.
8. Gottesman, Coons, and Donahue, Milieu Therapy and Long-Term Geriatric Patients.
9. Gottesman, Quarterman, and Cohn, "Psychosocial Treatment of the Aged,"
10. Bourestom, N., Tars, S., and Pastalan, L., Alterations in Life Patterns

Following Nursing Home Relocation, paper presented at 26th Annual
Gerontological Society, Nov. 9, 1973, Miami, Florida; Lawton, M.P. and
Nahemow, L., "Ecology and the Aging Process," in C. Eisendorfer and
M.P. Lawton (eds.), *The Psychology of Adult Development and Aging*,
Washington, D.C.: American Psychological Association, 1973, 619-74.
11. Folsom, J.C., "Reality Orientation for the Elderly Mental Patient,"
    Journal of Geriatric Psychiatry 1, (1968): 291-307.
12. Gottesman, Quarterman, and Cohn, "Psychosocial Treatment of the Aged."
13. Brody, E.M., Kleban, M.H., Lawton, M.P., and Silverman, H.S., "Excess
    Disabilities of Mentally Impaired Aged: Impact of Individualized Treat-
    ment," *Gerontologist* 2 (1971) 2: 124-33.
14. Glasscote, R.M., Cumming, E., Rutman, I., Sussex, J.N., and Glassman,
    S.M., in *Rehabilitating the Mentally Ill in the Community*, Washington,
    D.C., 1971, APA.

12

The Halfway House as an Alternative to Hospitalization
Mildred S. Cannon

Introduction

The management of patients suffering from chronic mental illness or problems with alcohol has undergone radical change in recent years. Innovations in physical, pharmacological, psychological, and social therapies have contributed to paving the way for many patients, who previously would have been condemned to lifelong custodial care in psychiatric hospitals, to be reintegrated into the community. The trend toward care outside the hospital has been accompanied by a diverse range of noninstitutional community services that provide support to patients. The halfway house represents one such service.

Definition and Purpose

There is no formal definition of a halfway house describing what this type of facility must or must not provide. A working definition developed by the National Institute of Mental Health (NIMH) defines halfway houses as residential facilities, in operation seven days a week, with around-the-clock staff supervision (or a staff member living in), and providing room, board, and assistance in the activities of daily living. The primary "problem group" served must be either the mentally ill or alcoholic, although persons with other problems, such as drug abuse, may be admitted on occasion. These facilities are differentiated from other mental health facilities in that the primary focus is on the provision of room and board and assistance in the activities of daily living rather than on the provision of a planned treatment program.

Apte[1] describes a halfway house or transitional hostel as fulfilling a rehabilitative function, focused on the reintegration of the handicapped person into the community that, from a public health standpoint, would be considered as a tool for tertiary prevention. Apte further describes the halfway house as a place where mentally ill individuals living in their own homes may go to avoid entering a mental hospital during a period of excessive stress or emotional crises.

This report, based on the most recent NIMH National Halfway House survey, is an abridgment of a forthcoming report on the halfway house as a community resource for persons with psychiatric and alcoholism problems, to be published in the National Institute of Mental Health Report Series on Mental Health Statistics.

In addition to the functions of "bridging the gap" between the hospital and the community and/or serving as an alternative to hospitalization, R.M. Glasscote et al.[2] cite other appropriate uses for halfway houses as follows:

1. To provide a more or less permanent placement for people who no longer need to be in hospitals, do not require the physical care of nursing homes, yet have little potential to become employed or to live in the community without supports.
2. To reach into the hospitals, to recruit people who remain there because of the lack of an acceptable release plan. These may be people without families, or with families unwilling to accept the patient back in the home.
3. To serve as a facility that has the potential to shorten the length of inpatient stay so that persons need only be hospitalized during the "crisis" phase of their illness.

Types of Halfway Houses

Halfway houses may be categorized by whether they provide transitional or permanent residence. Those considered as primarily transitional halfway houses provide a temporary residence for patients, either following hospitalization or in lieu of hospitalization. Other halfway houses provide long-term sheltered living arrangements that serve as a permanent substitute for hospitalization. However, no strict dichotomy can be made between these two categories of halfway houses, since many serve both a transitional and a permanent function.

Specialized halfway houses have been developed to serve the mentally ill, the mentally retarded, paroled offenders, delinquent juveniles, alcoholics, drug addicts, and groups of persons with a variety of other problems. A number of "multicategory" halfway houses have also been established that serve more than one impairment group. However, it is only those halfway houses serving primarily the mentally ill or alcoholics or combinations thereof with which this report is concerned.

NIMH Halfway House Surveys

With the movement toward increased community-based services accompanied by the necessity for planning for such services, there emerged an obvious need for various types of information regarding halfway houses: (1) their general characteristics; (2) whom they served; (3) their utilization; (4) their staffing patterns; and (5) their expenditures and funding. For this reason, the decision was made in 1969 to include transitional mental health facilities or halfway

houses among the universe of facilities covered by the NIMH National Reporting
Program for mental health facilities.

Since its inception the halfway house inventory has been a single-phase
survey encompassing all facilities of this type known to NIMH. The initial survey
was conducted in January 1970 and repeated in August 1971 and October 1973.
Findings from the first two surveys along with a description of the methodology
have been published.[3]

For purposes of analysis, halfway houses have been grouped into categories
based on the primary population group served. A total of 806 facilities were
identified in the October 1973 survey as meeting NIMH criteria for a halfway
house. Of this number, 209 halfway houses served the mentally ill and 597
served primarily alcoholics.

Data from the latest NIMH survey on which this report is based provide
perhaps the best available estimate of the status of halfway houses in the United
States today. The following sections describe differences between psychiatric
and alcoholism halfway houses in terms of their operating characteristics and
utilization patterns.

Operating Characteristics

Span of Operation

The halfway house movement is a comparatively new phenomenon reflecting
the changing trend toward treatment and rehabilitation in the community.
Table 12-1 indicates that only 2 percent of the psychiatric halfway houses and
4 percent of the alcoholism halfway houses were operating prior to 1955, the
year beginning the trend toward large numbers of discharges from the state mental hospitals. The median number of operating years for psychiatric halfway
houses, 5.4, is somewhat longer than that for alcoholism halfway houses, 4.4.

An explanation for this factor might possibly reside in the recent interest
and widespread publicity directed toward combating alcoholism at the national
level accompanying the establishment of the National Institute of Alcoholism
and Alcohol Abuse.

Distribution

There is a disproportionate distribution of the halfway houses with respect
to geographic location. While 71 percent of the psychiatric halfway houses were
located in states east of the Mississippi River, 54 percent of the alcoholism halfway houses were located west of the river. There were eleven states in which
no psychiatric halfway houses were identified, in contrast to only one state
(Mississippi) in which not one alcoholism halfway house was identified.

The uneven state distribution is also apparent when looking at the number of halfway house beds in relation to the general population. This ranges from those states with no halfway house beds, to one (Vermont) with as many as 29.5 psychiatric halfway house beds and 22.2 alcoholism halfway house beds per 100,000 civilian resident population. These data on the availability of halfway house beds do not necessarily imply that some states provide better community-based services than others. Additional factors to be considered include the availability of other types of residential-care programs such as foster- and family-care homes, rehabilitation centers, and also the possible existence of halfway houses that inadvertently may have been missed in the survey.

Type of Licensing

There is currently little consistency with respect to laws governing the licensing and regulation of halfway house programs from state to state. Among halfway houses responding to the question regarding types of license, only 26 percent of the psychiatric halfway houses, and 33 percent of the alcoholism halfway houses are actually licensed as halfway houses. A sizable proportion, including 29 percent of the psychiatric halfway houses and 41 percent of the alcoholism halfway houses reported not having a license. Still others are reported as operating under licensing categories that bear little resemblance to the type of service which they provide.

Ownership and Bedsize

Nonprofit organizations predominate in halfway house ownership, encompassing 59 percent of the psychiatric halfway houses and 90 percent of the alcoholism halfway houses. These facilities are established on the premise that residents pay for their keep, enabling the house to operate without a deficit (Table 12-1).

It is interesting to note, however, that while 59 percent of the psychiatric halfway houses are nonprofit, only 35 percent of the total psychiatric halfway house beds are contained within these facilities. On the other hand, 57 percent of all psychiatric halfway house beds are located in the 23 percent of the total halfway houses that come under proprietary ownership. Among alcoholism halfway houses, the distribution of facilities and beds within the facilities is nearly the same, with respect to ownership.

The optimum halfway house is, by intention, small in size, imparting a homelike atmosphere. The greater proportion of the facilities are small and indeed could fit this definition. Although the halfway houses ranged in size from those with five beds to others with over 300 beds, the median bedsize

Table 12-1
Distribution of Halfway Houses by Type of Halfway House and Selected Facility Characteristics, United States, October 1973[a]

	Type of Halfway House			
	Psychiatric		*Alcoholism*	
Facility Characteristics	*Number*	*Percent*	*Number*	*Percent*
Total, all facilities	209.0	100.0%	597.0	100.0%
Sex groups admitted				
Both sexes	140.0	67.0	134.0	22.5
Males only	31.0	14.8	390.0	65.3
Females only	38.0	18.2	73.0	12.2
Number of beds				
14 beds or fewer	89.0	42.6	225.0	37.7
15-24 beds	65.0	31.1	194.0	32.5
25-49 beds	25.0	12.0	137.0	22.9
50-99 beds	13.0	6.2	34.0	5.7
100 beds and over	17.0	8.1	7.0	1.2
Median bedsize	16.9		18.1	
Type of control				
Government	37.0	17.7	37.0	6.2
Proprietary	49.0	23.4	22.0	3.7
Non-profit	123.0	58.9	538.0	90.1
Years in operation				
Under one year	15.0	7.2	57.0	9.5
1-2 years	29.0	13.9	177.0	29.7
3-5 years	76.0	36.3	141.0	23.6
6-10 years	61.0	29.2	120.0	20.1
11-20 years	23.0	11.0	78.0	13.1
20 years and over	5.0	2.4	24.0	4.0
Median years	5.4		4.4	
Geographic region				
Northeast	49.0	23.5	63.0	10.5
North Central	69.0	33.0	127.0	21.3
South	68.0	32.5	186.0	31.2
West	23.0	11.0	221.0	37.0

[a]This table includes estimates for nonresponding facilities.

in the psychiatric halfway houses was seventeen beds, and in the alcoholism halfway houses, eighteen beds. The transitional psychiatric halfway houses, those where the average stay for residents was less than six months, were somewhat smaller, with a median bed-size of fifteen beds. In contrast, the nontransitional halfway houses that have an average stay of over six months tended to be larger with a median bed-size of twenty beds. This latter group of facilities includes a few exceptionally large hotel-like facilities considered to be operating a halfway house program. Among the alcoholism halfway houses there was no difference in bed-size between the transitional and the nontransitional types.

Expenditures and Funding

Salaries comprise the largest single expenditure in both the psychiatric and alcoholism halfway houses, 49 percent and 44 percent, respectively (Table 12-2). Food, the next largest expenditure, accounts for 14 percent of the total budget in psychiatric halfway houses, and 18 percent of the total budget in alcoholism halfway houses. The distribution of expenditures for other purposes (e.g., utilities, maintenance, supplies) is nearly the same proportionately between the two types of halfway houses.

In view of the close comparability of median bed-size between the psychiatric and alcoholism halfway houses, it is of interest to note that per facility expenditures in psychiatric halfway houses are on the average 76 percent higher than in alcoholism halfway houses (Table 12-3). Furthermore, costs are over

Table 12-2
Percent Distribution of Halfway House Expenditures by Type of Expenditure and Type of Halfway House, United States, 1973[a]

	Type of Halfway House	
Type of Expenditure	Psychiatric	Alcoholism
Total Expenditures	100.0%	100.0%
Salaries and employee benefits	48.8	44.1
Food	14.4	18.2
Rent or mortgage	11.0	10.6
Utilities	5.8	6.2
Maintenance, supplies, and fixtures	8.2	8.1
All other (including insurance, transportation, recreation, laundry, etc.)	11.8	12.8

[a]This table is based on reports from 111 psychiatric halfway houses and 280 alcoholism halfway houses.

Table 12-3
Average Annual Expenditure per Facility and per Admission by Type of Halfway House, United States, October 1973[a]

	Type of Halfway House	
Expenditure Ratio	Psychiatric	Alcoholism
Average annual expenditure:		
Per facility	$73,732	$41,977
Per admission	$ 1,644	$ 371

[a]This table is based only on reports from facilities responding to this item.

four times greater for the average resident admission to psychiatric facilities than for admission to alcoholism facilities. This latter difference might be attributed in part to large numbers of persons admitted to alcoholism halfway houses who return to drinking and leave after a few days' stay. (Due to reporting difficulties in this survey, estimates of per patient day expenditures are not available.)

Usually halfway house residents are expected to be employed and to pay their expenses from their earnings. Psychiatric halfway houses, however, reported welfare payments as the primary source their residents had for paying expenses. This was followed in frequency of reporting by vocational rehabilitation, with employment earnings reported third. In alcoholism halfway houses, employment earnings constituted the primary means by which residents paid their expenses, with public welfare second. No charge is reported for 15 percent of the residents in alcoholism halfway houses. Residents working in the halfway house in lieu of paying, or residents who leave after a short period without paying, might provide a possible explanation for this occurrence.

Staffing Patterns

Staffing patterns differ between the psychiatric and alcoholism halfway houses with respect to the occupations of the workers, their status (that is, whether full time, part time, or volunteer), the average number of workers per facility, and the number of staff members relative to the number of persons served.

The average psychiatric halfway house has eleven employees, seven of

Table 12-4
**Selected Halfway House Staffing Indices by Type of Halfway House,
United States, October 1973[a]**

Staffing Indices	Type of Halfway House	
	Psychiatric	Alcoholism
Average number staff per		
facility–total	11.6	5.8
Full time[b]	7.0	3.6
Part time[c]	3.3	1.2
Volunteer	1.3	1.0
Number staff per 100		
residents–total	40.1	34.2
Full time	24.2	21.1
Part time	11.5	7.2
Volunteer	4.4	5.9
Percent distribution of staff		
by discipline–total	100.0%	100.0%
Mental health professionals[d]	14.3	6.8
All other professional[e]	25.8	33.1
Paraprofessional	30.4	18.8
All other	29.5	41.3
Percent of total staff formerly		
in problem group		
Former mental patients	5.6%	0.6%
Recovering alcoholics	0.9%	60.2%

[a]This table includes estimates for nonresponding facilities.

[b]Employees working thirty-five hours or more per week.

[c]Employees working less than thirty-five hours per week.

[d]Includes psychiatrists, psychologists, social workers, and registered nurses.

[e]Includes nonpsychiatric physicians, counselors, therapists, and school teachers.

whom are employed full time, three are employed part time, and one is a volunteer. In comparison, the average alcoholism halfway house operates with about half as many staff members as the psychiatric facilities—a total staff of six, of whom four are full time, one is part time, and one is a volunteer (Table 12-4).

The employee/resident ratio for the two types of facilities indicates that psychiatric halfway houses have considerably more paid employees per 100 residents than do the alcoholism halfway houses. This pattern does not hold true among the volunteer staff, however, since volunteers are utilized more fully in alcoholism halfway houses than in psychiatric halfway houses. It is also interesting to note that 60 percent of the employees in alcoholism halfway houses are recovering alcoholics.

Unlike patients in the traditional mental health facilities such as psychiatric hospitals, halfway house residents usually obtain their psychiatric or medical care outside of the halfway house, a factor reflected in the staffing patterns within these facilities. As a consequence, many halfway houses provide only limited treatment and employ very few professional mental health workers, particularly those in the four core mental health disciplines: psychiatrists, social workers, psychologists, and registered nurses. This group of workers comprised only 14 percent of the total workers in psychiatric halfway houses and 7 percent in alcoholism halfway houses.

Services Provided

In response to the survey question regarding services provided within the house, those reported by the greatest proportion of psychiatric halfway houses were house meetings (89 percent), individual or group counseling (80 percent), and planned recreational activity programs (64 percent). Usually residents are encouraged, though not required, to participate in activities within the house. House meetings might often be little more than informal sessions during which menus may be planned, decisions may be made regarding allocation of household chores, or some problem that may have arisen in the house may be discussed. Individual or group counseling simply provides the opportunity for residents to discuss personal problems either with a staff member of a trained psychotherapist coming from the outside on a regular basis to serve as a consultant or a group leader. In response to the same survey question regarding services provided in the house, alcoholism halfway houses reported Alcoholics Anonymous services (87 percent), and also reported house meetings (87 percent), and individual or group counseling (84 percent).

Admission Restrictions

Most of the halfway houses observe one or more restrictions concerning who may be accepted with respect to sex, age, or diagnosis. Two-thirds of the psychiatric halfway houses accept residents without regard to sex, and the remaining facilities are about evenly divided between those that accept either males only or females only. Nearly two-thirds of the alcoholism halfway houses restrict their admissions to males. While 23 percent of the alcoholism halfway houses accept both sexes, only 12 percent of these facilities were specifically for the female alcoholic.

Of all facilities surveyed, only one reported that age was not considered a factor for acceptance. A greater proportion of psychiatric halfway houses impose age restrictions on admissions than do alcoholism halfway houses. Most of the psychiatric halfway houses imposing age restrictions reported having a minimum age for acceptance, with seventeen to eighteen years most frequently reported. All but one of the alcoholism halfway houses reported having a minimum age for acceptance, and two-thirds of these indicated seventeen to eighteen years as being the minimum age for acceptance. Among the facilities reporting a minimum age, only 45 percent of the psychiatric halfway houses and 29 percent of the alcoholism halfway houses reported having a maximum age also.

Nearly all of the halfway houses imposed some diagnostic restriction on acceptance. Only four of the psychiatric halfway houses and one alcoholism halfway house reported accepting all problem groups. About one-fourth of the psychiatric halfway houses reported that they would also accept alcoholics or mentally retarded persons as residents. Conversely, only 5 percent of the alcoholism halfway houses accepted the mentally ill, and even fewer accepted retarded persons. The second most frequently reported problem group accepted by alcoholism halfway houses are drug abusers (18 percent).

In addition to restrictions with respect to age, sex, and diagnosis, many of the halfway houses also imposed other restrictions on prospective residents. The three most frequently reported requirements for both the psychiatric and alcoholism halfway houses were that prospective residents (1) be able to benefit from rehabilitation; (2) be able to manage their personal needs; and (3) agree to share in housekeeping and maintenance tasks.

Length of Stay and Readmissions

Considering both psychiatric and alcoholism halfway houses, about one out of five reported having a policy regarding the length of time a resident could remain although the length of permitted stay varied greatly by facility type. Over half of the alcoholism halfway houses reported as having a maximum-stay policy do not allow residents to remain over ninety days, whereas the majority of the psychiatric halfway houses observing such a policy permit residents to remain longer. While the majority of alcoholism halfway houses permit unlimited readmissions for persons who have setbacks with their drinking problem, about 26 percent of these facilities reported limiting the number of times a resident could be readmitted. Only 11 percent of the psychiatric halfway houses reported having such a policy; of this group, 27 percent do not permit any readmissions and 50 percent permit only one readmission. Among the alcoholism halfway houses that limit readmissions, 42 percent permitted three or more readmissions, 34 percent permitted two readmissions, and 20 permitted only one readmission.

Characteristics of Residents

As of October 1973 there were 6,003 persons residing in psychiatric halfway houses, and 10,295 persons residing in alcoholism halfway houses. Males comprised a slightly larger proportion of total residents in psychiatric halfway houses (54 percent) and accounted for 88 percent of all residents in alcoholism halfway houses (Table 12-5). Eighty-five percent of all psychiatric halfway house residents lived in houses serving both sexes, while only 27 percent of alcoholism halfway house residents lived in coed facilities. Sixty-six percent of the alcoholism halfway house residents lived in houses that restrict admission to males, reflecting the circumstance that males comprise the overwhelming majority of residents in such facilities. The preponderance of males over females is not a phenomenon unique to halfway houses. Males exceed females among admissions with alcohol disorders to all psychiatric inpatient facilities.[4] Seventy-one percent of residents in psychiatric halfway houses lived in nontransitional-type houses in contrast to alcoholism halfway houses, where 85 percent of the residents lived in transitional-type halfway houses.

For both psychiatric and alcoholism halfway houses, the average number of residents was largest in the houses serving both males and females. In all likelihood this is due to the larger number of beds in these facilities created through the utilization of separate dwellings by members of each sex, which function together as one administrative unit.

The average number of persons residing in nontransitional psychiatric facilities is three times greater than that in the transitional type. Among alcoholism halfway houses, the length of stay category for the facility had no influence on the average number of residents.

Residents in psychiatric halfway houses have a median age of thirty-six years as compared to a median age of forty-four years for residents in alcoholism halfway houses. There is little difference in the median age of residents in psychiatric halfway houses with respect to sex of the residents. In comparing median age of residents by type of halfway house, residents in transitional houses are considerably younger than those in nontransitional houses: twenty-five years as compared with forty years, respectively. This difference might be expected in view of the many nontransitional houses that serve more or less as permanent residences for many persons who are either too old or too ill or who, for some other reason, can never be expected to live independently in the community. Male residents are generally older than female alcoholism halfway house residents, and this age differential is more pronounced in nontransitional than in transitional facilities.

While the vast majority of residents in psychiatric halfway houses are mentally ill and those in alcoholism halfway houses are alcoholics, a small proportion of residents in both facility types have a variety of other problems (e.g., mental retardation, drug abuses, paroles).

Table 12-5
**Selected Characteristics of Halfway House Residents by Type of
Halfway House, United States, October 1973[a]**

	Type of Halfway House	
Characteristics of Residents	Psychiatric	Alcoholism
Sex distribution		
Total, both sexes	100.0%	100.0%
Male	54.2	88.2
Female	45.8	11.8
Median age		
Total facilities	36.1 years	44.0 years
Transitional	25.4	43.5
Nontransitional	39.9	46.7
Number males per 100 females		
Total, all ages	116.0	751.0
Under 18 years	98.0	180.0
18-24 years	113.0	609.0
25-44 years	130.0	695.0
45-64 years	97.0	828.0
65 years and over	137.0	1,243.0
Percent of total residents in problem group[b]		
Emotionally disturbed	88.5%	4.7%
Mentally retarded	5.9	0.4
Alcoholics	4.5	96.2
Drug abusers	1.6	4.5
Maladjusted children	0.7	0.1
Parolees or ex-convicts	2.2	6.0
Homeless or transient	1.6	9.2
Other	0.6	0.4

[a]This table is based only on reports from facilities responding to the individual items.

[b]Figures shown do not add to 100 percent since the categories are not mutually exclusive.

New Admissions and Readmissions

Most persons admitted to both psychiatric and alcoholism halfway houses are new admissions. Among psychiatric halfway houses, greater proportions of readmissions were reported by facilities serving either both sexes or only females than those serving only males. Within these categories, halfway houses serving both sexes or females only, the percentage of readmissions reported by nontransitional facilities was higher than that reported by the transitional facilities.

Alcoholism halfway houses have nearly twice the proportion of readmissions as psychiatric halfway houses. In all likelihood this results from residents having to leave the halfway house because of having broken abstinence rules, and then returning to the program at some later time. Among alcoholism halfway houses, fewer readmissions were reported by facilities serving only women than for those serving only males or those serving both sexes.

Source of Referral and Prior Treatment

Over half of all residents in psychiatric halfway houses were referred by psychiatric hospitals or clinics. Vocational rehabilitation ranks second among referrals to transitional facilities for both males and females. This is not surprising in light of the fact that a major goal of these facilities is for residents to develop employable skills and to become employed in preparation for independent community living.

Alcoholism treatment centers are the leading source of referral to both transitional and nontransitional alcoholism halfway houses for both males and females. Alcoholics Anonymous ranks second as a referral source for nontransitional halfway houses for both males and females, and ranks third among males in nontransitional halfway houses and fifth among females in these facilities.

Table 12-6 shows that nearly 90 percent of all psychiatric halfway house residents have been hospitalized at some prior time. Seventy-five percent entered the halfway house directly from a hospital, while another 14 percent, although coming directly from the community, had a prior history of hospitalization. In contrast, only 30 percent of alcoholism halfway house residents entered the halfway house directly from a hospital, with a higher percentage of females coming via this route than males. The proportion of residents in alcoholism halfway houses, coming directly from the community, but having a prior history of hospitalization, is nearly as great as the proportion of residents in these facilities who entered the halfway house directly from a hospital. Twenty-two percent of the alcoholism halfway house residents had never been hospitalized, in contrast to only 8 percent of the psychiatric halfway house residents.

Utilization Indices

On the average, psychiatric halfway houses operated nearer to capacity than alcoholism halfway houses: 85 percent occupancy compared to 77 percent,

Table 12-6
Percent Distribution of Halfway House Residents by Type of Halfway House, Previous Treatment Category, and Sex, United States, 1973[a]

Previous Treatment Category	Type of Halfway House					
	Psychiatric			Alcoholism		
	Total Residents	Males	Females	Total Residents	Males	Females
	Percent Distribution of Residents					
Total	100.0%	100.0%	100.0%	100.0%	100.0%	100.0%
Entered halfway house on convalescent leave or discharge from hospital	74.3	75.3	73.6	30.1	29.0	37.7
Entered halfway house from community:						
—previously hospitalized	14.0	12.7	15.4	29.7	30.0	28.0
—never hospitalized	7.7	7.1	8.5	21.8	21.3	25.1
Entered halfway house on release from correctional facility	2.0	2.4	1.5	6.9	7.4	3.2
Other	1.8	2.5	1.0	11.5	12.3	6.0

[a]This table is based on reports from 141 psychiatric and 334 alcoholism halfway houses.

respectively, for the two types of facilities (Table 12-7). While there was only slight variation in the occupancy rate by sex served, this rate varied somewhat more by bed-size, ownership, span of operation, and geographic location. Among both psychiatric and alcoholism halfway houses, the facilities under government control had the highest occupancy rates. The effects of length of time in operation on occupancy rate, although apparent in both types of facilities, is more pronounced for psychiatric facilities. For both psychiatric and alcoholism halfway houses, the occupancy rate increases as the number of operating years increases, with the exception of those facilities in operation, the longest period, eleven years and over.

The average number of admissions per facility varied considerably by type of halfway house from forty-three admissions annually for psychiatric halfway houses to 116 admissions for alcoholism halfway houses. This disparity in the average number of admissions per facility indicates a much lower turnover rate in psychiatric halfway houses than in alcoholism halfway houses.

Median length of stay ranged from slightly over three months in the alcoholism halfway houses to nearly eleven months—over three times as long—in the psychiatric halfway houses. Among the nontransitional facilities, the range was from nine months in alcoholism halfway houses to over seventeen months in the psychiatric houses. The range was not nearly as great among the transitional type facilities, with the median stay being just one month longer in psychiatric halfway houses than in alcoholism halfway houses.

Table 12-7
Selected Utilization Indices by Type of Halfway House, United States, October 1973[a]

Utilization Indices	Type of Halfway House	
	Psychiatric	Alcoholism
Average number beds per facility	34	22
Average number residents per facility	29	17
Occupancy rate	85%	77%
Average number admissions per facility	43	116
Number admissions per 100 residents	178	737

[a]This table is based only on reports from facilities reporting this information.

Living Arrangements on Discharge

The goal set by most halfway houses is that its residents, on leaving, be capable of independent functioning and self-support in the community. With this in mind, then, success for the halfway house would be measured by its residents' subsequent resumption of normal life.

Overall, residents who leave the halfway house tend predominantly to move into independent living arrangements in the community, and a somewhat smaller proportion go to live with relatives or friends (Table 12-8). About one-fourth of the alcoholism halfway houses reported not knowing where their residents went on leaving the house.

While 15 percent of the psychiatric halfway house residents returned to the hospital, this could be a function of the initial selection process. If halfway houses selected only persons with high rehabilitative potential, perhaps a somewhat different pattern would emerge. Such a practice, however, would have the adverse effect of screening out those persons who initially show poor rehabilitative potential, yet could achieve considerable benefit from a halfway house setting.[5]

*Halfway House Availability in Relation to
State Hospital Location*

During 1971 nearly one-third of all inpatient admission episodes to mental

**Table 12-8
Percent Distribution of Halfway House Discharges by Where Residents
Go On Leaving the House, United States, 1973[a]**

	Type of Halfway House	
Place to Which Discharged	*Psychiatric*	*Alcoholism*
Total	100.0%	100.0%
Live with relatives or friends	21.6	21.2
Live independently	40.8	39.7
Return to hospital	15.0	4.9
Another halfway house or sheltered living arrangement	9.5	4.2
Living arrangement on discharge not known	8.7	25.3
Other	4.4	4.7

[a]Based on reports from 122 psychiatric and 249 alcoholism halfway houses.

health facilities were to state and county mental hospitals.[6] In addition, state and county mental hospitals account for almost two-fifths of all admissions diagnosed with alcoholism to mental health facilities, not including persons admitted with other diagnoses who are also alcoholics.[7]

Discharges from state and county mental hospitals create the greatest source of potential halfway house users. Therefore, it is of interest to relate the availability of halfway house beds per 1,000 additions (i.e., admissions, readmissions, and returns from long-term leave) to state and county mental hospitals. At the national level there are over six times as many halfway house beds available for persons with alcohol problems as there are available for persons with other mental disorders. This pattern is apparent although at differing proportions in each geographic region. The number of beds available in psychiatric halfway houses relative to the number of public mental hospital additions without alcohol disorder varies considerably among the states. There are some states with no halfway house beds, while Illinois and Wisconsin have as many as 122 and 117 psychiatric halfway house beds per 1,000 state hospital admissions with nonalcohol disorders.

The range of alcoholism halfway house beds available between the states is even wider. While only one state does not have any alcoholism halfway house beds, several states have more available halfway house beds than there were state hospital additions with alcohol disorders (Florida, Arizona, Utah). While these hospitals provide the major source of inpatient care for alcoholics in the United States, as mentioned earlier, halfway house residents come from a variety of other places as well.

Discussion and Implications

The foregoing discussion of the development, characteristics, and utilization of halfway houses indicates that they differ from one another in a number of ways. They are unevenly distributed geographically, have different staffing patterns, serve different patient populations, and have different utilization patterns. In spite of these differences, however, halfway houses share a number of common features.

The halfway house has helped to break the separation that has traditionally existed between the hospital and the community. The most difficult period of adjustment for the discharged mental patient or recovering alcoholic is the first few months. Readjustment to normal life in the community requires a set of skills, and perhaps more importantly the attitude that one can succeed in the process. The halfway house, with its small homelike setting and supportive living environment can provide an important resource for assisting in this transition. The experience of living together with others who share similar problems and experiences can serve to remove feelings of isolation and difference and allow for reestablishment of interpersonal relations and resocialization, one of the major functions of the halfway houses.

The halfway house movement seems in keeping with the current trend away from large impersonal organizations with highly structured programs toward decentralization and relocation of services in the community. The high expectations that these facilities have of their residents further serve to make them different. Although some state hospitals today are quite progressive and innovative in their treatment programs and goals, there are still those that promote dependence. One of the major goals of the halfway house is to encourage self-reliance. More importantly, the halfway house helps to reduce the stigma associated with institutionalization. Halfway houses are usually located in urban residential areas with no publication given to the type of service they provide or the status of their residents.

The advantages provided by these facilities seem numerous; however, the halfway house should not be viewed as a panacea for all those too troubled to live in the ordinary community. With their lack of highly trained professional staff, halfway houses are not designed to help persons needing intensive supervision. There is a need to guard against their being inappropriately used to assure that they do not become miniature hospitals in the community without the trained staff or facilities of a regular hospital.

The recent proliferation in numbers of halfway houses is an indication of their new-found popularity. No hard data exist, however, to validate the general belief that halfway houses are effective in their rehabilitative efforts and hence worth their expense. There is a confounding of personal enthusiasm and the financial and emotional investment of the innovators with the actual efficacy of the program. Further study is needed to assess the value of the halfway house facility. While the justification of these facilities seems logical, and this approach is in keeping with the cherished American values of peer group support and personal independence, controlled studies are needed to measure the success or failure of patients—with respect to remaining out of the hospital, employment patterns, and living status—when a halfway house is used, as compared with placement in other types of after-care settings or where no special service is utilized. Society needs to know if halfway houses are capable of advancing care and treatment, or are simply, at best, a means of delaying institutionalization or, at worst, a new form of institutionalization.

To date there have been no published results from controlled studies designed to measure halfway house effectiveness, which is understandable because of the newness of this approach to rehabilitation. However, this lack is felt to be one of the most important challenges facing researchers and professionals in this field today. The need for hard empirical evidence has been recognized, and several studies designed to measure the efficacy of halfway house programs are currently underway.[8]

Even with their recent growth, halfway houses are still small in number;

they are not distributed evenly throughout all geographic areas, and the numbers of discharged patients whom the houses have the capacity to serve is but a small fraction of the total numbers of patients discharged from mental hospitals. While there is no formula for determining what the actual number of halfway houses should be, certain assumptions could be made to estimate the potential demand for such services. Considering that 455,000 persons were discharged from public mental hospitals during 1973, and assuming that halfway house services would be appropriate for one-quarter of these persons, and that they would remain an average of six months, it is estimated that 56,900 halfway house beds would be needed, or nearly three times the number currently available (20,385). Such estimates suggest that current halfway house resources meet at best one-third of the potential demand.

Based on the rapid growth in the numbers of halfway houses in the past two decades, however, and the current trend toward community care for troubled persons, there is every reason to assume that the growth will not only continue, but will possibly accelerate. Expansion of other community services such as day hospital programs could necessitate an increasing need for and use of halfway house facilities as a place for participants in such programs to live.

In all likelihood, the trend in community care will continue regardless of the future role of the state hospital. While some groups argue that state mental hospital systems should be abolished, still others recommend their expansion in the research and training areas and integration with community functions. Nevertheless, the trend will undoubtedly remain to keep mentally ill or troubled persons in the community where they can derive greater meaning and satisfaction from life than they historically have been able to as permanent residents of state hospitals. The halfway house may represent important means for achieving this goal.

Summary

This report is based on information obtained in the third national inventory of halfway houses conducted in October 1973 by the Biometry Division of the National Institute of Mental Health. Of 806 facilities identified in the survey as meeting the NIMH criteria of a halfway house, 26 percent served primarily the mentally ill and 74 percent served primarily alcoholics. There is considerable variation between these two types of halfway houses with respect to their general characteristics and utilization patterns.

The halfway house as it is known today is a relatively new phenomenon. The majority have been in operation less than five years. Only 2 percent of the psychiatric halfway houses and 4 percent of the alcoholism halfway houses were operating prior to 1955, the year begining the trend toward large numbers of discharges from the state mental hospitals.

Halfway houses are not evenly distributed throughout the country. A considerably greater proportion of halfway houses for persons with emotional disturbances are located in the eastern part of the country while a somewhat larger proportion of halfway houses for alcoholics are located in the west. There is considerable variation between states with respect to whether these facilities are licensed and, if so, the type of license under which they operate.

With some exception, these facilities are small in size. About 74 percent of the psychiatric halfway houses and 70 percent of the alcoholism halfway houses have fewer than twenty-five beds. Most of the facilities are operated on a nonprofit basis.

The average annual cost to operate a psychiatric halfway house in 1973 was about $74,000 as compared with an average annual cost of $42,000 to operate an alcoholism halfway house. While psychiatric halfway houses are funded primarily by state or local government, the latter type receive the greater part of their funds from patient fees.

The average psychiatric halfway house has twelve employees while the average alcoholism halfway house has six. Professional workers comprise only a small proportion of the total workers in both types of houses. A possible explanation for the small staff size is that these facilities tend to operate on a rather informal basis with few services or activities offered within the halfway house itself. Halfway house residents are usually encouraged to utilize services provided in the community.

While most psychiatric halfway houses accept both males and females, the majority of the alcoholism halfway houses restrict their services to males. Almost all of the halfway houses reported a minimum age for acceptance while more psychiatric halfway houses than alcoholism facilities reported having a maximum age also. Nearly all of the halfway houses imposed some diagnostic restrictions on whom they would accept.

Only a small proportion of the halfway houses restrict the length of time a resident can remain and of those which do, alcoholism houses impose shorter periods than psychiatric houses. Although the majority of halfway houses do not impose readmission restrictions, such restrictions are reported by more alcoholism than psychiatric halfway houses.

While males comprised a slightly larger proportion of total residents in psychiatric halfway houses, in alcoholism houses they outnumbered females over seven to one. Among the psychiatric halfway houses there is little difference in the age distribution of the residents with respect to sex. In the alcoholism halfway houses, however, female residents tend to be younger than males.

While most persons admitted to both types of halfway houses are new admissions, alcoholism halfway houses have more readmissions than psychiatric halfway houses.

Mental hospitals and clinics are the greatest referral source for psychiatric halfway houses, with three-fourths of the halfway house residents coming directly to the halfway house from the hospital. Most alcoholism halfway house residents, on the other hand, are referred by alcoholism treatment centers.

Psychiatric halfway houses had a higher occupancy rate (85 percent) than alcoholism halfway houses (77 percent) and the turnover rate in psychiatric halfway houses was much lower than in alcoholism halfway houses. Median stay in psychiatric halfway houses (eleven months) was over three times as long as that in alcoholism halfway houses (three months). Most residents on leaving the halfway house go into independent living arrangements and a somewhat smaller proportion go to live with relatives or friends.

Notes

1. Apte, R., *Halfway Houses: A New Dilemma in Institutional Care*, London: G. Bell Ltd., 1968.
2. Glasscote, R.M., Gudeman, J.E., and Elpers, R., *Halfway Houses for the Mentally Ill*, Washington, D.C.: JIS-APA, 1971.
3. Cannon, M.S. and Witkin, M.J., *Halfway Houses Serving the Mentally Ill and Alcoholics, United States, 1969-1970,* DHEW, NIMH, Mental Health Statistics, Series A, No. 9; Cannon, M.S., *Alcoholism Halfway Houses — General Characteristics*, Statistical Note 73, Health Services and Mental Health Administration, National Institute of Mental Health, Rockville, Md.; _____, *Selected Characteristics of Residents in Alcoholism Halfway Houses*, Statistical Note 76, Health Services and Mental Health Administration, National Institute of Mental Health, Rockville, Md.; _____, *Psychiatric Halfway Houses — General Characteristics*, Statistical Note 80, Health Services and Mental Health Administration, National Institute of Mental Health, Rockville, Md.; _____, *Selected Characteristics of Residents in Psychiatric Halfway Houses*, Statistical Note 93, Health Services and Mental Health Administration, National Institute of Mental Health, Rockville, Md.
4. Redick, R.W., *Utilization of Psychiatric Facilities by Persons Diagnosed with Alcohol Disorders*, DHEW, National Institute of Mental Health, Report Series on Mental Health Statistics, Series B, No. 4.
5. Raush, H.L. and Raush, C., *The Halfway House Movement: A Search for Sanity*, New York: Appleton-Century-Croft, 1968.
6. Taube, C.A., *Utilization of Mental Health Facilities 1971*, DHEW, National Institute of Mental Health, Report Series on Mental Health Statistics, Series B, No. 5.
7. Redick, *Utilization of Psychiatric Facilities*.
8. Gurgevich, L., Petroni, R.A., and Beigel, A., "Overview of an Evaluation

to Assess the Therapeutic Effectiveness of a Psychiatric Halfway House Program"; Salem, R. and Roth, D., "Evaluation Design for the Columbus Halfway House"; Loeb, A., Vanna, S., and Rutman, I.D., "Focus on Long-Term Follow-Up: A Critical Step in Program Evaluation and Modification"; Papers presented at the National Conference on Evaluation in Alcoholism, Drug Abuse, and Mental Health Programs, Washington, D.C., April 1974.

13 Transitional Housing
Charles R. Orndoff

For the past fifteen to twenty years, the halfway house movement in the United States has shown a dramatic increase—both in numbers and quality of programs. Although the idea is not a new one (in England the approach has been used for many years) there were relatively few halfway houses in this country prior to the early 1950s. Indeed, their direct antecedents appear to be the settlement houses. The idea of providing housing, support, and social orientation for immigrants became readily adaptable to serving the mentally disabled. The needs of both groups are strikingly similar, being primarily those of community adjustment.

The model in greatest use in this country prior to ten years ago was the group home or extended family setting. Usually located in a residential neighborhood, the houses accommodated from five to twenty former patients, offered twenty-four-hour supervision, and provided meals and semiprivate sleeping arrangements. This simple approach was used with very little elaboration or modification.

Though the stated goal was to serve as a halfway step between the institution and community living, in reality the term has been misleading. Too many so-called halfway houses have, in effect, become mini-institutions in the community without effecting the transition implied in their name. Two main factors contribute to this failure: (1) the physical setting does not accurately reflect the kind of independent living arrangements to which the client will eventually return and thus does not lend itself to skill acquisition; and (2) program goals are not truly transitional in nature; residents are placed in the homes with very little planning or programming, few services, and low expectations of their eventual achievement of independent status. In the past ten years, new concepts have been introduced into the housing of former mental patients in the community, giving rise the transitional housing model.

This term is also somewhat misleading. For a significant percentage of the mentally disabled, a complete transition to the community may not be possible. But a greater percentage could make the transition regardless of length of institutionalization or severity of illness if those working in the field were to avoid their historical bias of low expectations and recognize and encourage their client's potential for full independent living. Many have been denied that degree of independence because of a lack of adequate programming resulting in part from the recent rapid developments in public and professional attitudes toward the traditional mental hospital.

The "warehousing" of mental patients in state hospitals is certainly no new phenomenon. The community mental health movement has helped to create a climate of distrust in such former practices, resulting in a perhaps too hasty move on the part of mental health professionals to empty the institutions of all but the most severely disabled. As a result the dumping syndrome has occurred. We appear to have rid ourselves of one evil—the institution, only to create another just as bad—neighborhoods oversaturated with the mentally disabled adrift in an alien environment without adequate housing, health care, or supportive services to aid their adjustment to the community.

In many cases it has been a disservice to discharge these unfortunates from the institution without adequate planning and programming. While this is not intended to imply support of institutionalization in any way—in most cases it is a totally unproductive process—it must be stressed that to initiate deinstitutionalization without an appropriate sequence of planning, programming, and service provision is self-defeating.

Institutionalization is a dehumanizing process where the patient's individuality is lost, his self-concept greatly lowered, and in many cases, his ability to make even the simplest life decisions seriously imparied. With this in mind, the goal of any community residential program must be to reverse the process. To deinstitutionalize people effectively, they must be given the self-confidence needed to enable them to make their own life decisions, build their self-image, and in effect make whole persons of patients.

Goals of Transitional Housing

The type of patient who can best be served in a community residential program depends to a large extent on the type of service offered and the expertise of the staff involved. Length of institutionalization and/or the clinical diagnosis is not a significant variable in the potential for making a successful community adjustment. Most community residential programs that are transitional in nature find the effects of institutionalization more long-standing than the effects of the illness. The psychosis originally diagnosed may have burned itself out years ago, leaving no symptoms, but the disability stemming from chronic institutionalization lingers. If for ten, twenty, or even thirty years a patient has been told what time to get up, what time to go to bed, what time to take his medication, what time to shower, and what time to eat, he becomes utterly dependent. When he moves into a community setting he discovers that he has lost the ability to make even these basic life decisions on his own.

The biggest challenge then facing the staff of a community residential program is dealing with the fear these people have in leaving a totally structured, dependent setting and trying to assume a quasi-normal role in the community.

The fear may manifest itself in many ways—hostility, withdrawal, or acting-out behavior. The staff and the program must confront that basic fear on the part of the patient—the fear that he is going to be ostracized from the community, that he is going to be lost, that he does not, in fact, have the ability to make his own decisions.

Programming in transitional residential facilities sometimes must start with very basic skill training, for instance, locking and unlocking a door; even the simple use of a key is a significant problem for many of the chronically institutionalized. The staff must tailor their community adjustment training to the individual needs of each client; not to do so is perpetuating the institutional system. Starting with the most basic decision-making processes, growth proceeds on a gradual, logically progressive track. One step at a time, the client is encouraged to adjust to the demands community living is placing on him.

The physical setting has a significant role to play in this gradual assumption of responsibility. One of the shortcomings of the traditional halfway house setting has been its inability to provide this gradual growth-producing process. Residents leaving a halfway house and moving into the community too often have experienced separation trauma and anxiety as severe as when they originally left the institution. Obviously, the most successful system of transitional housing would be one that offers settings appropriate for each stage of the growth process, a variety of facilities that offer progressively more freedom and more responsibility as the resident takes each transitional step.

Where most halfway houses have failed is in their assumption of the traditional institutional philosophy. For example, the emphasis on labels. One of the biggest hurdles to be overcome by those formerly hospitalized for mental illness is the label that was attached to them by the treatment system. This diagnostic label, while appropriate to the traditional clinical setting, is a tremendous disadvantage to the person trying to assume a normal role in the community. It is irrelevant to a community residential program, and in many cases can be destructive. It prejudices the way staff members work with a person. In effect, the staff help to perpetuate the label. The diagnosis, whether it be simple schizophrenia, chronic undifferentiated schizophrenia, or an IQ score in no way predicts that person's potential to assume an independent role in the community if adequate community services and programming are available.

This growing rejection of labelling per se is another result of the community mental health movement, and, truly, labels have proved liabilities not only to the client but to the working relationship established with him by staff members. For this reason, many transitional residential programs avoid a clinical diagnosis and instead try to consider only the functional abilities or potentials of their clients. Staff members need some degree of expertise in predicting the adjustment potential of the residents in the program, their ability to stay out of the institution once they have been discharged. Because of the variety of stimuli that bombard the newly released patient, there are no single predictors of success or failure as to his eventual adjustment. Rather, the whole person must be considered—his needs, aptitudes, and strengths—with particular concentration on his healthy characteristics rather those which might be termed sick. The goal of a residential treatment program should be not to deal with the illness but to nurture and develop the well.

The Transitional Services Model

As indicated above, the physical setting has a significant impact on effective service delivery; living facilities must be structured in a logically progressive sequence. One such model, which will be described here, is Transitional Services, Inc. of Buffalo, New York, an example of a graduated series of residential facilities utilizing a trilevel housing plan. The first level of the program is an Evaluation Center, which closely resembles the traditional halfway house. It is an extended family setting with resident counselors available twenty-four hours a day; a cook prepares the meals and professional staff are there during the normal work week and in crisis situations. The Evaluation Center accomplishes two main purposes: (1) to ease the transition from institutional to community living for the most severely regressed and withdrawn patients with which the program is working; and (2) to give the agency a period in which to assess the level of functioning shown by the patient.

The principal difference between this facility and most traditional halfway houses is that the average duration of residence is anticipated to be between one and two months, in order to avoid institutionalization of the client at this level. As rapidly as possible, the agency wants to move the residents of this facility to their second level—the supervised apartment building.

At present the agency operates three supervised apartment buildings. One has twelve units and a capacity for thirty residents; the other two have eight units, each with a capacity of twenty and twenty-two residents. One apartment unit in each building is occupied by resident counselor staff who offer twenty-four-hour supervision and support to the residents. The other units are shared by residents. Two to four residents, sharing an apartment, are responsible for maintaining that living unit completely, with continuous support and supervision from the resident counselor staff. The professional staff work a staggered work schedule covering the period from 9 A.M. to approximately 8 P.M. and are also on call for crisis situations.

After an indeterminate period at the second level, the resident is moved to the third level—the independent apartment program. (There are no rigid time limits on the length of stay at each level, it depends on each resident's individual adjustment. An attitude of movement is constantly stressed from the first day the client moves into the program until he leaves). The third level utilizes a number of independent apartment units scattered throughout the community.

Usually four residents share a two-bedroom apartment, taking full responsibility
for maintenance, meals, etc. There is no twenty-four-hour supervision at this
level; a staff unit visits the apartments possibly once a week or as often as twice
a day depending on the individual needs of each living group.

The emphasis on this final phase of the program is to approximate living
in the community completely independently. Agency staff feel that they should
gradually withdraw services at this level and make the client more independently
responsible for his own life decisions. Although there is no twenty-four-hour
supervision, there is a twenty-four-hour on-call phone system, so that residents
can receive assistance at any time.

From the independent apartment level residents move on their own into
the community and a significant percentage of staff time and effort goes into
trying to find them adequate housing. Once a person has moved on his own
into the community the agency provides follow-up services for a period of six
months. Subsequently, there is no planned follow-up but the agency does try
to respond to crisis situations involving former consumers of the service as
they arise.

Operating Procedures

The intake staff at this time consists of three full-time professionals. They
act primarily in a liaison relationship between the referral sources and the agency
itself. Their job is to screen potential applicants for the program and to coordinate their entry into the program. The intake staff is geared to look at
strengths, not weaknesses, and to assess an applicant's potential regardless of
his diagnostic label. At the point of intake, a Resident Program Chart is completed by the intake worker. This chart follows the client through the program
with each individual staff member making entries as appropriate. The intake
worker attempts initially to assess the client's functional abilities in each of ten
areas: environmental skills; personal hygiene; daily grooming; medication;
money; mobility; cooking; nutrition; motivation; and communication skills.
This initial assessment determines at which level the client will be placed.

Each client is rated weekly by a counselor on a zero through five scale for
each of the above categories—five being mastery of that particular area. The
agency feels that mastery of these survival skills is essential for every resident
of the program prior to their moving into the community on a completely
independent basis.

The agency draws its staff from various disciplines but job descriptions are
of a generic nature. All staff members are called counselors regardless of their
professional background, training, and/or experience. Because of the generalist
nature of the service provided: that is, community adjustment, it is important
for staff members to be able to assume the generalist role. Services provided

include a variety of community adjustment exercises, for example, personal adjustment counseling, mobility training, work with budgeting, job procruement, interpersonal relationships, and the complete area of home mangement training. This last segment is handled by a group of home economists who are the only "specialists" on the staff.

One of the major functions staff members perform is an advocacy role, helping the client obtain needed services from other specialized agencies and institutions in the mental health system. These services include a medical/psychiatric follow-up, usually obtained from the referral source. The agency feels that establishing these vital links while the person resides in the residential program helps bridge the gap when he leaves to move on to independent community living. One of the keys to the program's success is the cooperation shown by referral sources in terms of referring and backup support. With the referral source or some other community agency providing medical/psychiatric support the agency is able to concentrate on skill training to a greater degree, thus keeping the program from developing into a medical model. The agency does employ consultant services as needed.

This is a high expectation program not only for the clients but also for the staff. The pervading emphasis on movement out towards independent living is a strong motivating force for both elements to make the concept work. Over its two years of existence, the agency has had a success rate of approximately 85 percent placement and stabilization in the community. At present, it operates at a capacity of close to 165 persons in the three different levels of the program.

Handling Community Resistance

In the wake of national trends towards increased residential living programs, many communities have become alarmed at the influx of mentally disordered people in their midst. In part this is the fault of the mental health system for not providing adequate services and, in effect, oversaturating particular areas. Community resistance can be extremely detrimental to any program attempting to move people back into the mainstream of society. Certain considerations should be taken into account before any community residential program is attempted.

The socioeconomic makeup of a neighborhood, as well as the way in which a program is administered, all have direct effects on its success. The kind of community most adaptable to phasing people back into the mainstream is one that has a balanced socioeconomic mix and a highly transient nature. However, even this type of neighborhood has a saturation point and any program should be aware of this. Great care must be taken that even the most ideal neighborhoods not get "turned off" by the influx of residents connected with transitional housing facilities.

In their book, *The Halfway House Movement—A Search for Sanity*,[1] Raush and Raush point out two alternatives for administrators preparing to move a residential program into a community: (1) conduct a public education promotion program to prepare the neighbors for what is coming; (2) move quietly into the community and handle public resistance later. Although the former may seem the most logical approach, experience has shown that it meets with limited success. It may be possible to interpret the program effectively to a majority of residents in the area but there will still be a highly vocal minority who will be strongly opposed to the program when it opens. Moreover, if one of the goals of a community residential program is to minimize labeling, to broadcast your intention to open a residential program for the mentally disordered seems to be perpetuating the label.

The Transitional Services program of Buffalo, which assumed a posture of moving into a neighborhood and handling the resistance later, opened their first facility and were in operation for eight months before there was any local resistance. Even that was a minor incident and was handled in a relatively swift manner with no ultimate harm done to the program. A community adjustment program must assume as low a profile as possible in any location. At all costs it must try and avoid publicity, especially the kind that publicizes addresses and emphasizes the type of clientele being served.

One especially effective technique in handling community resistance is to invite the protesting neighbor to come in and see the program work, and meet with staff members in order to get a full, concise picture. In some cases, people who have initially resisted a program later become advocates of the service and sometimes even volunteers. The key to handling community resistance is to take each complaint on an individual basis; even the most trivial must be attended to and disposed of. If each case is not dealt with quickly and efficiently a snowballing effect can take place and the resistance, instead of dissipating, can grow to destructive proportions.

As briefly mentioned earlier, the ideal community for a transitional residential program is a highly transient, mixed socioeconomic area with, if possible, a mixture of residential and commercial property. Real estate acquisition has been a problem for some programs. Facilities have been purchased in marginal neighborhoods that two or three years later have deteriorated, burdening the program with structures in the wrong part of a town. A more reasonable approach is to lease all real estate on a one to five year lease with renewal options. This gives an agency the flexibility to leave a neighborhood that may not be conducive to accomplishing its goals. Although some landlords are not particularly supportive of the movement, a private agency leasing facilities has certain advantages to offer that make them desirable tenants: (1) the rental is steady, amounting to guaranteed income for the landlord, who does not have to worry about vacancy and loss rate; (2) the agency is able to lease the building as a whole and provide minor maintenance of the facilities, which again is an economic advantage to a landlord.

Zoning, particularly restrictive zoning, has also been a problem for some agencies. There have been cases where facilities were purchased or leased in areas zoned to prohibit the operation of transitional housing programs. Zoning ordinances should be carefully checked before leasing or puchasing agreements are entered into. Obtaining a variance from the local zoning board may be difficult and will most certainly raise the visibility of the program, and thus is not recommended.

Fiscal negotiations are important for any program. In most cases an agency or lessor will have to pay at least fair market value and in some cases in excess of fair market price for properties to be used in such programs. There are all kinds of landlords with motivations varying from altrustic to materialistic. It is fortunate when an agency encounters a civic-minded property owner who is willing to lease to a nonprofit agency for a small margin of profit through understanding the program's goals and the long-term positive results it will have for the community.

Staff Considerations

The staff of a residential program differ in many essential ways from the traditional mental health professional. More importance is given to a generalist philosophy and role in comparison to the specialized training which has hitherto been required. Many professionals who have had prior experience in traditional psychiatric settings feel uncomfortable in the more informal atmosphere of the transitional program and are unable to adapt to the generic model. Younger staff who have just received their degrees have more to offer in this type of setting. They are not so dismayed by the bureaucratic strictures under which they must work, or by the chronicity of the clientele. They bring to the program a considerable measure of enthusiasm and energy, obviously needed in such a setting, although they may lack experience. One obvious advantage, from an administrative standpoint, in hiring younger staff is that it becomes unnecessary to untrain them in the traditional ways of viewing the mentally disabled.

Other key staff members in a residential program are the live-in resident counselors. These persons have, in essence, the most difficult job in the program. Certain kinds of strengths are needed rather than particular academic skills and training: the ability to relate to people as people and be willing to dedicate a major portion of their waking hours to the rehabilitation process. Experience has shown that on the whole untrained people are best in this role. They do not have the traditional stereotyped ideas of the mentally ill in terms of their limitations or capabilities. It is essential, if the residential program is to be a mirror of the community, that these key resident counselors be able to relate to the residents in the program as people who are assuming a normal role in the community rather than as clients or patients.

At present there appears to be no training program that adequately pre-pares good resident counselors. On-the-job training and in-service training seminars run by the agency itself have been found most effective in increasing the competence of the resident counselor staff. Human qualities such as patience, warmth, understanding, empathy, and the ability to relate to people have been found more desirable qualifications than academic training. Experience has also shown that having the staff spend 100 percent of its time in the facility is not the ideal situation. A five day week, with two days off, is more conducive to overall program goals. Resident counselors need to get completely away from the facility and its clientele for at least two days a week to allow them to renew their dedication and insure their efficiency. This system is also sounder, thera-peutically, for the residents. By forcing them to identify and relate to different counselors two days a week the dependency syndrome is reduced.

Age considerations are also a factor. We have found that the person over thirty-five has more to offer in terms of life experience for this job. Some pro-grams have experimented with using graduate students as resident counselors, and although advantageous in some respects this policy tends to perpetuate the traditional treatment approach as opposed to the interpersonal benefits implied in the generic model.

In this type of program, where the degree of success depends primarily on the individual nature of the service, the size of the program is obviously a key factor. The optimum size for a residential program of the kind described here is probably between 175 and 250. To run a program any larger than this necessitates administrative controls that may, in effect, decrease the quality of the service. It then takes on an institutional character which is the direct antithesis of the environment we are attempting to create.

Funding Considerations

Residential programs in most cases should be performance contract funded (unit cost funded) for program costs. The unit cost on a daily basis depends on the richness of the staffing pattern. An adequate staffing pattern for the kind of program described here would be one counselor and one home eco-nomist for every twenty residents. In addition, support personnel such as resi-dent counselors, supervisors, administrative/clerical staff are needed. For an adequately staffed program, the daily unit cost should be in the vicinity of $11 per day. Compared to institutional care, the costs for this program are rela-tively low.

Real estate costs can be offset by the rent charged to residents. This method is convenient for existing programs, but with new programs deficit funding may be necessary. Performance contracting does not allow for start-up costs prior to the first residents being placed. Local funding sources should be consulted prior to any detailed planning. In most cases, the local tax base must support a large part of the cost of this kind of program. For this to happen, the mental health community must be convinced that a community-based system of service is better than an institutional base. Most institutional programs are funded by state monies and have very little if any effect on the local tax structure. Third party payments may also have some effect on reducing the amount of local monies that must be contributed.

The unique aspect of a residential treatment program is the prime role of real estate; in effect, it is "real estate therapy." The movement toward residential facilities in the community is growing steadily across the country, as another paper in this section documents. The rationale and the philosophy creating the impetus are laudable; however, caution must be urged. Without proper planning and implementation the backlash created by this movement can have catastrophic effects on the community mental health system. Only with systematic prior investigation and enlightened direction can the residential facility movement succeed in reducing the patient load of inpatient facilities and preventing inappropriate hospitalization.

Note

1.   Harold L. Raush and Charlotte L. Raush, *The Halfway House Movement: A Search for Sanity,* New York: Appleton, 1968.

Part IV
Internal Pressures for Change

Introduction to Part IV

The history of medicine for the past 150 years is impressively highlighted with major advances in the treatment and prevention of disease. Generally, mental health has not shared in this dramatic progress. However, many professionals now feel that there is a strong prospect for improving the bleak record of mental health. This optimism is based on the belief in the new social therapies, a community-based health delivery system, and the use of behavior-controlling drugs. The social therapies were first introduced during World War II. As a result of wartime demands for resources, especially personnel, it was necessary to "make do" with patients performing tasks traditionally performed by staff. Dramatic improvement in the behavior of patients was noted when they were required to be more self-reliant. There was little in the mental health literature of that day to warrant this approach to the mentally ill; it was a wartime necessity.

Traditionally, it was assumed that while the specific causes of the different forms of mental illness were not known, they had a biophysical origin. Such a view is not without merit when one considers that before the introduction of penicillin, syphilis was one of the major causes of mental illness. However, if one does assume that an unidentified agent, or agents, is the cause of a disease, it follows that there is little that can be done to reverse the basic disease process in those affilicted until the causal agent is identified. How can one be expected to actively intervene when the cause is still a mystery? Humane custodial care of the afflicted becomes a reasonable option.

With the increased use of social therapies after World War II, numerous reports began to appear in the literature which showed that many of the well-established symptoms of the various types of mental illness as seen in institutions were, in fact, not symptoms of mental illness at all, but rather a result of institutionalization—iatrogenic disease.

At about the same time that social therapies were gaining wide acceptance, new behavior-controlling drugs with the potential for eliminating many of the more bizarre forms of behavior were introduced. Thus, for the first time in well over 100 years, mental health professionals were faced with the real prospect of making major advances in the treatment of the mentally ill.

A major question facing mental health professionals and policy makers in the early 1960s was how to incorporate this new knowledge into a mental health care delivery system. In the United States, the decision was made at the national level that this would be accomplished through community mental health centers

233

(CMHCs). These were to be new facilities, located in communities throughout the country, each serving a relatively small population limited geographically. This legislation has provided major financial incentives to state and local governments to develop these totally new institutions for the implementation of community approaches.

At the time the legislation was passed, it was already widely recognized that there would be no continuing need for large custodial institutions. However, the legislation does not suggest an alternate role for state hospitals, nor does it suggest how state hospitals are to relate to the new community mental health centers. In fact, the new legislation largely ignores state hospitals altogether, even though they are the single largest provider of mental health care in the United States. Rather than viewing state hospitals as a reservoir of ready-trained personnel, or as established mechanisms for the administrative implementation of the new mental health approaches, the legislation—by omission implied that state hospitals were suitable only for custodial care.

Although the basic theory underlying community mental health centers preceded the legislation by a full decade, community approaches are now so closely associated with CMHCs in the view of many professionals and the general public that they are seen as synonymous. It may be peculiarly American to assume that new ideas require new institutions for their implementation. In any case, the message of the federal legislation is clear—it is the responsibility of the CMHCs to provide mental health care using the community approaches, not that of the state hospitals. Understandably, to whatever degree state hospitals now adapt to the new community approaches it is seen as something done in imitation of CHMCs rather than as part of the "natural" evolution of state hospitals.

The link between custodial care and state hospitals is now so firmly fixed in the minds of many that not infrequently the question of the future role of the state hospital becomes the question of whether or not there will continue to be a need for large custodial care institutions in the future.

That state hospitals and custodial care are inseparably linked in dramatically demonstrated by Ethel Bonn in Chapter 14, as she reviews the history and present status of the Fort Logan Mental Health Center. Fort Logan has long been nationally recognized as a model mental health facility. Built at a time when it was already acknowledged that custodial care facilities no longer needed to be emphasized, it adapted its programs and trained its staff to provide a mix of community and residential programs. However, today its continued support is in doubt, and the staff of Fort Logan is being seriously questioned by the state legislature and local CHMCs as to whether it is appropriate for it to offer community outreach programs.

The profound impact of the community mental health center legislation and the wide acceptance of the new treatment approaches by professionals and public alike required the states to change their mental health delivery systems. The first state to attempt a total community approach to mental health care was California. Dr. William Beach played a major role in developing the California plan and implementing it in its early stages. In Chapter 15 he describes how the plan was developed and how problems encountered in the legislative arena were met.

The California plan calls for a shifting of basic responsibility for the mentally ill from the state level of government to the county level. The counties were accustomed to relying on the state government to care for their mentally ill citizens. It was necessary for each county, therefore, to face the task of identifying local needs and developing programs to meet them. Dr. Ernest Klatte describes how Orange County, California, met this task (Chapter 16). He gives a detailed account of the administrative structure the county developed for this purpose and discusses the effects of the county's utilization of state facilities in the early stages of the program. In 1972-73, Orange County negotiated an agreement with the state as a result of which the county agreed to discontinue the use of state hospitals altogether. This agreement had far-reaching immediate effects, including the substantial increase in total cost for mental health services in Orange County. The reasons for this phenomenon are examined by Dr. Klatte and will be of interest to those now considering county-based mental health programs.

Building on the California experience, New York State has recently enacted a unified services act. Through financial incentives, this legislation encourages counties to assume primary responsibility for service to their mentally disabled citizens. In Chapter 17 Mr. Hyman Forstenzer, consultant to the New York State system, and Dr. Alan Miller, commissioner of mental hygiene for New York, provide detailed descriptions of the legislation and its intent. Two options provided in the unified services legislation are of particular interest. One provides for counties, participating in the unified services plan, to assume control of state facilities within their boundaries. This feature permits counties to determine how state hospitals and state schools for the retarded might best be utilized to meet local needs. The second feature relates to the funding incentives under the legislation.

In the early version of the California plan, each county was eligible for a certain amount of state reimbursement for mental health services based on the percentage of the total cost to the county. It was recognized in New York that such a plan might not create the desired financial incentive for rural counties that now make relatively small financial contributions to their mental health programs, relying instead on state facilities in the vicinity to provide such care. At the same time, a system that would provide reimbursement for a fixed percentage of the cost would give undue advantage to large metropolitan counties that already have highly developed programs, now reimbursed at only the 50 percent level. In order to provide the necessary incentives to rural counties to join in the unified services plan without giving undue advantages to the large metropolitan areas in New York State, a system was devised through

which the state reimbursement to counties choosing the unified services option
was based on the combination of population and the amount of money committed by each county.

In Chapter 18 Dr. John Talbott provides a picture of the demands made
on a metropolitan state hospital in New York, attempting to gear up for the
unified approach to delivery of service. He describes the intricacies of administering a facility serving multiple catchment areas, both with and without
community mental health centers, while at the same time trying to respond
to the demands made from within the New York State Department of Mental
Hygiene.

A major problem facing state hospitals, in part as a result of the federal
community mental health centers legislation, is that they are viewed only as
physical plants, too frequently located in isolated rural areas. They are not
often enough viewed as a configuration of service providers capable of mounting a community program.

Perhaps the most stereotyped view of the state hospital is that of a large
custodial institution located in a small rural community. In Chapter 19
Dr. Roger Mesmer, director of Warren State Hospital, in Warren, Pennsylvania,
demonstrates how a state hospital in such a rural setting can be adapted to
provide an active community-based treatment program for a large rural population. He demonstrates how the state hospital has been used to provide community programs in many small rural communities that might otherwise be
totally without mental health services. Of particular interest is the heavy
use the Warren State program has made of volunteers within each town and the
dedication of these volunteers to the programs.

In Chapter 20 Carl A. Taube and Richard W. Redick of the NIMH Division
of Biometry, look at the utilization of mental health facilities since the advent
of the out-of-hospital care trend in mental health. Their report shows an
increase in the number of episodes of mental illness being treated since the
introduction of this new approach. There is also a dramatic increase in the
use of general hospitals for inpatient psychiatric care. Generally, it appears
that outpatient treatment for mental illness is preferred over inpatient care,
with the switch from inpatient to outpatient care being particularly marked
in the treatment of those over age sixty-five. Their report also shows an
increase in the number of younger people seeking mental health care as compared to 1966. It is not yet clear whether this is a reflection of the drug culture
of the early 1970s, or if it will be a continuing trend that will require a shift
in program emphasis.

In Chapter 21 Dr. Jonathon Cole shares the pressures experienced by the
director of a large state hospital as he attempts to respond to the various forces
demanding change. The doubt now common among state legislators as to
whether or not state hospitals should continue to be funded are translated into
program effects by Dr. Cole. Not only must the state hospital director redirect

his basic program, he must do so with reduced budgets and archaic buildings while responding to public demands for better service in more areas. The public shows little recognition of the conditions under which a state hospital director must perform. In addition to being an excellent review of the many pressures faced by directors of state hospitals, Dr. Cole's account is warmly personal.

The response that has been made in the United States to the new directions set for mental health may be unique to this country. In France, rather than attempting to implement the new community approaches by creating a second mental health system in competition with the existent system, they have chosen to convert the established mechanism to the new community approaches. In Chapter 22 Dr. Gittelman et al. review the success of the French effort to redirect the established mental health delivery system. The reader is given the opportunity to compare the benefits and liabilities of the French approach of trying to redirect a large bureaucracy with the American approach of creating an entirely new system which is then left to "fight it out" with the established one.

There is a tendency for mental health professionals to assume that the merit of the new community approaches is self-evident and that they are therefore being implemented universally. Dr. Jimmie Holland, in Chapter 23, describes the system of care for the mentally ill used in the USSR. Dr. Holland, for reasons she explains, was afforded a unique opportunity to work in the Soviet system for the better part of a year. Mental health professionals in the USSR are much more organically oriented in their view of mental illness, a bias reflected in their classification of mental disorders. Some indication of how this organic view of mental illness effects treatment programs is illustrated in Dr. Holland's chapter.

14

Evolution of a Modern State Hospital: The Fort Logan Mental Health Center Experience

Ethel M. Bonn, Paul R. Binner,
and *Helen M. Huber*

In the late 1950s there was growing awareness in Colorado that conditions in the public mental health system had reached a crisis point. The state's total population was approaching two million. To serve it, a single state mental hospital (located at Pueblo) had become overburdened with more than 6,000 patients, more than half of whom had been in residence for over ten years. Patients continued to be admitted—often under court order. Only small numbers of patients left the hospital.

A campaign of publicity about conditions at the state hospital was waged by the Mental Health Association and other groups. The governor and legislature brought in consultants to study the problems and make recommendations for reform. The consultants recommended that (1) a new state hospital, embodying modern concepts of treatment, should be established in Metropolitan Denver to serve that population center of the state, and (2) a reorganization of the Colorado State Hospital at Pueblo, with the necessary additional funding, was needed in order to convert the Colorado State Hospital programs from custodial to actively therapeutic.

The state hospital for Metropolitan Denver was located at Fort Logan on the grounds of a former Army cavalry post. Some of the old buildings were retained, while many were razed; some new buildings were constructed. The planning group proposed to the legislature that if sufficient numbers of trained staff were provided, a minimum number of buildings would be needed, thus saving millions of dollars in construction and maintenance costs. Because an active treatment program could be instituted, with shorter lengths of stay and successful return of the vast majority of patients to the community, the number of twenty-four-hour-care beds needed would be less than the 3,500 ordinarily planned for such a facility to serve a population of 1,000,000. The planners proposed 379 total beds, to provide treatment services for all age groups with the major mental illnesses. Thus, over $25,000,000 in construction costs, plus additional millions for maintenance and staffing were saved.

The planners of Fort Logan created a system of transitional forms of treatment providing continuity of care and relationships from maximum intensity to minimum intensity. To meet the needs of the patients, there would be inpatient, day patient (also evening and night patient), halfway houses, family care, and outpatient follow-up statuses available to each of a number of administratively and geographically decentralized teams to use in providing entry and exit for patients. All patients applying for admission would be evaluated clinically prior to admission. Admission and treatment or referral elsewhere would be planned by the teams. Thus, Fort Logan Mental Health Center's treatment resources would be utilized for treatment and not simply utilized for persons requiring social and economic assistance. The exit system for patients would depend heavily on continuing supportive relationships with center staff, the patient's family, friends, etc., the use of sheltered workshops, sheltered living situations (cooperative apartments, family care, group foster homes, and nursing homes), and other rehabilitation opportunities.

To carry out modern concepts of community-oriented and community-based treatment, the new facility would be based on new knowledges from the social sciences about institutions and their inhabitants; use of the open hospital and group approaches; and use of the psychotropic drugs. World War II had spurred awareness of the need for better treatment of the mentally ill and better training of practitioners in the field of mental health. Publication of the Report of the Joint Commission on Mental Health and Mental Illness[1] in 1961 provided a series of recommendations for public mental hospitals, all of which came to fruition at the Fort Logan Mental Health Center except for one, a chronic disease hospital.

To help the new state hospital get started, massive transfer of the long-term Metropolitan Denver patients, then at the state hospital at Pueblo, was ruled out. The new state hospital was named Fort Logan Mental Health Center, not "state hospital," as a way to distinguish it from a "traditional" state hospital.

Fort Logan Mental Health Center opened its doors to patients in July, 1961. First day hospital and later inpatient services for adult psychiatric patients (age eighteen and up) were started. The alcoholism division opened in September 1961. By 1963 Fort Logan began to receive many visitors, the number increasing when it was named one of eleven "model mental health centers" by the Joint Information Service of the American Psychiatric Association and National Association for Mental Health.[2] The National Institutes of Mental Health awarded Fort Logan a grant for a full-time staff member to accommodate the large numbers of professionals who would want to visit Fort Logan. In 1964 the APA awarded Fort Logan Mental Health Center its Hospital Achievement Award for "imaginative uses of partial hospitalization." Visitors, professional and nonprofessional, totalling 3,000 to 5,000 per year, have continued to come from all over the world.

In 1964 and 1965 a Children's Psychiatric Division and a Medical-Geriatrics Division was established. The total number of children's treatment units needed has been four, instead of the planned six, and the Geriatrics Division has required only two teams, instead of the planned three. The inpatient medical unit proved to be underutilized and was discontinued in 1967. A medical consultation capability for specialized examinations and treatment, mostly on an outpatient basis, and the use of other hospitals for medical and surgical treatment beyond our capability, proved adequate. Only ten, not the fourteen originally planned adult psychiatric teams were established.

A crisis intervention unit was established in 1967 and discontinued in 1971, its functions being assumed by local community mental health centers when Fort Logan Mental Health Center's funding was reduced. At the same time one of the Children's Division teams was reduced in size and its treatment program changed from residential inpatient to home treatment of children and their families. The reduction in funding in 1971 for Fort Logan reflected a growing trend to fund with state moneys the community mental health centers in metropolitan Denver and the rest of the state. Meanwhile in 1969 an Adolescent Division had been established at Fort Logan Mental Health Center and a closed unit (for runaway delinquents and predelinquents) was established three years later at a nearby institution. The needs for public sector psychiatric services for adolescents far exceed the capacities of these two units. Requests for funding for additional capability for adolescents have been turned down but will be resubmitted again in the coming year.

In 1973 and 1974 the legislature discontinued certain adult psychiatric services at Fort Logan and transferred them, along with funds that provided not only those direct services but also administrative and supportive services. This resulted in a weakening of the program base for the remaining services. The long-term patient and those under court orders remained the continuing responsibility of Fort Logan. The shift in funding from state hospitals to community mental health centers seen in other parts of the country was being repeated in Colorado.

Fort Logan is one of at least forty-three new state hospitals that have been opened in the United States since the 1961 Report of the Joint Commission on Mental Health and Mental Illness. While a number of facilities have developed along similar lines, no other single facility has embodied the same features as this modern state hospital.

The following sections will review some of the evidence of how the program has worked, what its cost picture has been, and why we think the program is currently contracting and not expanding, nor being sustained at its maximum level. Much of what we have to report is still unfolding and only future reports will be able to provide an historical perspective on these events.

Evaluation of the Program

The Fort Logan program was built on a series of assumptions and hopes that were appealing and logically compelling to its founders, but had not previously been put together into a single, viable program. Certainly, there were many misgivings among the members of the mental health establishment at the time of its opening.

Foremost in the minds of many was the question, "How well will it work?" In this section, we will review some of the answers to that question over the thirteen years of the center's operation. These answers cover the general topics of (1) the patient population served, (2) the ability to return people to the community, and (3) the ability to help patients improve.

The Patient Population Served

One of the main questions in the minds of many as the plans for the center crystallized was, "Can such a state hospital treat the full range of patients?" The question was a natural one in view of the plans for a completely open setting within a heavily populated major metropolitan area. Concerns about patients "escaping" or causing commotion in the neighborhood were common. There were questions about the staff's ability to control disturbed patients within the program. No one knew how far the concept of a completely open setting with controls based mainly on adequate staffing levels, the proper use of drugs, and the social pressures generated by the patient group could be extended.

The design and intent of the program was to treat the full range of patients needing state hospital services. A group clearly excluded from these services were those mentally ill individuals who had committed crimes that required their incarceration in a locked correctional facility. These people continued to be served at the Forensic Unit of the Colorado State Hospital at Pueblo.

This is an important exclusion, since it was part of the effort to change the identification of a state hospital from "a place where troublesome people are locked up" to "a place where people receive help for their problems." It is, after all, no more appropriate to identify all the patients seeking mental health help as people needing to be locked up than it would be to identify patients in a general hospital that way. A similarly small percentage of people who need help with mental and physical problems also engage in dangerous criminal activity. They are locked up because society believes this is the most desirable manner in which to control such criminal activity. They are not locked up because they have a mental or a physical problem.

The traditional identification of state hospitals as places where dangerous or troublesome mental patients are locked up is a very unfortunate one. It is greatly and unjustly damaging to the public image of the patient seeking help in such a facility as well as to the patient's already uncertain self-image. We felt it was a major step forward to separate the correctional incarceration function from the mental health function.

This still left open the unanswered question of those patients who might be regarded as "too disturbed" to function in an open setting. The experience of the center indicates that in a setting with adequate numbers of staff who are well-trained, the percentage of patients who fall into this class is very small.

Over the past thirteen years of operation, we estimate that less than 1 percent
of the patients admitted each year have been referred from Fort Logan to a
locked facility. Many of these cases stayed in these locked facilities only
short periods before they were returned to an open program at the center or
elsewhere.

From our experience, it seems a much wiser policy to build the program
that suits the vast majority of patients and to provide some "safety valves" for
the few extreme cases than to characterize the entire population as violent,
uncontrolled, or in need of locked facilities. The amount of damage saved for
the vast majority of patients is enormous.

The center's success in dealing with a state hospital population with minimal
use of physical restraint has sometimes led to the conclusion that the patient
population is not representative of a "true" state hospital population. This
conclusion is contradicted by several lines of evidence.

First, a substantial proportion of the patients receiving services at Fort
Logan have been judged seriously enough disturbed in the past to need inpatient
services. Many of these have been in locked wards. For instance, for the years
1961-62 through 1972-73, 79 percent of the admissions to the Adult Psychiatry
Division had been inpatients elsewhere prior to admission.

Second, the diagnostic composition of the patients admitted is comparable
to those reported for admissions to state and county hospitals by the National
Institutes of Mental Health. In 1969-70 Fort Logan admitted 24.4 percent with
psychotic diagnoses, 14.3 percent neurotic, 10.1 percent personality disorders,
37 percent alcoholism, and 14.2 percent all other diagnoses. Admissions to
state and county hospitals for the same year were 34.3 percent psychotic, 8.5
percent neurotic. 7.4 percent personality disorders, 25.7 percent alcoholism,
and 24.1 percent all others.[3]

Finally, the organization of mental health services in the state is such that
patients from the Denver metropolitan area requiring state hospital services
are virtually all referred to Fort Logan. With the few exceptions already mentioned, the center serves the wide range of mental health problems ordinarily
seen in a large metropolitan area. A comparison of the ethnic characteristics
of the patient population and the metropolitan area population also tends
to indicate that the population served is representative of the base population.
The center admits 78.5 percent whites, 5.8 percent blacks, 12.3 percent
Chicanos, and 3.3. percent others. The 1970 census figures for the Denver
metropolitan population are 83.2 percent white, 4.1 percent blacks, 11.3
percent Chicanos, and 1.4 percent others.

The Ability to Return People to the Community

The center's main goal for its patients is to assist them with their problems
as much as possible in order to help them return to living in the community as

independently as possible. The center's ability to meet this goal has been evaluated from a number of vantage points over the years.

First, each patient upon discharge from the center's program is evaluated by a clinical staff member on that treatment unit as to improvement in nine areas of functioning, as well as an overall judgment of improvement. Table 14-1 summarizes the findings based on the judgments of overall improvement for discharges from the center from 1965-73.

Over all these years, an average of 84 percent of the patients discharged have been rated as improved at the time of their discharge. It should be noted that this rating does not refer only to improvement in an inpatient setting but is based on the patient's ability to function in a variety of partial hospitalization statuses or as an outpatient in many cases. As such, it is a much more broadly based rating than the more commonly reported improvement within an inpatient state hospital setting.

Admittedly, ratings provided only by the treatment staff could be suspect of a positive or self-serving bias. However, independent ratings of improvement obtained from community members and patients both tend to support the positive results reported by the staff.[4] More important, there is also evidence that the improvement seen at the time of discharge persists over time. Follow-up studies, using a variety of methods, have indicated that the patients discharged from Fort Logan continue to show improved functioning six months to a year after discharge.[a] These follow-up studies support the clinician's impression that

---

[a]The studies, most of which are unpublished research reports and papers generated by the Ft. Logan professional staff, include the following: Impact Indicators Report (tables showing impact of FLMHC programs), October 1973; Wanberg, K. Treatment Impact for Alcoholism Programs, FLMHC working paper, September 1973; Esty, J.A. and Briggs, B. A Follow-up Study of Children Discharged from Children's Division—July 1, 1972 to June 30, 1973, Unpublished manuscript, 1974; Christopher, B. and Esty, J.A. Follow-up Study of Children Discharged from Children's Division—July 1, 1971 to June 30, 1972, Unpublished manuscript, 1973; Esty, J.A. and Christopher, B. A Follow-up Study of Children Discharged from Children's Division—July 1, 1969 to June 30, 1971, Unpublished manuscript, 1973; Keepers, T.D. Follow-up Study of Children Discharged from the Rene' A. Spitz Children's Division of the Fort Logan Mental Health Center—January 1, 1968 to June 30, 1968, Unpublished manuscript, 1969; Keepers, T.D. Lives in Progress: A Follow-up Study of Children Discharged from the Rene' A. Spitz Children's Division of the Fort Logan Mental Health Center—July 1, 1968 to June 30, 1969, Unpublished manuscript, October 1971; Brittain, J. Community Informant Method: Part I, II, and III, FLMHC research reports, 1964-65; Berry K.L. Community Respondent Method: Part IV. FLMHC research report, 1966; Gordon, H.G. The Measurement of Treatment Impact on Patients of a Comprehensive Mental Health Center. Presented at Rocky Mountain Psychological Association Convention, Denver, May 1974; Gordon, H.G. Employment of Patients after Hospitalization at Fort Logan Mental Health Center and at Other Hospitals, FLMHC research report, December 1973; Gordon, H.G. Response to Treatment at Time of Discharge and Readmission Rate, FLMHC research report, February 1973; Gordon, H.G. Evaluation of the Community Informant Method, Part I. FLMHC research report, October 1971; Gordon, H.G. Percentages of Improved and Regressed Patients among Discharged Patients as Shown by Returned Questionnaires

Table 14-1
Overall Response to Treatment, 1965-73

---

[*] 84% of those discharged from the center were judged as benefiting from treatment at the time of discharge.

91% of those discharged from Children's Division benefited.

86% of those discharged from Adolescent Division benefited.

81% of those discharged from Adult Divisions benefited.

83% of those discharged from Geriatric Division benefited.

86% of those discharged from Alcoholism Division benefited.

---

[*] 1965-73 averaged, except Adolescent Division, which is 1969-73.

patients generally tend to improve in the program and also show that they are usually able to sustain that level of improved functioning.

Another line of evidence that supports the contention that patients are able to maintain their improvement in the community is the center readmission rate. Whereas, it is not uncommon to find readmission rates of 30 to 50 percent in the literature,[5] the center has experienced a readmission rate of only 24.7 percent readmitted within the first year after discharge over the past eleven years. Admittedly, an index such as a readmission rate is an imperfect indicator of successful community functioning.[6] However, when combined with the evidence from the ratings at time of discharge and the follow-up evidence, there is a convergent picture of positive and sustained response to the center's programs.

Perhaps an even more fundamental challenge to a new state hospital than achieving a reasonable rate of improvement for the patients served is to serve them in a way that avoids the inducement of the chronic institutionalization that filled the back wards of so many hospitals across the country.

Fort Logan invoked a number of strategies in attempting to reach this goal. First, by having available within the program a wide variety of partial hospitalization and outpatient options, it minimized the program's dependence on inpatient treatment. Second, by being completely open and accessible to the community, it minimized the development of an institutional culture. And, third, by stressing an active program throughout all its divisions, it attacked the natural tendency of some patients to "settle in" and try to find a home within the confines of the institution.

---

of Community Informants, Part II. FLMHC research report, December 1971; Wanberg, K.W. Pilot Follow-up of Alcoholics, *Journal of the Fort Logan Mental Health Center*, Fall-Winter 1968, Vol 5(2), 101-106; Foster, F., Horn, J., and Wanberg, K. Dimensions of Treatment Outcome: A Factor-Analytic Study of Alcoholics' Responses to a Follow-up Questionnaire. *Quarterly Journal of Studies on Alcohol*, 1972, 33, 1079-1098.

That the center's program achieved the goal of returning patients to the community rapidly is supported by the length of stay patterns over the years. Table 14-2 summarizes the median length of stay of discharged patients over the past twelve years. Note that these length of stay measures cover all enrolled time from admission day until discharge, including inpatient, partial hospitalization, and outpatient status.

Even the very short lengths of stay achieved in the early years of the programs have been progressively shortened for several of the divisions in more recent years as the comprehensive community centers have been able to accept responsibility for much of the outpatient follow-up care.

Even with short median lengths of stay, it is still possible to have some patients who become chronically dependent on the institutions. However, investigation of all the patients admitted to the center from 1961 until 1971 revealed that only 28 or 0.2 of 1 percent met the usual criterion of chronic institutionalism, that is, of two years of continuous inpatient hospitalization. Stated positively, 99.8 percent of the patients admitted had not reached the minimum criterion of chronic institutionalism. Since the program has many options for treatment, we thought the requirement for continuous hospitalization might be understating the case. Therefore, the number of patients who had accumulated two years of inpatient care during the course of a single admission was investigated. Even counting discontinuous inpatient time, only 0.3 of one percent of admissions reached the minimum criterion of chronic institutionalism.

Table 14-2
Median Total Length of Stay (in Days)

	Children's Division	Adolescent Division	Psychiatric Division	Geriatric Division	Alcoholism Division
1961-62			273		41
1962-63			156		64
1963-64			130		50
1964-65	889		160	101	42
1965-66	954		153	156	44
1966-67	533		132	170	44
1967-68	296		147	213	53
1968-69	312		120	173	60
1969-70	201	105	101	175	59
1970-71	283	103	90	146	50
1971-72	189	139	83	170	47
1972-73	207	188	83	174	27

In no sense does this mean that the program has found the cure for the chronically disabled individual. After these individuals have been helped as much as possible by the inpatient or partial hospitalization components of the program, supportive community placements for these individuals are developed. For some, this may mean placement in a family care home or in a group living and working situation. For others, it may mean a nursing home or boarding home, with supportive follow-up visits.

Whatever the vehicle, the goal is to provide the patient with the maximum possible degree of independence, while giving the support needed to maintain an acceptable level of adjustment in the community. These continued care situations hold great promise for avoiding many of the negative results of institutional care. However, as has been reported,[7] they also hold great danger for becoming the back ward simply moved to the community. One of the next great challenges in the evolution of mental health services is the development of truly constructive placements in the community for patients needing extended periods of support. Because of their relative invisibility, such services must be regularly monitored and supported in order to avoid the creation of a new generation of neglected and debilitated patients.

In summary, we think the answer to the question, "How well did Fort Logan work?" is that it worked very well indeed. It was able to handle all but a very small percentage of those patients ordinarily seeking state hospital treatment. It was able to treat them rapidly and effectively and return most of them to adequate community living. And, perhaps most important of all, it was able to provide these services without allowing chronic institutional dependence to develop in all but a fraction of one percent of the clients served.

We recognize full well that much progress is still needed in the treatment of the kind of clients ordinarily seen in a state hospital. We believe our experience has shown that an effective job of helping these clients, while avoiding the danger of institutional dependence, can be done even within the limitations of our current state of knowledge. One of the major challenges now facing state hospitals and the comprehensive community centers is the development of truly constructive and supportive community placements for those clients who continue to need some degree of support in order to maintain an adequate adjustment in the community. Failure to do so can only lead to another version of the back ward tragedy. Even within the limitations of our current knowledge, provision of constructive supportive placement seems well within our grasp. Most important, we need to maintain a sense of urgency that the task must be done. We cannot allow the apathy and lack of public support that ordinarily occurs when a problem has low visibility to develop.

Assessment of Cost Factors

As has been described, the program must be considered well staffed by state hospital standards. Moreover, the staff has been well trained . This is especially true of the psychiatric technicians or mental health workers who make up a large proportion of the direct treatment staff. Given these considerations, it has been commonly assumed that the program must be very expensive and therefore not suitable as a general model for the state hospital.

This assumption is as incorrect as it is logical. However, in order to demonstrate this fact, it is necessary to discard some of the conventional methods used to measure the cost of programs and to accept other measures as being more relevant. In order to give an adequate understanding of the cost of the Fort Logan program, then, it is useful to first review briefly several measures that should not be used.

Misleading Measures of Program Cost

Perhaps the most common measure for estimating state hospital expense is the cost per day. This is ordinarily computed by dividing the total costs of a given program by the number of treatment days provided. The assumption is that as this cost rises, treatment is getting more expensive and as it falls, treatment is getting less expensive. This may, of course, be true. Equally likely, however, is the possibility that the obvious conclusion is completely false. The truth is that it is impossible to tell from the cost per day alone whether treatment is getting more or less expensive. This is because the cost per day is essentially an installment payment and unless one knows the number of payments to be made, it is impossible to know what the total cost of the service will be.

The distinction between an installment payment and a total cost may not have been critical for analyzing the costs of a state hospital prior to 1950 or 1960, because the bulk of the costs were related to the chronic patient population that was largely destined to spend the rest of its days in that hospital. A relatively small part of total costs were being expended on that part of the population that moved through the hospital and returned to the community. Within that context, the size of the installment payment was a relatively informative number.

In a program dedicated to the active treatment of all its patients, however, the installment payment by itself is not only uninformative, it may be seriously misleading. It becomes misleading if high daily costs are coupled with short lengths of stay, thereby giving a low total cost for a given course of treatment. The more active and intensive a treatment program is, the higher its daily costs tend to be. Thus, the average cost per day tends to be systematically biased against an active treatment program. This is a serious flaw and one that works against the development of a progressive treatment program, if this measure is used to gauge program costs.

A closely related cost factor that is sometimes used is the cost per the average daily attendance (ADA) in an agency. This cost factor tends to give the impression of enormous program costs, since it loads all costs on the average number of patients who attend per day. At the very least, this factor should be divided by either 365 or 252, depending on whether the program is available seven or five days a week, in order to place its magnitude in proper perspective.

It may be tempting to argue that the higher this cost ratio is, the better the program is performing. However, it seems likely that at some point the cost would be so high that program costs have indeed gotten out of hand. Since it is not obvious how that point could be identified, it might be better to avoid using this cost factor altogether and to turn, instead, to a more direct approach to cost monitoring and cost containment.

Useful Measures of Program Cost

One useful measure of program costs is the cost per patient treated during a given time period. By taking into account all patients treated, this cost factor recognizes that costs are generated by all these patients and must be spread across all these patients, whether they are discharged or not. This measure tends to give equal recognition to a program that treats large numbers of patients on an ongoing basis with little turnover as well as a program that treats large numbers of patients through rapid turnover. Before valid interprogram comparisons can be made, of course, it would be necessary to establish the comparability of the programs both in regard to their turnover factor as well as the composition of the patient population treated. The significance of any differences in this cost factor should also be related to the relative effectiveness of the programs compared.

A more stringent measure of program costs is the cost per patient discharged. It is more stringent than the cost per patient treated in that it loads all program costs on the product of the system, the discharged patient. This means that a low turnover program treating many patients but discharging few would have a high cost factor relative to a high turnover program. Whether this cost factor should be given primacy over the cost per patient treated would be determined by management aims and philosophy.

As a cost factor, it is also paradoxical in that the better the program gets, the worse the factor looks. This can be demonstrated in the following simplified illustration of the interaction between admissions (Adm.), length of stay (L.O.S.), average daily attendance (ADA), discharges (Dis.), program costs, and the costs per ADA and per discharge. Assume a program has been running steadily for some time and has the characteristics listed in Table 14-3. The hypothetical example illustrates a program that has 100 admissions a year, an average length of stay of twelve months, which results in an ADA of 100 and 100 discharges

Table 14-3
Interaction Among Admissions, Length of Stay, Average Daily Attendance, Discharges, and Program Costs

	Admission	Length of Stay	Average Daily Attendance	Discharge	Cost	Cost / Average Daily Attendance	Cost / Discharge
Year 1	100	12	100	100	1,000,000	10,000	10,000
Year 2	100	6	50	100	1,000,000	20,000	10,000
Year 3	100	3	25	100	1,000,000	40,000	10,000
Year 4	100	24	200	100	1,000,000	5,000	10,000

each year. In the second year, if the average length of stay is cut in half, this also drops the ADA in half and doubles the cost /ADA. In the third year, the length of stay is again cut in half and the ADA drops again and the cost per ADA again doubles. Note that during all these changes, the program cost and the cost per discharge has held constant. If all other things are equal, treating the patients and returning them to the community more quickly is ordinarily considered desirable. However, the better the program gets in this respect, the worse it looks on the cost/ADA ratio. It is only in the fourth year, when the length of stay is doubled over year one, that the cost/ADA ratio drops. This logic could be extended further, with lifetime stays for all the patients giving the most "favorable" ratio. Either measure, however, seems more useful than the cost per day or cost per ADA reviewed above, in that they take into account both the cost per day and the number of days involved in providing a given service.

How Expensive is Fort Logan?

Now we can return to the question of how expensive Fort Logan is compared to the other state hospitals in the country. Table 14-4 summarizes cost indicators and patient/staff ratios for state and county mental hospitals in the United States and for Fort Logan Mental Health Center for the years 1969-72.

Note that the crude workload measure, the average number of patients attending each day divided by the full-time equivalent staff, (ADA)/(FTE), indicates that Fort Logan is relatively well staffed compared to other state hospitals. For instance, in 1969-70 Fort Logan had only 0.62 patients attending per full-time staff member compared with 1.54 patients attending per full time staff member in other hospitals. This was only 40 percent of the national average. Obviously, the cost per day and the cost per ADA at Fort Logan would be relatively high.

Note, however, that the productivity measures, the number of patients discharged per full-time staff (Dis)/(FTE), and the number served per full-time staff (Served)/(FTE) show quite the reverse picture. That is, Fort Logan staff produced many more discharges and served many more patients per staff member than the average for staff of other hospitals. That is, they had a higher level of productivity, running 159 percent and 137 percent of the national average on the number of patients discharged and the number of patients served per FTE in 1969-70 and even increased their relative productivity in subsequent years.

The impact of this greater productivity is seen in the cost per patient discharged and per patient served. These figures are $2,630 per patient discharged by Fort Logan in 1969-70 as compared with $3,842 for other mental hospitals. That is, Fort Logan's cost per patient discharged was only

Table 14-4
Workload, Productivity, and Cost Indicators: U.S. State and County Mental Health Hospitals[a]—Fort Logan Mental Health Center, 1969-72

	Workload Indicators			Productivity Indicators						Cost Indicators					
	ADA/FTE	ADA/FTE	% U.S. Average	Dis./FTE	Dis./FTE	% U.S. Average	Served/FTE	Served/FTE	% U.S. Average	Expend./Dis.	Expend./Dis.	% U.S. Average	Expend./Served	Expend./Served	% U.S. Average
	US	FL		US	FL		US	FL		US	FL		US	FL	
1969-70	1.54	.62	40	2.17	3.45	159	3.79	5.19	137	3842	2630	68	2204	1746	79
1970-71	1.40	.63	45	2.21	3.80	172	3.70	5.80	157	4064	2610	64	2436	1711	70
1971-72	1.29	.67	52	2.15	3.96	184	3.52	6.20	176	4543	2569	57	2773	1642	59

[a]Source: Statistical Note 40 (1969-70, January 1971), Note 60 (1970-71, January 1972), Note 77 (1971-72, March 1973), Survey and Reports Section, Biometry Branch, NIMH.

68 percent of the national average. The cost per patient served was only 79 percent of the national average.

These figures indicate clearly that a well-staffed treatment center can be a more economical operation than a more conventional state hospital, in spite of the better staffing ratios and the higher daily costs. While it may seem less painful to pay the lower installment payments demanded by the more conventional operation, the total cost per product produced or per person served is clearly lower in the kind of active treatment system Fort Logan provided.

Are Mental Health Expenditures Good Investments?

If it is granted that Fort Logan has been able to demonstrate the economy of an active treatment approach for a state hospital population, it might still be questioned whether even this level of expenditure is a good investment. By "good investment" is meant an expenditure of funds that results in a positive return for the investor. Some funders suspect that money spent on mental health services is simply consumed and little return is realized by the funding source. Consequently, there is a reluctance to spend any amount on mental health services.

The center has been engaged in a benefit/cost analysis of its services aimed at providing an answer to this and other questions. This line of analysis, called output value analysis,[8] estimates the benefits produced by the program by placing a value on each discharged patient. This value is a function of the patient's estimated economic productivity and the value of the amount of response to the program. The value ascribed to each discharged patient is then related to the program costs involved in treating that patient. This gives a kind of benefit/cost relationship called the output value index in this line of analysis.

While output value analysis concerns itself with many more program indicators than the output value index, this benefit/cost relationship does speak most directly to the question raised. And, while the methodology and the measures currently used will undoubtedly continue to undergo refinements and improvement, the consistent impression gained thus far from this line of analysis is that Fort Logan's services do return more in value to the patient and society than it costs to provide those services. Fort Logan's rate of return on investment of treatment dollars has been shown to vary for different diagnostic groups,[9] groups that differ in age, education, or socioeconomic characteristics,[10] and groups treated with differing levels of intensity or extensiveness of treatment.[11] Even when discounted to allow for the fact of readmissions,[12] the results still show more than a dollar return for each dollar invested.

While these early results can hardly be regarded as definitive or final, they are encouraging in view of the substantial amounts of money spent on mental health in this country. Of course, as we have seen, Fort Logan is more productive than the average state hospital and has a lower cost per discharged patient. More conventional programs might not show as favorable a return on their program investments. If this were found to be true, this would be one more reason to support the active treatment model for the state hospital.

Rationale for Program Reduction

When a program has been shown to be effective in treating its patients, less expensive than the conventional model, and returns more in value than its costs, one might expect that the program would be looking forward to a bright future. Instead, its services are being cut back and in many respects it is fighting to avoid being forced back into the conventional more custodially oriented model. How could such a state of affairs come about?

Such happenings are, of course, the result of a complex interaction of many forces. Included in the matrix of forces are such factors as (1) the local political power base of the center, (2) the lingering stereotype of the "state hospital," (3) the political spirit of the times, and (4) internal divisions within the center. All these have played a part.

The Local Political Power Base

In the beginning Fort Logan enjoyed widespread support from the executive and legislative branches of the state government. There was a general recognition for the need to change from the previous state hospital model and the plan proposed for the center seemed to incorporate the best available thought on what the new model should look like.[13] There was, therefore, an initial honeymoon period during which funds were available, criticism was minimal, and support for the center's plans was very strong.

In addition to the local support, national recognition came early[14] to the center and a steady stream of visitors came from all over the country and around the world. Again, the reaction of the visitors was generally positive, and the center staff felt further validation was given to their belief that they were doing a good job.

The staff was generally young, enthusiastic, newly trained, and determined to make the program a success. Extra effort and overtime were the norms for most staff, but everyone gave willingly in the belief that what they were doing was important, and it was appreciated.

Perhaps the very ease and quickness with which success and recognition came to the center helped to determine some of the weaknesses in its present position. Success is said to breed success, but it also breeds jealousy and competition. Other mental health agencies have felt that Fort Logan was the "favorite child" and that their own considerable contributions were not being adequately recognized. The pride that Fort Logan staff took in their work could easily be taken as conceit or intolerable brashness. The inevitable failures or troublesome patients could be taken to prove that the program really could not take all the responsibilities expected of a state hospital. Differences in professionals' interests in the short-term and the longer-term patients produced differences in the interests of the center's staff in the value of the organization. Whatever the reason, even the early successful years of the center's operation could easily have spawned the seeds of later criticism.

Because of the considerable momentum of the early years, however, no great anxiety was felt about these criticisms at Fort Logan. The forces supporting its development were simply too strong to be deflected. No great urgency was felt to develop some powerful political friends who would help to protect the center when the inevitable periods of criticism would come. Further, the center, being the state hospital for the entire metropolitan area, did not "belong" to any political group or person in particular. As a state facility, it was not the property of the county officials in the counties it served. As a metropolitan facility, it was not the sole property of any state representative from the districts it served. And, as a metropolitan facility, it did not belong to those legislators who represent areas of the state outside of the Denver metropolitan area. Most important, perhaps is that most legislators in the metropolitan area have a clinic or comprehensive center in their district that is clearly part of their political constituency. The result is that the center has had a relatively weak political base compared to many other local mental health agencies.

Given the early momentum that minimized the need for building a political power base and given the circumstances that operated against close identification with any specific representative's district, this still leaves the question of why more effective action was not taken to overcome this situation when its importance was finally recognized. The most direct answer to this seems to be that, given the obstacles to be overcome, the center could not muster sufficient skills and strengths to overcome them. By the time the center ceased believing that the virtues of its program would speak for themselves, the tide was running so strongly that the available skills were insufficient to reverse the situation. Needless to say, publicly funded facilities are, by definition, affected by political forces, and are, therefore, "political."

Because psychiatric treatment resources at the local level were meager and often so expensive, Fort Logan adult psychiatric teams found themselves treating some patients whose problems did not fit in the category of "major mental illness." There were many patients who needed short-term crisis intervention and/or insight-oriented therapy competing for treatment with the patients who needed long-term, supportive, social rehabilitation. Highly qualified professionals, who really wanted to work with insightful, motivated, neurotic patients, were recruited because of their competence in various verbal therapies. Unfortunately, many of these had neither interest nor skills in working with the long-term patient. Their status on the treatment teams lent support to emphasizing the short-term acute patient's needs at the expense of the chronic patient. This group supported the affiliations of Fort Logan with local clinics to deliver the range of services required for comprehensive community mental health centers. For a time this group also naively believed that their own "excellence" was demonstrated by their concern for the shorter-term patients. Those staff members who had invested their energies in chronic patients were welcome to do so, but from many staff, there was little support or recognition for those efforts.

It is important to acknowledge the relationship of the decentralized administrative structure to the evolution of the process, as well as the mood of the 1960s and its impact. At the time Fort Logan came into being in 1961, there were no other hospitals, to our knowledge, operating on such a decentralized model.

The Lingering Stereotype of the State Hospital

One of the ironies of our history is that one of the most unexpected sources of difficulty for Fort Logan turned out to be the lingering stereotype of the classical state hospital. For many people, the label "state hospital" conjures up an image of the large, dismal, understaffed, overcrowded, custodial hospital far removed from the population centers of the state. Because Fort Logan had provided such a radical departure from this model, we often had difficulty in convincing people we were a "real" state hospital. We did not anticipate that at a later date we would have difficulty because we were seen as a classical state hospital.

This phenomenon could be observed among people who had not visited Fort Logan and had great difficulty in grasping the program description or the conditions described once they were informed that Fort Logan was a "state hospital." However, in the last few years, it could also be observed among some local individuals, who were familiar with the program and had visited the center.

While part of this difficulty in shaking the stereotype of the classical state hospital could be ascribed to the same forces that made it difficult for individuals who had not seen the center to fully grasp the new concept, it was also an exceedingly convenient stereotype to maintain. There was much talk around the country about phasing out the "state hospitals," and a number had been closed down. As it turned out, it was a very effective banner under which to propose the redeployment of resources then used at Fort Logan in order to move treatment "close to the community" and to help rid the mental health system of some of the evils of another "classical state hospital."

The fact that Fort Logan had pioneered community-oriented treatment did not deter use of the slogan nor did it appear to strike mental health officials and legislators who were the main beneficiaries of this line of reasoning as incongruous. Nor did the fact that Fort Logan delivered many of its services in the community, often in conjunction with other mental health agencies, seem to undermine the line of argument. Fort Logan was to be partially dismantled in order to "modernize" the mental health system.

What seems to have happened, then, is the reaction of individuals facing a threat to their own survival (due to the declining federal support for community mental health centers). Naturally, the mental health authority did not want to see the comprehensive centers having to cut back their services severely or to go under entirely. They had been providing large amounts of vitally needed services. If redeploying funds from the state hospital could save these centers, it must have seemed like an admirable solution. The fact that Fort Logan would be severely damaged because of the concurrent erosion of its remaining direct and supportive services was not accepted. Just what the long-term effects of the redeployment will be remains to be seen.

The Political Spirit of the Times

The solution for the funding crisis sought by the mental health authority was, of course, extremely congenial to the political spirit of the times. Legislators are rightfully reluctant to increase expenditures for public services by large amounts. Many are very concerned with avoiding duplication of services and promoting economy and efficiency in government. Claims could be and were made that the redeployment was furthering these virtues too. Evidence Fort Logan presented to the contrary was either seen as not sufficiently convincing or as probably self-serving. Again, only time and a wholly impartial analysis of the situation can determine the truth.

While the political spirit of the times certainly provided a favorable climate for the redeployment, and a few of the actors involved had personal constituents that felt strongly they would gain through it, it was not the political process that was the prime mover in this drama. In this drama, the prime mover for the dismantling of Fort Logan was the state mental health system itself. If this should ever be judged in history as the outrageous event many of us within the organization now feel it is, it is sobering to realize that it was done by the mental health community itself and was not completely forced on the mental healther by the politician.

Internal Divisions Within the Center

Given the external forces described, the center might still have withstood these pressures successfully if it had been internally united on some critical issues. Unfortunately, it was not.

First, there were divisions among the clinical staff as to the desirability of redeploying responsibility for services to community centers. Many close working relationships had been formed with the comprehensive community mental health centers over the years. Cross-staffing had not only allowed for maximum continuity of care for patients, it had given Fort Logan staff some exposure to the treatment of the less chronically and less seriously disturbed patients seen by these community centers. When the proposals were made to redeploy the responsibility for adult services to the community centers, some staff saw this as a favorable opportunity to work with a more responsive mix of clients. Consequently, there was a division of opinion on the desirability of the redeployment plan within the clinical staff.

Second, there was a division of opinion among administrative staff as well. Some felt the redeployment was an acceptable idea but that the poor planning and the excessive withdrawal of supporting resources was damaging to the program. Others felt redeployment was not the logical next step but rather that greater integration of all services in the Denver Metropolitan area would serve patient as well as administrative needs better. Generally, however, this was seen as not practical in view of the strong preferences for local autonomy by the community centers.

Epilogue

The struggle and drama and turmoil described are still very much in the process of unfolding, and it is much too soon to take a dispassionate view of the situation. However, perhaps it is not too early to draw two conclusions: (1) cannibalism can be a compliment, and (2) a return to the old state hospital model is unthinkable.

Cannibalism Can be a Compliment

Individuals generally feel that their entire identity is coming to an end if they are ingested by cannibals. An organization, however, need not feel that way. Organizations are, after all, simply social entities constructed to carry out some socially desired purpose. If the entities that cannibalize its resources seek to carry out that same purpose, then the reason for its existence is not being repudiated. The responsibility for carrying out that purpose is simply being transferred to another organization.

It is important that the dismantling of Fort Logan not be seen as a repudiation of the values and goals of the organization. It has been a highly successful organization, doing an effective job. Others now will be given an opportunity to show if they can do as well or better. To the extent that we believe firmly in the values exemplified by the organization, we can only hope that they succeed. To the extent that we are human and feel a considerable investment in what is now being dismantled, we wish the relay-runner had taken only the baton and had left the arm.

Return to the Old State Hospital Model is Unthinkable

If Fort Logan has accomplished anything at all in its brief existence, it has provided abundant evidence that there is a practical and viable alternative to the classical state hospital. Not only does it provide effective services, it does so at a cost lower than the average for the conventional model. Most important, it provides these services in a way that avoids inducing chronic institutional dependence in its clients. It has shown clearly that there is no excuse for continuing to act as if there were only one "classical" model for the state hospital.

Fort Logan has received many rewards for its accomplishments. We can only hope that it does not also become the first state hospital that both demonstrated a viable alternative to the old model and was then forced to return to that model. That is what the struggle and turmoil are all about, not the wish to maintain an exclusive franchise on community-oriented treatment. We are assured that no one intends this fate (of returning to the old model) for us, but the road paved with good intentions may lead precisely there.

Notes

1. *Action for mental health*, Final Report of the Joint Commission on Mental Illness and Health, 1961. New York, Basic Books, Inc., 1961.
2. Glascote, R.; Sanders, D.; Forstenzer, H.M.; and Foley, A.R., *The Community Mental Health Center. An Analysis of Existing Models.* 1964 by American Psychiatric Association. Library of Congress Catalog Card No. 64-8013.
3. National Institute of Mental Health, Socio-economic Characteristics of Admissions to Inpatient Services of State and County Mental Hospitals, 1969, DHEW Publication No. (HSM) 72-9048, Superintendent of Documents, U. S. Government Printing Office, Washington, D.C. 20402, 1971.
4. Coates, C.J., Incorporation of Goal Attainment Treatment Effectiveness Measures in an Output Value Mental Health Evaluation Model. FLMHC working paper, April 1974.
5. Anthony, W.A.; Buell, G.J.; Sharratt, S.; and Althoff, M.D., "Efficacy of

Psychiatric Rehabilitation." *Psychological Bulletin*, 1972, 78, 447-556; Odegard, O., "Pattern of Discharge and Readmission in Psychiatric Hospitals in Norway, 1926 to 1965. *Mental Hygiene*, 1961, 45, 185-93.

6. McPartland, S. and Richart, H., "Analysis of Readmissions to a Community Mental Health Center." *Community Mental Health Journal*, 1966, 2, 22-26; Rutledge, L. and Binner, P.R., "Readmissions to a Community Mental Health Center." *Community Mental Health Journal*, 1970, Vol. 6(2).

7. Murphy, H.B.M., "Foster Homes: The New Back Wards?" *Canada's Mental Health*, bimonthly journal of the Department of National Health and Welfare, Ottawa, Canada, September-October, 1972; Chase, J., "Where have all the Patients Gone?" *Human Behavior*, Vol. 2, No. 10, 14-21, October 1973; Lamb, H.R. and Goerzel, V., "The Demise of the State Hospital—A Premature Obituary?" *International Journal of Psychiatry*, Vol. 11, No. 2, 239-55, June 1973.

8. Halpern, J. and Binner, P.R., "A Model for an Output Value Analysis of Mental Health Programs." *Administration in Mental Health*, Winter 1972.

9. Binner, P.R., An Output Value Analysis of Schizophrenic Patients at the Fort Logan Mental Health Center. Paper prepared for the Institute on Research on Psychosocial Treatment of Schizophrenia, American Orthopsychiatric Association, May 28-June 1, 1973, New York City.

10. Wilderman, E., Summary Statistics six-year Output Value Analysis—Adult Psychiatric Division. Unpublished manuscript, FLMHC, June 1973.

11. Binner, P.R., Halpern, J., and Potter, A., "Patients, Programs, and Results in a Comprehensive Mental Health Center." *Journal of Consulting and Clinical Psychology*, 1973, 41(1), 148-56.

12. ____, Readmission Discount Factors in Program Evaluation: An Output Value Analysis. Unpublished manuscript, FLMHC, May 1974.

13. Joint Commission on Mental Illness and Health, Action for Mental Health.

14. Glascote, et al. (1964), *The Community Mental Health Center;* Glasscote, R.M.; Kraft, A.M.; Glassman, S.M.; and Jepson, W.W., *Partial Hospitalization for the Mentally Ill. A Study of Programs and Problems.* 1969 by American Psychiatric Association. Library of Congress Catalog Card No. 69-20395.

15

An Assessment of the California Unified Services Plan with Reference to State Hospitals
William B. Beach, Jr.

California's mental health program is the product of many years of community development and services. To understand how it reached its present level requires both a knowledge of the history of mental health services in California, and a knowledge of those characteristics of the state that contributed to the development of the community health program.

Until after World War II mental health services in California, as in most states, were provided by state mental hospitals, plus a few outpatient clinics operated by the State Department of Mental Hygiene. In addition, there were private agency facilities, private practitioners, and several private inpatient institutions. However, considerable interest was generated for the establishment of public community services for those who could not afford private care, an interest encouraged by the federal mental health grant-in-aid program that followed World War II. These funds were used in California primarily as seed money to establish or expand outpatient types of mental health service in new or already established agencies in the community, including those under private auspices, as well as those operated by city and county governments.

As an approach to developing community services, this use of federal grant-in-aid mental health funds involved the statewide Governor's Advisory Committee on Mental Health. Committee members were asked to review applications from the various community agencies. Their review included site visits and interviews with the applicants and their boards. Funds were allocated only as "start-up" or "seed" grants, usually for a five-year period with the amount gradually declining over each period, making it necessary for the applicant to secure his own sources of other funding as the federal funds declined. A very careful assessment of applicant agencies was therefore needed beforehand as to their potential for raising their own financial resources. In many instances, additional resources came through the United Fund, or, in some instances, through local tax dollars when the applicant was a local government agency.

In the utilization of the Hill-Burton program, the state also used a one-third, one-third, one-third formula of funding where the applicant, the state, and the federal government each provided one-third of the dollars used for construction. A condition for the one-third state funding was a requirement that any general hospital construction would include inpatient facilities for the psychiatric patient. Since there was considerable new hospital construction

261

in California following World War II, a large number of psychiatric inpatient units evolved throughout the state as a result, including the development of many such units in county hospitals.

By the mid 1950s, California sought to establish a community program closely paralleling the plan evolved in New York State. The first attempts in 1955 to pass a community mental health act were unsuccessful, but, finally, in 1957 the Short-Doyle Act was enacted and went into effect in January 1958. This initial legislation provided for a 50 percent reimbursement program matching local city or county tax dollars with state dollars. One major difference between the New York and California programs at the outset was that funding and local administration of the program was by county or city government, rather than by administrative boards. Also, with one exception, only local tax dollars were matched, not private sources of funds, and no per capita limitation on funding was established. Local mental health boards were strictly advisory in nature and advisory to the local governing body. The dollars to be matched not only had to be local tax dollars but matching occurred only after other sources of funding, such as insurance and private funds, were utilized. The one exception mentioned above is that initially federal mental health grant-in-aid dollars could be used as the local matching funds. In addition, reimbursement initially was only for services provided patients who sought care on a voluntary basis. All forms of involuntary care originally were excluded from reimbursement.

The first programs to begin under the new law were primarily those that had initially been funded through local government agencies, using federal grant-in-aid moneys and local tax dollars. These groups immediately expanded their programs in almost every instance, and services continued to grow but rather slowly.

By 1963 the Short-Doyle Act was amended to provide greater incentives for the development of locally governed services through expansion of the funding mechanism to include involuntary care. The funding formula was simultaneously changed to 75 percent state funds and 25 percent local tax funds for all new and expanded programs, while maintaining a 50-50 funding ratio for existing programs. This provided incentives to local government to expand services, by placing traditional involuntary nontreatment detention services for those awaiting commitment proceedings under the community services program. These detention programs could be funded on a 75-25 basis only if an active treatment program were provided.

The choice of local government as the funding avenue relates to a characteristic of California that would not be applicable in most other states. In California, county government is very strong, very well-organized, and very effective in its lobbying activities with the state government. County boards of supervisors, elected locally, number five for every county, with the exception of San Francisco, which is a combined city-county government. Local government has long been the chief service provider in California, particularly in the health field. County public health departments have been the principal public health agencies, with the state health department primarily providing policy, direction, regulations, and funding.

This was true for many years and was readily seen, for example, in the care and treatment of the tuberculous patient. California never had a state-operated tuberculosis sanitarium; all such facilities were county-operated under state regulations and subvention.

The local mental health program continued to grow and expand and by 1967 plans had proceeded to provide the 75-25 funding ratio across the board for all services to be rendered in the community, thus totally eliminating all 50-50 funding, and legislative studies were initiated to assess the entire system and to recommend changes. A major study was undertaken by a Mental Health Sub-committee of the Appropriations Committee under the leadership of Assemblyman Frank Lanterman of the California Legislature. This committee was a very active bipartisan group that also included consultation with key senators. As a result, a new revised Short-Doyle Act evolved that was passed in 1969 along with a major new act called the Lanterman-Petris-Short Act.

Some of the main thrusts of this new legislation were directed at a revision of commitment procedures, at a spelling out of patients' rights, and at a new funding structure that emphasized even more the role and responsibility of community programs. Most of the impetus for this came from Mr. Lanterman, a very dedicated, humane legislator who was always very concerned about the care and treatment of the mentally ill and the mentally retarded.

By this time there had been a decline, as in most states, in the population of the state mental hospitals. Prior to this, a major decline had already occurred in the over sixty-five population in the state hospitals. This was accomplished through major efforts to develop alternatives to state mental hospital care for the aged in state institutions, and to put into operation specific screening programs for the care and treatment needs of the geriatric patient so that these people would not be committed automatically to state institutions in lieu of other more appropriate resources. A pilot geriatric screening program developed in San Francisco, where the commitment rate of geriatric patients had been high, served as a model for other parts of the state. Another contributing factor was the rapid and extensive development of nursing homes in California.

The state had long had an excellent family care program that provided for the placement of patients from mental hospitals into small community home settings of no more than six per family home. Supervision was provided through a social work staff that helped provide a continuity of observation once placement had been made. This served to reduce the hospital population and to insure that services were provided after release from the hospitals. However, responsibility was later given to the local mental health programs for providing needed after-care services and for follow-up of the patient who had left the institution.

During the review by the legislature of the Short-Doyle legislation and the state hospital program, there was considerable discussion as to the pros and cons of increasing local government responsibility for community operations or developing local services as a state responsibility. Contributing to the problem was the planned closure of some of the state hospitals, notably Modesto State Hospital, and later DeWitt State Hospital. Both of these institutions had been World War II Army Hospitals, semipermanent structures, primarily wooden, with a life expectancy of approximately twenty-five years. The critical problem with these institutions was their unsuitability for patient use from a safety standpoint, and the decision to be made was whether to close or reconstruct them. The decision finally made was to close these facilities.

It is noteworthy that long detailed studies were carried out by the legislature in connection with this movement, involving all key people and organizations in the state with an interest in the area of mental health. Numerous public hearings and many legislative hearings were held about various aspects of the legislation. Finally, through the concerted effort of the legislative committee, with executive branch help and with marked input from local groups, the new legislation was adopted—specifically, a revised Short-Doyle Act and a new Lanterman-Petris-Short Act. It was Mr. Lanterman's strong intent that any major new legislation should be exhaustively reviewed and input solicited from any and all interested groups or individuals.

Politically, the approach was non partisan. The new Short-Doyle and Lanterman-Petris-Short Acts had the support of a Republican governor, Ronald Reagan, the Democratic leader of the assembly, Jesse Unruh, and bipartisan support in the authorship, with Mr. Lanterman being a Republican and Senators Short and Petris being Democrats.

One of the major effects of this legislation was to insure patients' rights in California. Prior to the legislation, a person committed to a state mental hospital in California lost more of his personal rights and freedom than a person convicted of a felony. This new legislation constituted a major step forward. Another major aspect of the legislation was to place time limits of commitment for the mentally ill. Every form of involuntary care, except for sexual or criminal offenders, would have a time limit that, in some instances, could not be renewed; and, in other instances, could be renewed only after specific actions were taken and needs demonstrated to the satisfaction of all concerned.

Throughout these involuntary procedures, full access to courts was always available to protect the individual's rights. The imposition of a time limit on involuntary care automatically resulted in a reassessment of a patient's needs the moment he entered the state hospital. What could be done and how quickly had to be determined, and whether it could be done in the community or needed to be carried out in a state institution. For those who required long-term custodial care, a form of guardianship known as conservatorship was set up involving a court action. Even in this instance a time limit of one year was imposed, and the conservatorship had to be renewed annually with justification shown as to the need and degree of such action. Varying degrees of conservatorship could be provided relating to the facts of each individual situation.

Obviously, these kinds of limitations imposed requirements for careful review and assessment of all state mental hospital patients and their treatment programs, and did much to eliminate unnecessary commitments to state mental hospitals. These aspects were coupled with a financial arrangement, whereby all care was funded on the basis of 90 percent state funds to 10 percent county funds after all other sources of revenue, such as third party payments, medical assistance, and private funds had been utilized. The 90-10 state-county funding applied not only to community programs, but to the state mental hospital programs as well; so that, in effect, the state mental hospitals became agencies providing services under contract to counties with the counties being the responsible agencies for the patient's care and his program.

The state mental hospitals thus provided services much as any other vendor contracting with the county for provision of services, with the county now paying 10 percent of the cost of patient care in the state hospital. This represented a strong inducement and encouragement for the county to develop alternatives to state mental hospital care, using such care only when definitely required, and for such length of time as was needed. Through this legislation, the counties receive a budget each year that includes a state mental hospital portion, as well as funds for services provided locally by community agencies.

The law also stipulated that no person could be admitted to a state mental hospital unless he had been screened and approved for admission by the county from which he came. This then imposed another area of restriction. The responsibility for planning a program of treatment for patients was clearly that of the county, and it was for the county to determine whether someone should be admitted to the state mental hospital, not the state hospital. In some instances, particularly in rural areas where counties do not have the capacity to make these determinations on a twenty-four-hour a day, seven-days-a-week basis, they can contract with the state mental hospital in their area to provide this service for them, much as they would contract with any other agency; but the responsibility was still that of the county and they paid for care and treatment. Likewise, the continuing after-care needs of the patient were definitely and firmly fixed as the responsibility of the county.

Another feature that evolved in the funding mechanism was the setting of priorities for allocation of new funds for mental health. In the new legislation enacted in 1969, traditional inpatient services were given the lowest priority for funding of new programs. Receiving higher priorities were those services that provided alternatives to a twenty-four-hour care, such as crisis intervention (which again might be on a twenty-four-hour basis), partial hospitalization, outpatient services, or other alternatives that eliminated or reduced the need for continuing twenty-four hour inpatient care.

Many problems develop when such a program is instituted, but, again, because of the uniqueness of different states, there are different problems for California than there would be for Pennsylvania or other states. One of the features, for example, that helped deinstitutionalization in California and that is not possible in many other states, was the fact that the Civil Service mechanisms in California were very extensive in county government, as well as in the state. For years there had been an ability to transfer from state employment to county employment or between counties without losing retirement benefits and longevity. Salary scales might be different, (although, because of competition, they usually tended to be somewhat similar) but moves were possible from one county to another or from state to county government or vice versa, without sacrificing benefits. This made it easier for employees to move from state hospital employment to community mental health program employment. Taking the most advantage of this were psychiatrists, psychologists, and social workers; nursing staff and psychiatric orderlies were less able to do this since their numbers were greater compared to relatively few openings locally.

In addition, there were not as many institutions to deal with in California as there are in many other states. California, with 20 million people, originally had ten state mental hospitals, including one exclusively for the criminally insane. In contrast, Pennsylvania, with 12 million population, has nineteen hospitals for the mentally ill. The more hospitals there are and the more intimately they are related to the community, the greater the difficulties in deinstitutionalizing, particularly if the facility has been the primary resource for an adjacent community.

Institutions in California were also largely under centralized direction and there had been frequent shifts of superintendents and other professional personnel among them. As a result, there had been a constantly changing pattern with respect to many of the personnel who had not been located in one place their entire lifetimes. However, there was great resistance to deinstitutionalization, particularly from psychiatric aide professionals, many of whom were husband and wife and who had spent their whole career in one particular institution or location. The other professionals, particularly social work psychologists, psychiatrists, and physicians more readily moved into community activities of one sort or another.

It has been determined in California to try and eliminate the state hospital system and replace it with a community-based program. Recent announcements have indicated a proposed timetable for eliminating all state mental hospitals within five years. Dr. Ernest W. Klatte discusses this in the following chapter, indicating where, as the head of a county agency, he sees the county fitting in with these plans and activities. Dr. Klatte was formerly superintendent of a state mental hospital and is in an ideal position to look at this subject from more than one viewpoint, and certainly to assess where it is today. It is most important, however, to look at California for what can be learned from that state with the understanding that not all its ideas or concepts can be transferred elsewhere. This is readily apparent in the development of community mental health programs in Pennsylvania. There are features similar to California, approaches that are applicable, but there are many contrasts and many differences, as there are among other states. A uniqueness of approach is required to fit the situation in any particular state.

Several problems are now facing California as a result of the rapid growth of the community program and decrease in size of the state mental hospital program. These programs seem to relate to challenges as to the effectiveness of the community program, and expressions of concern that state hospital closures are being planned without adequate concern for the effects of closing. In general, there seems to be a conflict between the two segments—community mental health programs and state mental hospital programs, and patients could get lost in the struggle.

To relocate patients out of hospitals into inadequate settings with no program could be harmful. The need for good aftercare programs and continuity is essential, and has been voiced loudly and clearly in California, along with a condemnation of any policies that would just place patients in boarding homes or other settings with no supervision and no program to meet their needs. It is becoming increasingly obvious that any mental health system must be developed adequately to guarantee that appropriate supervision and programming are available in whatever setting the patient is in. It is also obvious that a patient can "fall between the cracks" without services when he moves from an inpatient setting to another setting, or from a state program to a local program unless programs are structured and planned according to his needs.

It would appear that in California the unified system has accomplished an intensive review of the state hospital structure, not only by state officials but also by legislative committees and local community mental health programs who hold the key to their utilization. By placing fiscal, screening, and after-care responsibilities on the local counties, an involvement with the state hospital is forced. A particular incentive, of course, is the fiscal incentive. However, there are concerns of problems of premature release of patients from state hospitals, inadequate aftercare services, and inappropriate posthospital placements.

The announcement that many state institutions would be closed has accomplished one desirable feature—that is, specific planning with respect to the closing of specific facilities according to a prescribed timetable. The tremendous concern being expressed by some groups, however, around these closings raises the question as to whether or not adequate consideration and planning were given to patient care, patient needs, and community needs that would be affected by the closing of specific hospitals on specific dates, as well as to whether or not certain community programs have the capability and potential for assuming the responsibility for long-term care of patients currently in state hospitals or those in the community who may require long-term care. It again emphasizes the need to look at programs completely and totally with respect to patient and community needs, as well as to fiscal aspects.

There is tremendous concern on the part of the State Employees Association, which is very critical of this program. Here again, one must consider whether or not the criticism is justified, or whether it is seeking to maintain institutions for the benefit of staff rather than patients. Obviously, there is no easy answer. There are personnel whose primary interest is not whether patients need hospital care to the degree that it is now available; rather, they see the institution as necessary to their job survival. Some of this is understandable, but much bitterness, anger, resentment, and criticism occur, often directed at the wrong people and for the wrong reasons. These problems obviously show the necessity for careful, meticulous planning with respect to the future of the state mental hospital in relationship to the growing and rapidly developing community mental health programs.

Summary

The decline in state hospital populations has created many problems as to the role of the state hospital in any unified system. The experiences in California identify the many factors that must be dealt with as changes in hospital use occur. These include the following:

1. Disposition of buildings and grounds
2. Utilization and future of career state employees employed in state mental hospitals
3. Adequacy of the community to provide for all its own needs in the absence of the state mental hospital
4. Most important of all—what happens to the patient now in the state mental hospital and the patient in the community who may need long-term care such as was provided in the state hospital

Projections on the actual future role of the state mental hospital vary from state to state. State mental hospitals will probably exist in most states for many years to come—but probably not as many as there are currently nor as big. These should be mental hospitals that are better staffed and better utilized, and, most importantly, *used as an integral part of the community program.* Large boarding home situations without any program for patients do not appear to be valid substitutes for good programming in state mental hospitals. At the same time, good programming in state mental hospitals is not a proper substitute for *adequate* alternatives to hospitalization when hospitalization is not needed, nor should institutions be maintained for the benefit of staff rather than for the patient.

A patient should be treated as early in his disorder as possible, as intensively as possible, and with as little dislocation from his home, his family, his community, and his job as is possible. By adhering to those concepts, appropriate roles can be found for the state mental hospital, for the community mental health program, for trained manpower, and for other kinds of services that an individual needs. The program must be developed to meet the patient's needs, rather than trying to fit the patient into existing structures because they are there.

16

The Orange County Experience
Ernest W. Klatte

Orange County, California, with a population of approximately 1.7 million people, has committed itself to stop using state hospitals except for penal code and retardation cases, through the development of community alternatives by January 1975. This chapter describes one community's experience with the California Community Mental Health Services Act, including immediate plans and projected results and problems.

Orange County adjoins Los Angeles and is California's most rapidly growing metropolitan county, with a population increase approaching 100,000 per year. Geographically, the county is relatively small for California, so that it can be traversed in any direction in considerably under one hour. The distribution of population by age is typical of high-growth urban areas, with 40 percent of the population being under twenty years of age and with a median age of 26.2 The ethnic and racial composition is atypical for large urban areas, with the largest ethnic minority group being Mexican-Americans and representing approximately 11 percent of the population. Racial minorities in 1970 comprised about 3 percent of the population compared with 11 percent for the state as a whole. The mean income of residents is somewhat above the statewide average. Politically, the county has a history of conservatism. The political mix, however, has changed considerably in recent years with the influx of new people, so that at this time, three of the five members of the County Board of Supervisors are registered Democrats.

Prior to implementation of the California Community Mental Health Services Act in July 1969, the county had not been a heavy consumer of mental health services, either locally or at the state level. As most counties in the state, it was not conceptually, administratively, or financially equipped to deal with the increased responsibilities demanded by the new act. From a conceptual standpoint, the county's mental health services had been elective and small. The professionals in the program had never assumed a basic responsibility for making mental health services available as needed, since this basic responsibility had previously rested with the state. Since the county had little concept as to the complexity of the mental health services that were to evolve, it failed to set up an administrative structure that could deal effectively with the new responsibilities. Financially and programmatically, the county had to continue its dependence on the state hospital system for the majority of its services.

271

Organization

In the ensuing four years, the county's program has grown tremendously, albeit painfully, from a conceptual, programmatic, administrative, and financial point of view. Administratively, the program was developed on a matrix table of organization, establishing deputy directors responsible for the various special functions of the department. These included administrative services, general direct care services, childrens, drug abuse, alcoholism, training, and research and evaluation. Each deputy had countywide responsibility for his particular function. The county was then divided into six catchment areas of from approximately 200,000 to 300,000 population each. Regional deputy director level positions were established to direct and coordinate the overall mental health services in each particular region. The regional deputies are responsible to the special deputies for the various special functions within their regions. By the same token, the special deputies, who have responsibility for developing budgets and overall county policies in their particular special areas, have a responsibility to each of the regional deputies to see that resources are available equally in each of the regions. Originally, as special services such as alcohol and drug abuse programs were developed, the dearth of available funds required them to be centralized in nature. Gradually, as the programs have enlarged, they have decentralized.

Since most of the deputy directors had not previously assumed this type of responsibility, nor had worked in this organizational framework, they tended to look for structure and programmatic guidance that were not readily available. The result seems to have been development of a high degree of autonomy at the deputy level, with each feeling increasingly more comfortable with his expertise in his personal area of responsibility. An overall policy has been that program development would not include bricks and mortar. Community services were developed in leased space rather than county-owned space, or by contract with private providers; and any needed residential services over and beyond that provided by the county medical center would be on a contract basis with private providers.

Patient Population

Some had expected that as local programs were developed, there would be a concomitant decrease in admissions to state hospitals. Table 16-1 demonstrates that in Orange County, as with most counties that had an underdeveloped local mental health program before the initiation of the Community Mental Health Services Act in 1969, admissions to the state hospital increased for a time as the local programs developed. This appears to be a result of the case-finding effect of new community programs. As new needs become apparent

that the local program could not meet, the state hospital was encouraged to
develop appropriate programs and patients sent there. In 1968-69, before the
initiation of the act, Orange County admitted 1,106 patients to the state hospital, exclusive of the retarded and penal code type cases. In 1969, because of
the obvious need for drug detoxification and long-term family-type drug abuse
programs, as well as residential treatment programs for disturbed but nonpsycho-
tic adolescents, the state hospital developed the appropriate programs, and
admissions soared. By 1970-71 they had peaked at 2,889. Last year they
decreased to 2,232, still over twice that of the year preceding the act. They
are continuing to decrease this year.

There was an immediate, rather precipitous decrease in the number of
state hospital patient days utilized by residents of the county immediately
after the act was passed. This seemed to have been the result of the limitations set on the length of hospitalization under the new act rather than on the
provision of local alternatives for treatment. In 1968-69 there were 161,526
patient days used. The first year following the act this had decreased to
137,056 patient days. By 1972-73 this had decreased to 99,836. The decrease
between 1970 and 1973 seems to have been primarily the result of local alternatives to state hospitalization.

Although there was some anxiety that the limitations set on civil commit-

Table 16-1
State Hospital Utilization for Orange County

	Total	LPS	Non-LPS
Res. Pop.			
6–30-69	602	504	98
6–30-70	497	293	204
6–30-71	502	396	106
6–30-72	365	367	98
6–30-73	361	273	88
Admissions			
68-69	1,260	1,106	154
69-70	1,845	1,755	90
70-71	3,011	2,889	122
71-72	2,311	2,231	80
72-73	2,307	2,232	75
Patient Days			
68-69	196,326	161,526	34,800
69-70	174,983	137,056	37,927
70-71	174,174	136,879	37,295
71-72	155,833	117,541	38,292
72-73	130,784	99,836	30,948

Table 16-2
Local Program and State Hospital Costs for Orange County

	Actual 68-69	Actual 69-70	Actual 70-71	Actual 71-72	Budgeted 72-73
Local programs adjusted gross	$1,987,896	$3,362,182	$4,677,765	$ 6,433,883	$ 8,743,346
State hospital adjusted gross	(N.A.)	$3,612,013	$4,092,674	$ 3,905,436	$ 3,447,780
Total adjusted gross		$6,974,195	$8,770,439	$10,339,319	$12,191,126

ments would precipitate an increased number of penal code commitments, where there were no limitations on length of hospitalization, this does not seem to have occurred in Orange County. The year prior to the act there were 154 penal code and retardation commitments from the county. By 1972-73 these had decreased to 75. Some are of the opinion that a larger number of individuals who might otherwise have been handled by the mental health system are now retained in the correctional system. Certainly, there is a large number of disturbed individuals in the county jail; and because of this, a full-time mental health team headed by a sophisticated psychiatrist has been assigned to the jail. Whether the number of such disturbed people has increased since initiation of the act cannot be determined, since this type individual was not identified prior to the act and there were no local services available. It may very well be that persons who always made up a large percentage of the correctional population are now being identified and treated.

Costs

The total cost of mental health services has rapidly expanded. The year preceding the act, expenditures for local mental health services in Orange County were $1,987,896. No figures are available for state hospital services for Orange County in that year, since they were not tabulated by county. As Table 16-2 demonstrates, in 1969-70, the first year of the act, local program costs were over $3,300,000, and state hospital costs for the county were over $3,600,000, with a total just under $7,000,000. The state hospital costs continued to rise until the third year, at which time they started to decrease. By 1972-73, local costs had increased to $8,700,000, and state hospital costs decreased to $3,400,000, for a total of over $12,000,000
In the fall of 1972 the State Department of Mental Hygiene proposed

that Orange County develop a plan to discontinue completely the usage of the state hospital system for nonjudicially committed patients (noncriminal commitments). The state agreed to fund the necessary local program. Since it appeared that the state was going to close the nearby state hospital in any case, the county agreed, as a way to assure the necessary funding at the local level.

What evolved were six months of negotiations during which, at first, both state and county made what later seemed unreasonable demands on the other. The state was anxious to prove that mental health needs could be met without the utilization of any hospital beds, including those at the county medical center. The county, on the other hand, felt that not only did it need the medical center beds, but it needed the ability to contract for acute inpatient psychiatric services with private providers in each of the six regions. In addition, the county was acutely aware of the case-finding effect of transferring state hospital services to the local level and demanded program approval for caseloads far in excess of that previously cared for at the state hospital.

By July 1973 the state and county reached tentative agreement on a local program and budget that would allow the county not to utilize state hospital services. Since it would take some time to implement the local program, the county agreed to purchase state hospital services out of its local budget rather than have a separate allocation for the state hospital. This meant that the county had to be quite careful in phasing in its increased local program so that it could make concurrent cuts in state hospital usage to meet the local budget needs.

The following is a description of the "get out of the state hospital" package, which is euphemistically referred to as GOSH.

Local Services Agreement

The county agreed not to increase expenditures locally for acute psychiatric hospitalization. Since the county medical center was to be the only resource for intensive inpatient service, only the most seriously disturbed and those cases that had a major medical complement to their psychiatric illness could be hospitalized there. This demanded intensification of staffing that was precluded by the budget agreement. Therefore, a decision was made to decrease the number of adult psychiatric beds in the medical center, in order to provide more intensive staffing for the remaining patients. The budgetary and programmatic controls remained at the regional level, and no patient was to be admitted to any service without prior approval within the region of his residence. The regional service deputy was given authority over all staff in his region as well as contract services provided to his region by other agencies. In addition to their pro rata inpatient services at the Orange County Medical Center, each region was promised the following:

Outpatient services: for children and adults (now in existence).

Emergency services: crisis intervention services to be available around the clock, seven days a week.

Therapeutic residential centers: Adult therapeutic residential centers would be the treatment facilities for those patients needing somewhat less intensive care than at the Orange County Medical Center but otherwise in need of hospitalization. Currently in Orange County there is a relatively large number of such private facilities that resemble convalescent hospitals but deal with chronic mentally ill and retarded patients. Operators of such facilities can collect through Medi-Cal, California's Medicaid program, for board, room, and general program costs for this type of patient. They are not staffed adequately to provide intensive treatment. In order to have this type of facility function as an active psychiatric treatment facility capable of handling the majority of patients requiring twenty-four-hour residential care, additional staff would be provided by the regional service.

Intermediate residential centers: In addition to the therapeutic residential centers, each region would have funds to support the cost of fifteen intermediate care placements at any one time.

Day treatment services: Each region would have an active intensive day treatment program. It was anticipated that a large percentage of the patients who in the past have been hospitalized may be able to remain at home and be cared for in the day treatment programs. Those who require residential services may be transported to day treatment programs through transportation services which are included in the budget. The use of day treatment services is expected to avoid the patient transferring his dependency needs to his particular residential facility.

Social rehabilitation centers: Each region currently has a well-staffed activity center that is geared to that patient population which, as the side effect of chronic mental illness, never developed or lost basic social skills necessary for community existence and self-support.

Halfway Houses: Each region would have funds to support approximately seven patients in a halfway house "lodge" program for the chronic mentally ill.

Drug abuse service: Currently the county has fairly well-staffed outpatient drug abuse services in each region, in addition to operating two methadone maintenance clinics. Large numbers of addicts have been admitted to the state hospital for the Family Residential Treatment Program. These latter two services would be transferred to the community, partly funded by this budgetary package and partly funded by new legislation in California providing for drug abuse treatment programs. An average of twenty patients per drug center is expected, to be paid for on a contract basis at any one time. In addition, there are funds to maintain 100 patients in residential drug-free therapeutic community-type programs.

Adolescents: Two therapeutic residential centers would be developed in the county for intensive treatment of disturbed adolescents. One would serve twenty adolescents who are disturbed but not psychotic; the other would serve eight psychotic youngsters. Both of these would be on a contract basis. In addition, there would be ten temporary foster home slots and one day treatment program for this age group. The county currently operates one twelve-bed adolescent ward for the most seriously disturbed at the Medical Center and this would continue.

Children's service: In addition to the existing twelve-bed intensive treatment children's service at the Medical Center, and the existing outpatient services, a total of four satellite homes, each of which can house five or six children, are being developed on a contract basis. In addition, day treatment programs for children are being initiated. The total amount of services for children will obviously be inadequate, but more than replaces the children's services currently available from the state hospital.

Since the county had not used the state hospital system for alcoholics since October 1971, no augmentation in the local program was included in this particular package.

In addition to the program elements, the package included additional administrative costs as well as costs for expansion of the management information system and for outcome evaluation.

The net budget of identified mental health dollars was not expected to increase with the "get out of the state hospital" package. The gross budget would have a rather marked increase, as Welfare and Medicaid programs pick up a large percentage of board and room and treatment costs. It is not possible at this time to report the gross local program costs for 1973-74, since the final allocations provided by new legislation for alcoholic treatment programs and drug abuse programs have not been negotiated. It appears that the gross budget for all mental health services in Orange County will be between $17,000,000 and $18,000,000.

In no way should these cost figures be compared with costs prior to the enactment of the Community Mental Health Services Act. In recent years there has been a huge increase in the demand for various types of local mental health services, particularly in the area of drug abuse and alcoholism, with concomitant legislation to provide for these increased services. It is apparent that the state hospital system was treating only a small segment of those in need of services in the past. At this time, although state hospital admissions are still in excess of those prior to the act, they represent approximately 10 percent of the total patients seen in public mental health programs in Orange County.

At present contracts are being developed with private providers for various types of residential programs; and as decreased state hospital utilization is demonstrated, local staff will be augmented.

Conclusion

In summary, the following are some points of change noted in the past four years at the local level that may or may not be directly related to the California Community Mental Health Services Act of 1969:

From a Socioeconomic Point of View

There is much greater concern with patient rights. Professionals are more concerned with protecting themselves legally in some instances, rather than using their clinical judgement. (Most patients are released after fourteen days). There has been some anxiety expressed on the part of the public, the judiciary, and law enforcement agencies that dangerous patients are being prematurely released. For various reasons, the ninety-day commitment proceedings for dangerous patients are not being used.

There is much more awareness of mental health problems and acceptance of treatment at the local level on the part of the public, resulting in a huge amount of case-finding in the local program. There is much more demand for public mental health services. Local governmental agencies are becoming more aware of mental health problems and the need for services.

Social problems that precipitate emotional illnesses are getting more attention. Perhaps some chronic mentally ill patients are getting less professional care than when they were in the hospital, but most seem happier; and almost no requests to return to the hospital have been received. All in all, more people are being treated without developing primary identification as a "mental patient."

From a Fiscal Point of View

The total cost for mental health services has risen. Much of the increase has been borne by federal programs. More sources of funds have been developed.

Administrative Changes

Administrative change is the area of most problems and one that conceivably could be responsible for the demise of local, county-operated mental health programs. Administrative procedures had gradually matured and developed over the 100-year history of the state hospital system. The new system does not have that degree of administrative sophistication, and many problems have yet to be resolved, for example:

1. The role of the state and counties is still confused. Although the law
    implies that the basic responsibility for the provision of mental health
    services now rests with the county, the state in discovering local prob-
    lems tends to react by developing more state regulations and controls.
    Clearly, both levels of government feel responsible.
2. County administrative regulations and budgeting cycles often conflict
    with those of the state.
3. The demands of bureaucracies on three levels of government often make
    for long delays in starting and implementing programs.
4. Both the state and the counties were understaffed to efficiently admin-
    ister the law or to push for needed changes in the law.
5. The counties had no consistent medical records system or management
    information reporting system, although these are gradually being
    developed.
6. The development of adequate after-care services for patients leaving state
    hospitals seems to have been delayed by the continued availability of
    regional state-operated social services offices with which counties were
    encouraged to contract for aftercare services. As a result, counties fre-
    quently did not know when patients left state hospitals and did not
    develop adequate aftercare services for them. As counties are gradually
    stopping their contracts with the state social service offices, this problem
    seems to be lessened.

In spite of the many problems enumerated here in the development of local
services under the California Community Mental Health Services Act, the act is
basically sound and other states should be encouraged to proceed in this direction. It has required, and will continue to require, modification as various problems are met. It has resulted in improved treatment services for individuals
previously identified as mentally ill; has decreased the chronic dependency of
those who would otherwise have become institutionalized; and it has aided
many to return to productive lives. Of perhaps equal significance has been its
indirect support of the development of mental health treatment programs to
deal with various types of emotional problems that often resulted in social
problems which had previously been dealt with by other parts of the human
service system.

17

Unified Services in New York State
Hyman M. Forstenzer and *Alan D. Miller*

On June 12, 1973, a unified services bill was signed into law in New York State.[1] In an informational brochure introducing the new law, Governor Malcolm Wilson called it the culmination of long efforts on the part of the state legislature, the Department of Mental Hygiene, and the executive branch to provide the best possible services to the people of New York State. The new law enables the state and its communities to jointly plan, finance, and deliver all mental health, mental retardation, and alcoholism services, he added, giving added impetus to the state's policy of promoting coordinated, comprehensive, community-based services for all the mentally disabled and removing cost differences as a major obstacle to the development and operation of effective local mental hygiene services.

In the same brochure, the commissioner of mental hygiene stated that the concept of the mental institution as an isolated community was obsolete, and that the state had recognized its responsibility to help the mentally disabled in such a way that their dependence was progressively reduced rather than heightened. The new law, he added, was designed to make better use of combined state and local resources to complete the development of a single system of mental hygiene care throughout the state, turning what had been a cooperative relationship between state and local governments into a full partnership. He called this approach in sharp distinction to previous attempts to deal with mental illness by setting up a separate isolated way of life that obscured the problem, anesthetized the discomfort of those responsible for solving it, and denied to the individuals most affected the chance to participate in its solution.

Like any change in a human service system, New York State's unified services law has many antecedents. It evolved from other laws enacted at both federal and state levels. It developed from the political system of New York State, especially the relationships between state and local government as mandated by the state constitution and by the many state laws that govern those relationships. In addition to describing the unified services law, this chapter will attempt to highlight the antecedents of the law and the conditions that shaped it.

Historical Background

World War II produced mounting public concern over mental illness because of the astounding number of draft rejections and service discharges for mental

281

disability.[2] At the same time the social and economic causes of mental illness were pyramiding in the immediate postwar years. New York State was confronted with a 3,000 annual growth in its mental hospital population, with its institutions already dangerously overcrowded.

The first governmental reaction was the National Mental Health Act of 1948.[3] This was the first major move to reexamine the century-old concept that responsibility for mental illness belonged exclusively to state government. The act emphasized community mental health services by providing, under a matching formula, grant-in-aid to states to develop mental health services other than the mental hospital. It established the National Institute of Mental Health and thus provided a focus of responsibility within the Public Health Service for mental health concerns. The administration of the grant program authorized by the act, especially in its early years, evidenced a strong bias against state mental hospitals. The availability of federal funds for the first time made it possible for most states to undertake extrahospital services.

Partly in response to the need to establish a way of administering the federal grant program, but primarily in response to the steady rise in hospital population and dissatisfaction with the state's mental health program as expressed by a Governor's Commission in 1944,[4] New York State established the interdepartmental Mental Health Commission in 1949.[5] The commission's assignment as stated in the law was:

> The commission shall have the duty and is empowered to initiate, formulate and coordinate a master plan for the promotion of mental health programs which may include but not be limited to the following:
>
> a. Provision for recruitment, training and education of professional and other personnel for psychiatric work.
>
> b. Development, expansion and coordination of psychiatric facilities of general hospital bed and psychiatric clinics and also provide for child guidance and adult mental health clinics for outpatient care, and such other mental health facilities as the commission may deem necessary or desirable.
>
> c. Development of a state-aided program or programs for such expanded mental health in general hospital, clinic and mental health facilities.
>
> d. Development and correlation of mental health activities of public and private agencies operating on the local community level in health, welfare, penal, judicial and other fields.
>
> e. Development of programs for research activities in the causes, diagnosis, prevention, treatment and cure of mental illness including those in conjunction with medical schools, the Psychiatric Institute and the State University of New York.

The composition of the commission reflected a beginning realization that control of mental disorders required cooperative efforts by all human service agencies and could not be accomplished by traditional mental health departments alone. The commission consisted of the state commissioners of mental hygiene, health, education, social welfare, and correction. This was also reflected in the charge to the commission (item no. d above). The various projects undertaken by the commission staff contributed to a fund of information, the selection of issues and alternative solutions, and the formulation of concepts essential to the development of a long-range plan for community mental health services. It is significant that from the very beginning of its work the Mental Health Commission established the first mental health epidemiological research unit in the nation. Findings and conclusions were submitted in June 1953 and were embodied in the Community Mental Health Services Act of 1954, the first in the nation.[6]

Community Mental Health Services Act

The act established a permanent system of state aid in localities for the operation of community mental health services. Perhaps its most fundamental principle was its placing of operating responsibility on local governments, with the state paying half the cost. For New York State it marked the first move away from the "state ward" concept embodied in the State Care Act of 1890. This emphasis on local responsibility is consistent with the "home rule" principle embodied in much of New York State law. It was based on the professional conviction that a local mental health program can succeed only to the extent that local citizens accept it and identify with it.

The act recognized the need for a new agency at the local government level. Parts of a mental health program were provided in many communities by education authorities, welfare officials, public health departments and courts, but nowhere was there a central planning body for mental health services. It was felt that comprehensive programming required the combined efforts of health, education, welfare, judicial, and correctional agencies, both public and private. A new agency of local government was authorized, the Community Mental Health Board. Of the nine members of this board, two had to be the ranking local health and welfare officials and two others had to be physicians. The other five were left to local choice with the recommendations that they include a member of the governing body of the city or county, an official or an employee of a school district; persons familiar with practices in courts of criminal jurisdiction or children's courts; and members of voluntary agencies.

The units of local government eligible for participation were determined in part by the nature of the program and in part by existing state statutes and precedents. Other factors weighed were the high costs of mental health services and the shortages of trained personnel. These made it necessary to plan services for fairly large population groups. Eligibility was, therefore, extended to all counties and to cities with populations of 50,000 or more.

The important role of voluntary organizations and nongovernmental groups in the development and support of most then existing mental health programs other than the state hospitals could not be overlooked. Reimbursement to local governments was, therefore, extended to include not only expenditures incurred through direct operation of services, but also payments on contracts for the purchase of services from approved service agencies or qualified personnel.

The intent was to write broad enabling legislation to permit maximum flexibility of development and to allow for the differences among the state's communities. In essence, the act provided state fiscal support for a permanent field trial of methods for the control of mental disorders. Because of the pervasiveness and diffusion that characterized mental illness and mental health, some limits had to be set. To get the law passed the program had to be fitted into the overall pattern of state services and a realistic limit set on the financial obligation the state was undertaking. The state's financial obligation in the original act was limited by a ceiling of $1 of state funds per year per capita of population. Over the years this ceiling was raised several times and finally eliminated.

To define the program further and to differentiate the responsibility of mental health agencies from other human service organizations, the act required that a qualified psychiatrist be appointed as director of the local mental health program and four types of services were declared eligible for reimbursement. These were (1) outpatient psychiatric clinics; (2) inpatient psychiatric services in general hospitals; (3) psychiatric rehabilitation services for persons suffering from psychiatric disorders; (4) consultant and educational services. In practice the first two were quite specific; the third had few clear-cut precedents; and the fourth provided an avenue for involving other human service agencies.

The community mental health board was empowered to review and evaluate services and facilities and to submit a program to the appointing officer and governing body. Within the amounts appropriated, it was authorized to execute the program and to maintain services and facilities. It could enter into contracts for services and facilities, establish rules and regulations for the various parts of its program, and appoint a psychiatrist as director.

The director serves as chief executive officer of the board. He exercises general supervision over the services rendered and facilities operated or supported by the board, and over the treatment of patients in these services and facilities. He recommends programs to the board, and carries on such studies as may be appropriate for the discharge of his duties or the promotion of mental health or prevention of psychiatric disorders.

Implementation

Although the "home rule" policy of the state required the program to be permissive rather than mandatory, all sixty-two counties of the state (five are subsumed in New York City) are now in the program. Within three years after passage of the law 90 percent of the state's population was covered. The sixty-second county (with a population of about 5,000) joined the program in 1970. Over the years as the state legislature enlarged the options under which counties could reorganize their own governments; many of the more populous counties changed over to a county executive form of government. Under new charters they were permitted to change the role of the community mental health board from administrative to advisory and the director became a commissioner of a department of county government, appointed by the county executive.

The state commissioner of mental hygiene was empowered to review the work of all boards and directors, advise them in the performance of their official duties and promulgate regulations governing the granting of state aid. He was authorized to formulate standards of service, personnel, administration, and equipment, and to approve fee schedules. He could withhold state reimbursement, in whole or in part, for failure to comply with the law or the regulations.

In the fiscal year that ended March 31, 1974, state aid for community mental health programs operated by local mental health boards and departments amounted to $64 million. The total spent was more than $200 million, counting contributions to local programs by voluntary agencies and third party payments. Included were 784 facilities with a wide range of service programs, such as general hospital inpatient psychiatric units (65), outpatient clinics (418), day hospitals (66), halfway houses and hostels (30), and twenty-one mental health centers. In that year there were 400,000 admissions, over six million outpatient visits and over one million inpatient days. Thus, over a twenty-year period the Community Mental Health Services Act produced a substantial community-based community-operated mental health program—substantial but not yet comprehensive, unevenly distributed throughout the state, and not yet adequately covering the full range of mental disabilities, and all segments of the population.

In 1959, five years after the Community Mental Health Services Act went into effect, its then director, in discussing problems in relating community programs to state hospitals, commented:

> Are our present efforts to develop community mental health programs more a protest against the state hospitals of the past than an attempt to meet the present and future needs of the mentally ill? I believe that our most immediate need is to develop a working partnership between community services and facilities and the state hospital systems. Unless this is accomplished, I fear that we run the risk of solidifying two separate and distinct programs, both operating at less than optimal levels, each handicapping the other and each presumably concerned with different portions of the range of mental illness and possibly with different segments of the total population. An adequate system for the control of mental illness in populations cannot be developed with the present dichotomy of community and state hospital services.[7]

Not all of the efforts to change came from outside the mental hospitals. In the middle 1950s the hospitals added the newly developed psychotropic drugs to their treatment armamentarium. At the same time they began to change over from locked to open institutions. Without these two intrahospital changes a shift in the locus of treatment might not have been possible and certainly would have been delayed. In the 1960s widespread acceptance by mental hospital administrators of the disability-inducing effects of long-term continuous hospitalization[8] reduced the length of stay and sharply increased the rate of release. All of these changes generated pressure for the development of community services. As in all human service systems, changes in one part inevitably produce change in the rest of the system.

Pressures for Change

In 1955 Congress authorized and appropriated funds for the first national assessment of mental health efforts in the United States.[9] In 1961 *Action for Mental Health* was published—the final report of the Joint Commission on Mental Illness and Health,[10] which had been given the task of carrying out the assessment. The Joint Commission's letter of transmittal to Congress of its final report stated in part:

> This study, while comprehensive, is not exhaustive because of the nature of the problems involved. Mental illness involves so many complexities—biological, chemical, psychological, and social—that we do not presume to present wholly definitive conclusions or universally approved recommendations. . . It remains for legislators and leaders in the mental health field to select for implementation those recommendations that seem immediately practicable and to press for the realization of others so far as they appear urgent and attainable.

In spite of the self-admitted limitations, the Joint Commission's report facilitated the process of change in New York State's mental health program. Its emphasis on major mental illness as "the core problem and unfinished business of the mental health movement" helped move community services toward involvement in the full spectrum of mental disabilities. Its call to general hospitals to provide services for mental illness, if they were to be truly general hospitals, helped reduce a longstanding resistance of general hospital boards and administrators. The commission's recommendation that state hospitals be limited to 1,000 beds or less helped bring about such a reduction in new construction in New York where fiscal authorities had for so long insisted on a minimum size of about 3,000 beds. Its recommendation that custodial care no longer be a function of a specialized mental hospital made it

easier to initiate an appraisal of the role of the state hospital. Its recommendation that rehabilitation be regarded as part of a comprehensive program of
patient services led to changes in both community and hospital programs.
Finally, its call for vast increases in expenditures for public mental services and
its emphasis on the need for increased fiscal support by the federal government
paved the way for a major expansion of federal funding.

The first response of the federal government to the Joint Commission's
report was the authorization and funding of a large grant program to the states
for mental health planning. In New York State these grants underwrote a two-
year planning effort by a state committee and ten regional committees composed
of 800 lay and professional citizens, with staff provided by the Department of
Mental Hygiene. A seven-volume report was published in 1965 under the title
"A Plan for a Comprehensive Mental Health and Mental Retardation Program
for New York State." Major recommendations were made on: Responsibility
for Control of Mental Disorders; Financing; Manpower and Training; Law and
Psychiatry; Facilities Construction; Community Mental Health Centers; The
State Hospitals; Prevention; Rehabilitation; Services for Children; Services for
the Aged; The Addictions—Alcohol and Drug Dependence; General Hospitals;
and The Private Sector.

Among the recommendations made by this planning committee to the
Governor, the following provided significant emphasis toward the unified services concept:[11]

1. Primary responsibility for planning, administering, and coordinating a
mental health and mental retardation program should be carried by a community
mental health board or department.

2. Area advisory committees on mental health and mental retardation
should be appointed composed of representatives of the broad spectrum of
agencies and organizations, the community mental health boards or departments,
the state institutions serving the area, and members of the public as consumers
and representatives of other planning organizations.

3. State aid should be extended to provide reimbursement to mental health
boards for the construction or acquisition of approved facilities, and the state's
Facilities Improvement Corporation should be permitted to fund and construct
community facilities.

4. The choice of treatment facility should be based on the needs of the
patient. To minimize the making of such choice on the basis of differences in
cost sharing between state and local government, exclusive state fiscal responsibility for state hospital care should be ended. A study of the impact of shared
financing of state hospital costs on state-local fiscal relations should be initiated
at once by the Department of Mental Hygiene in cooperation with other appropriate state and local agencies. By 1967 a beginning should be made on cost
sharing for state hospitals care, limited to patients admitted to a state hospital
after July 1, 1967.

5. No new state hospital should be built with accommodations for more than 1,000 patients. The size of each new facility should be appropriate to the size and needs of the population of the area it is to serve.

6. The staffing patterns and ratios of state hospitals should be reorganized to make it possible for them to provide treatment and rehabilitation programs for all of their patients designed to ameliorate or overcome the specific disability of each patient. Sharing of staff between the state hospitals and other community services is strongly recommended as a means of improving all of the services and of attracting staff.

7. Each state hospital should be related to and affiliated with the community mental health centers of its area.

8. In recognition of the present status of our technical ability to control mental disorders, the highest priority should be given to the development of rehabilitation programs in all state hospitals and community mental health centers.

9. There should be a planned and orderly transfer to community mental health boards and departments of mental health of responsibility for aftercare of patients released from state hospitals. Staff sharing for after-care is strongly recommended. The Area Advisory Committee, as soon as they are appointed, should address themselves to this recommendation. After-care should include active follow-up referrals to social, educational, vocational, employment, and public welfare agencies as well as for medication and supportive therapy. It should be made available to all patients regardless of how they were admitted or discharged from inpatient care.

10. Services and facilities for children with mental disorders, even more than in the case of adults, should be located in the communities in which they live, and should be part of a wide range of basic health, education, and welfare services. It is our consensus that the full range of services for children should become the responsibility of the community mental health boards as rapidly as possible. A wide range of alternative services to twenty-four-hour inpatient care should be developed.

11. The concept of the community mental health center should be predicated on the involvement in partnership of the private, voluntary and governmental sectors of the health economy and on the integration of mental health services with the total health field.

The 1964 Hospitalization Act

A study that began in 1959 at the request of the commissioner of mental hygiene culminated in the passage in 1964 of a new Hospitalization Act, a landmark in the history of mental health reform.[12] The principles of the new act are stated in the study committee report[13] as follows:

Every person with serious mental illness needs some care and in many cases must go to a hospital, even if he does not want to.

Mental hospitals are not prisons, but they do, by force on body or mind, deprive patients of some freedom.

Rapid, noncompulsory admission to mental hospitals is good for most patients and helps in allowing effective treatment and early release.

When a person must be sent to a mental hospital against his will, he should not be treated like a criminal and be tried and convicted of being sick. Procedures for his admission are only stepping-stones to treatment.

Any person hospitalized against his will is entitled to watchful protection of his rights, because he is a citizen first and mental patient second.

The principal changes effected by the new act follow:

1. Involuntary civil judicial certification is abolished.
2. All involuntary civil admissions will be based on medical certification.
3. The rights of patients will be protected by a new arm of the court to be known as the Mental Health Information Service.
4. Continued hospitalization of involuntary patients must be authorized periodically by the courts.
5. An informal admission procedure (established by legislation in 1963) is reaffirmed and its use encouraged, together with a requirement for the conversion of all involuntary patients who are suitable to a voluntary or informal status.
6. With only minor variations the new admission procedures are made applicable to all treatment facilities—state hospitals, licensed private institutions, city and county inpatient psychiatric units, and voluntary general hospital psychiatric units.
7. No person shall be deprived of any civil rights solely by virtue of entering a mental hospital as a voluntary or informal patient, nor shall a voluntary or informal admission modify or vary any civil right of a patient so admitted, including but not limited to civil service ranking and appointment or rights relating to the granting, forfeiture or denial of a license, permit, privilege or benefit pursuant to any law.

Perhaps of even greater significance than the elimination of judicial commitment is the requirement for court authorization of continued hospitalization of involuntary patients. The entire statutory base on which rested the system of continuous long-term custodial care was wiped out. Important, too, in the movement toward community-based programs, was the application of this law to all treatment facilities including voluntary general hospital psychiatric units. One other significant accomplishment of the new legislation was the removal of the exclusion of hospital psychiatrists from the decision-making process in connection with hospitalization. Not only were admissions facilitated when indicated, but also inappropriate admissions could now be prevented. Thus, the new Hospitalization Act quickened the pace of change in the mental hospitals and made comprehensive mental health services in communities more feasible.

The Mental Retardation Facilities and Community Mental Health Center Construction Act of 1963 and the 1965 amendments[14] constituted another major antecedent of unified services in New York State. Not only did these federal acts provide a substantial federal fiscal contribution to the development of community services, but they also provided a major impetus toward more comprehensive local programs to provide greater continuity of care and to involve community services more fully in the major mental illnesses.[15] Another federal assist was the Comprehensive Health Planning and Services Act of 1965.[16] This act included mental health as part of comprehensive health planning and required that no less than 15 percent of the funds allocated to each state for planning be devoted to mental health planning. Among other major federal contributions toward the unified services concept were the Medicare/Medicaid Acts, which extended federal health care coverage to the mental disabilities. The huge growth of third party payments for mental disability services made possible by these acts now provide a major funding source for comprehensive programs for the control of mental disorders.

As essential preconditions to unified services, two changes had to be effected in the state institutional system. The first was "unitization."[17] All institutions have been subdivided into units with each unit serving a specific geographic area. Depending on population size, the unit serves a county, a portion of a county, or a part of a city. Each unit relates directly to the local mental health program serving its area. The second change is twofold: sharing of staff with local programs and the use of institution staff for noninpatient services within and without the institution. To illustrate the latter, in the month of April 1974 state institution staff provided a total of 722,736 noninpatient services, which included 81,820 outpatient visits, 18,079 home visits, 49,757 visits for partial care, serving a total of 35,998 individuals in that month.[18]

Another change within the hospital system that contributed to the unified services system occurred in 1968. The Department of Mental Hygiene, utilizing the new admission laws passed earlier and implementing those sections that gave the hospital control over its own intake, announced a new policy on geriatric admissions. Only those elderly patients would be admitted who were in need of psychiatric care and treatment. Patients were not to be admitted when their problems were primarily social, medical, or financial, or for the convenience of some other care facility. In announcing this policy it was recognized that it would force a change in other human services for the elderly.

Another precondition for unified services was the creation of area committees throughout the state, an implementation of one of the recommendations
of the 1965 State Planning Committee. These committees consist of directors
of state institutions serving the area and the directors of the community mental
health boards and departments in each area. They were given responsibility for
making recommendations for programs, advising on construction, developing
methods for sharing staff, and making intercounty arrangements for specialized
services and for assisting smaller counties. A representative of each area committee serves on the department policy committee. The area committees also relate
to the mental health subcommittee of the Area Comprehensive Health Planning
Councils; the "B" agencies of the Federal Comprehensive Health Planning Act.

A final precondition to unified services was accomplished on May 9, 1972,
when Governor Rockefeller signed into law a Recodified Mental Hygiene
Law.[19] It became effective January 1, 1973, and repealed the old Mental
Hygiene Law that had been in effect since 1927 and that had retained most
of the original State Care Act of 1890. The recodification contributed to the
feasibility of unified services legislation by putting into a coherent whole what
had previously been an unwieldy accretion of separate laws. By defining
responsibility for quality of care and by its generous interpretation of the
rights of patients and residents, the recodification provided a sounder foundation for the unified services legislation.

The Advent of Unified Services

On June 12, 1973, a unified services bill was signed into law.[20] It took
effect immediately but the earliest that local government can take advantage of
the plan is July 1, 1974, for New York City and January 1, 1975, for other
counties. At this writing fifteen counties have signed letters of intent to enter
the plan on January 1, 1975. Counties that elect to stay in the present local
services program will continue to receive state aid according to the present
statutory formula of 50 percent for net operating costs, with counties under
200,000 population receiving 75 percent of the first $100,000 of such costs.

The unified services legislation has as its basic intent the development of
a single, integrated system of services to the mentally disabled, actively related
to all other human services in a population area required on behalf of the mentally disabled.

The legislation enables the mental hygiene system to be more capable of
achieving this goal by establishing the following objectives:

1. establish mechanisms through which the most appropriate treatment for
    individual clients can be satisfied, regardless of who provides or pays for it
2. improve planning and use of available resources by mandating joint and
    continuous planning between state and local governmental units

3. set program priorities within an entire geographical area that affect both
    state and local services
4. equalize fiscal support by shared funding of services regardless of sponsor-
    ing governmental level
5. provide for greater economy and effectiveness with greater flexibility in
    use of personnel across payroll jurisdictions
6. build in a requirement for fiscal and programmatic evaluation by both
    state and local authorities
7. establish accountability to consumers of services and encourage participa-
    tion by consumer, consumer representatives, and citizen interests in the
    planning and evaluation processes that determine mental hygiene policy[21]

The fiscal provisions of the law can be summarized as follows:

1. The aggregate costs (the sum of local net operating costs and unreim-
bursed charges for state facility services) will be apportioned between the state
and local government on the basis of the population of each local government
as determined by the last preceding federal census.

2. A local population credit of $10 per capita will be given for the first
100,000 population and $5 per capita for the remaining population of the local
government unit.

3. If such aggregate costs are less than the local population credit, the state
finances the service 100 percent.

4. If the amount of such aggregate costs exceeds such local population
credit, the balance over the local credit, up to $13 per capita, will be financed
on the basis of 80 percent state funds and 20 percent local contributions with all
remaining such costs financed 65 percent by the state and 35 percent locally.

5. Aggregate costs will not include the cost of services to any patients in
a state facility a) who are not residents of the local governmental area or b)
whose last date of admission or readmission to such facility was earlier than five
years prior to the first day of April next succeeding the date on which the first
unified services plan for such local government becomes effective. In 1974 the
law was amended so that the state will pay 100 percent of the costs of mental
hygiene services provided to persons released or discharged from state institutions after December 31, 1973, who had been continuously hospitalized for
five years or more. In addition, social services, medical assistance, and public
assistance provided by social service departments for such persons will also be
a 100 percent state charge—in this case, however, only for a period of five
years following discharge or release.

6. The state will pay 50 percent of all capital costs (excluding federal
aid) incurred by a local government or voluntary agency included in a unified
services plan.

7. The state will pay 100 percent of all capital costs incurred by the
department for state facilities.

8. To reduce any adverse fiscal impact either on local governments or the state, provision was made in the law for a five year phasing-in of local contribution decreases and a six year phasing-in of local contribution increases.

Other important provisions of the law include the following:

1. A unified services plan is a plan for the rendition of unified services designed to provide a broad range of services for all the mentally disabled of the area of local government jurisdiction, whether provided by public or private agencies and whether funded from local, state, federal or private sources.

2. It must arrange for the most effective and economical provision of services allowing for integration, to the extent possible, of all public and private facilities serving the area.

3. Such a plan must be developed by the joint and continuous planning of the local governmental unit, the department, and the directors of department facilities concerned.

4. The plan must be developed with suitable involvement of consumer groups and providers of services.

5. The plan must have the concurrence of the directors of department facilities serving the area and the local governmental unit.

6. It must contain adequate provisions for review and evaluation of the services covered by the plan.

7. The plan must establish priorities for the next local fiscal year in its first submission and long-range goals for a five-year period beginning with the submission of the plan for the second and all subsequent local fiscal years.

8. The department will regularly conduct evaluation studies to determine the relative costs and effectiveness of different types and patterns of service under these plans.

The central office of the department is being reorganized to function more responsively within the unified services system. A major objective is to remove the artificial organizational barriers between state and local efforts on behalf of the mentally disabled. To this end, the department will continue to strengthen its leadership resources to enable it to give the necessary guidance and support to all the components of the system.

A network of regional offices is being established. The central office, working with the regional directors and their staff, will approve plans and budgets and evaluate programs submitted by the regional directors for the geographic units within their responsibility. The regional office network is designed to decentralize the operation of the department in ways that will place management decision making as close as possible to the point where services are provided to clients and will facilitate staff and technical assistance to and cooperation between counties and voluntary agencies in the unified services planning process.

The program divisions are being reorganized to make their structures compatible with the new decentralized emphasis. The central office will play a leadership role in the preparation of regulations and guidelines for the development of unified service plans; in the definition and continuing setting of standards and evaluation of performance; in the review of plans and their approval; in certification and inspection of mental hygiene facilities as required by the law.

Planning Guidelines

The first set of guidelines[22] developed for unified services planning delineated a set of appropriate goals and suggested strategies designed to meet them:

GOALS	STRATEGIES
Broaden the scope of concern in planning and implementing services to focus on whole populations and target groups within them.	Establish responsibility of local govenmental unit for services to all clients from a defined population.
	Require regional offices to facilitate unified services plan development and implementation.
	Require community mental health service directors and D.M.H. facility directors to enter agreements for coordinated services.
Assure *responsiveness* of the unified service system to the needs of target populations.	Require identification of needs and objectives in unified service planning.
	Foster increased attention to citizen's rights and to citizen participation in the planning, implementation, and evaluation of programs designed to meet the needs of the mentally disabled.
Provide the mentally disabled with *appropriate* service.	Require unified service systems to provide a "minimum range of services" by direct service, contract, or intercounty arrangements.
	Require D.M.H. program divisions to develop statewide service plans and models for systems of service for the mentally ill, mentally retarded, and alcoholics.

Provide service with least possible *disruption* of individual and family living.

Establish criteria that interprovider arrangements maintain patient in setting that maximizes his level of functioning.

Require individual determination of appropriateness for inpatient admissions.

Establish *equity* in allocation of resources among different client groups

Require priority be given to populations and conditions involving greater handicap or risk of disability.

Prohibit discrimination against persons with disorders not easily treated or prevented or disabilities that evoke low level of professional interest.

Assure *continuity* of care among providers

Require interprovider arrangements that facilitate client movement and delineate responsibility for service delivery.

Require mechanisms to monitor "continuity."

Increase accountability (fiscal and programmatic) of mental hygiene structure.

Require development of management information system and ongoing programs evaluation efforts as a basis for analyzing effectiveness and efficiency.

Derive maximum benefit from fiscal and personal resources.

Require unified services plans to be based on defined populations and target groups and expressed in terms of dollars and personnel assigned to specific client service to be provided, thereby facilitating staff and space sharing.

Improve the *capacity of communities* to support the mentally disabled.

Encourage advocacy on behalf of the mentally handicapped with other human service systems responsible for the provision of housing, financial assistance, employment, transportation, correctional programs, recreation and socialization, medical care, education, and vocational training.

Reduce the number of *institutionalized* persons capable of protected community living.

Require the development of a variety of alternative sheltered living arrangements such as coop apartments, family care, and hotels.

Implement D.M.H. institutional treatment programs conducive to optimum functional growth.

Provide intensive, sophisticated care to current admissions to state institutions, enabling them to return to their normal pursuits as soon as possible and provide the most humane and modern care possible to those who must remain in department facilities for longer periods of time.

Planning Requirements

A significant section of the unified services law is the one setting forth the requirements for unified services planning. It states (in part) as follows:

(a) A unified services plan shall set forth priorities for unified services for the next local fiscal year and, commencing with plans to be submitted subsequent to the first approved plan, the long-range goals for such services and priorities for the five-year period commencing with the next local fiscal year.

(b) The development of each unified services plan shall be a continuous planning and evaluation process among the department, the department facilities providing services to the area, and the local governmental unit. Such process shall involve the providers of services and representatives of consumers of services and non-governmental organizations and groups concerned with mental disability. The director of any department facility providing services pursuant to such plan shall submit a copy of such plan to the department as part of the justification for such facility's annual budget. After approval by the commissioner, a unified services plan shall be a joint commitment between the department and the local governmental unit, subject to state and local legislative appropriations, for services to be provided pursuant thereto.

(c)   A unified services plan shall (i) arrange, in accordance with
the plan's priorities for unified services to the area, for the most effective and economical provision of such services and (ii) provide the
basis for state and local government financing of such services pursuant
to this article. To this end a unified services plan shall allow for the
integration by mutual agreement of all facilities serving the area, whether
publicly or privately operated and shall include participation as appropriate by all department facilities and local governmental facilities
serving the area. The services rendered by general and psychiatric
hospitals, city, county and state health and social services agencies,
facilities offering mental retardation services and alcoholism programs,
probation departments, physicians, psychologists, social workers, public
health nurses, and other public and private agencies and personnel may
be included in such plan.

(d)   The unified services plan shall provide an inventory of all
public and private resources for the mentally disabled serving the local
area.

(f)   The unified services plan shall specify all unified services and
the estimated operating costs of such services for the next local fiscal
year. Such unified services may include any of the following:

(1)   Inpatient services
(2)   Out-patient services
(3)   Patient hospitalization services, such as day care, night care, or weekend care
(4)   Emergency services
(5)   Consultation and education services to community agencies and
professional and associated personnel and information services to
the general public
(6)   Preventive services
(7)   Diagnostic and referral services
(8)   Rehabilitative services, including vocational, educational, and training programs
(9)   Precare and aftercare services in the community, including foster
home placement, home visiting, and halfway houses
(10)   Staff training
(11)   Research and evaluation
(12)   Activities involved in bringing the needs of the mentally disabled to
the attention of governmental and private providers of services
(13)   Such other services as may be approved by the commissioner

(g)   The unified services plan shall set forth a program for the acquisition, construction, renovation, rehabilitation, and improvement of local

and state facilities used for provision of services pursuant to such plan.

(h) The unified services plan shall include provisions for evaluation of programs together with detailed descriptions of persons to be served, priority of target groups, direct service programs, indirect and supportive services and methodology for monitoring and evaluating costs and effectiveness of different types and patterns of service.[23]

Another significant provision relates to the use of state facilities and makes possible the turning over of these facilities to the localities:

After approval of a unified services plan, services for the mentally disabled of the area served by a local governmental unit which are provided by such local governmental unit or any of the department's facilities shall be in accordance with and pursuant to such unified services plan. Services (including both inpatient and out-patient services) provided by department facilities pursuant to a unified services plan shall be provided pursuant to contracts between the department or its facilities and the local governmental unit. Alternatively, if the department and a local governmental unit agree, state facilities may, in whole or in part, be used by or leased, rented, or sold to such local governmental unit or to a voluntary agency, in accordance with applicable state law, for operation by or through it pursuant to a unified services plan.[24]

Summary and Conclusions

In principle, the unified services act has been hailed by most provider and consumer organizations in the state as a major step forward in the effort to control mental disorders. However, because it represents a major shift in public financing of mental disability programs it is being carefully scrutinized by local government. For the most part, the question local government is asking is, "Will this cost us more or less local tax dollars immediately and in the future?"

Under the unified services fiscal formula, and based on present program levels, forty-three counties and New York City would pay less than they pay under the local services program and fourteen counties would pay more.

If a county will be required to spend more money under unified services, a six-year phase-in provides that there will be no additional cost to the county in the first year. In the following years, any increased cost to the county will be phased in at 20 percent of the increase per year until the full increased cost is met over six years.

If a county will be paying less under unified services than under the present local services program, there will be a five-year phase-in. In the first year, the county will be required to spend 80 percent of the savings, 60 percent in the second year, and so on, until the full savings are realized at the end of five years.

Other issues that have been raised concerning the act include (1) Should a local government be permitted to change its mind after it has opted to enter the program? (2) Does the act still reflect too much state control over programs, especially the commissioner's power to approve or disapprove plans and to decide when there are differences of opinion between state, local, and voluntary providers in a given area? The attitude of the Department of Mental Hygiene is that neither the law nor the first regulations and guidelines are unchangeable and that changes should evolve from the first few years of experience under the act.

Finally, consistent with governmental responsibility for the care of the mentally disabled and for the protection of society, the unified services act of New York State neither freezes nor closes out the state hospital system. It provides for changes in the extent to which it can be used, the manner in which it can be used, and the ways in which hospital staff can be used—all of these on a county-by-county basis and with the full participation of local public and private providers, citizens, and consumers.

Notes

1. N.Y. Mental Hygiene Law, Article 11.
2. Senate Report #1353, May 16, 1946, 1946 U. S. Code Congressional Service, page 1260.
3. The Public Health and Welfare Law, U. S. Code Annotated, Title 42, Sec. 201, 209, 210, 215, 218, 219, 232, 241, 242a, 244, 246.
4. *The Care of the Mentally Ill in the State of New York*, 1944, N.Y.S. Legislative Document.
5. THE LAWS OF NEW YORK STATE, Chapter 733, 1949.
6. Community Mental Health Services Act, Article 8-A, N.Y. Mental Hygiene Law, now incorporated in Article 11 of the Recodified N.Y. Mental Hygiene Law.
7. Forstenzer, H.M., *Problems in Relating Community Programs to State Hospitals,* AMERICAN JOURNAL OF PUBLIC HEALTH, 51:1152, August, 1961.
8. AMERICAN PUBLIC HEALTH ASSOCIATION, MENTAL DISORDERS—A GUIDE TO CONTROL METHODS, New York, A.P.H.A., 1962.
9. Mental Health Study Act of 1955, Sec. 242b, U.S. Code Annotated, Title 42, The Public Health and Welfare Law.
10. JOINT COMMISSION ON MENTAL ILLNESS AND HEALTH, ACTION FOR MENTAL HEALTH, Basic Books, Inc., New York, 1961.

11. A Plan for a Comprehensive Mental Health and Mental Retardation Program for New York State, Volume 1, Report of the Mental Health & Mental Retardation Sections of the State Planning Committee, N.Y.S. Department of Mental Hygiene, Albany, New York, 1965.
12. Chapter 738 of the New York State Laws of 1964, now Article 31 of the Recodified N.Y. Mental Hygiene Law.
13. BAR ASSOCIATION OF THE CITY OF NEW YORK, SPECIAL COMMITTEE TO STUDY COMMITMENT PROCEDURES, AND CORNELL LAW SCHOOL, MENTAL ILLNESS AND DUE PROCESS, New York, Cornell University Press, 1962.
14. The Public Health and Welfare Law, Sec. 295, 2661-67, 2682-87.
15. Ibid., Sec. 2683, and Regulations for Community Mental Health Center Grants, NIMH.
16. The Public Health and Welfare Law, Sec. 242g-247.
17. Proceedings of the 38th Annual Conference, MILBANK MEMORIAL FUND, DECENTRALIZATION OF PSYCHIATRIC SERVICES AND CONTINUITY OF CARE, Milbank Memorial Fund, New York, New York, 1962.
18. N.Y.S. Department of Mental Hygiene, Statistical Report for April, 1974.
19. Chapter 251 of the Laws of 1972 of New York State, now known as the New York State Mental Hygiene Law.
20. Ibid., Article 11.
21. Preliminary Guidelines for Unified Services Law and the Planning Process, New York State Department of Mental Hygiene, Division of Unified Services Management, Albany, N.Y., 1973.
22. Ibid.
23. Unified Services Law, Section 11.21.
24. N.Y. Mental Hygiene Law, Section 11.19, paragraph e.

18 Developments in Metropolitan State Hospital Services

John A. Talbott

While the future role of the state hospital in large metropolitan areas is unpredictable, the complexity of problems in the big cities, the diversity of their population, and the massiveness of the state's resources combine to suggest numerous possibilities.[a] A large metropolitan area *is* different from a small town or city. Its population is more concentrated, poorer, blacker, and less educated; its streets teem with activity, crime, pathology, and energy; and its mentally disturbed citizens are more suicidal, more schizophrenic, and more likely to abuse drugs and alcohol. The big city's problems are greater, partially because of their large bureaucratic governmental structures, which are impersonal, unresponsive, and self-perpetuating; because societal problems surface rapidly in a pressure-cooker atmosphere; and because the identification of issues, isolation of contributing variables, and assignment of accountability are so difficult.

In spite of this tumultuous matrix, state hospitals in urban areas are probably more open to imaginative options than those located elsewhere because the land they occupy is valuable, their budgets are ample, their staffs diverse and multidisciplinary, and their mandate comprehensive, flexible, and public health oriented. And, at least in New York State, a new breed of directors has begun to implement progressive changes in the state facilities and to link their efforts to those of county or city mental health providers.[1]

What makes the role of the metropolitan state facility different from other state hospitals is its relationship to these population, problem, and potentiality factors. Because of the *number* of agencies, funding sources, population groups, and individual service providers; the *fragmentation* of health, mental health, and social services; and the *complexity* of problems seen in the urban population, there is a *multiplicity* of choices for alternate solutions—a potential cornucopia of permutations of people, problems, services, and service-providers. This leads to a more difficult problem on a different level—that of *coordinating* a comprehensive network of services within and between agencies and superagencies encouraging maximum

---

[a]Since my own professional experience has been largely limited to New York State and New York City, I will be using them as the basis for my observations in this chapter. However, most developments I discuss are common to other areas of the country, and New York City still has more similarities than differences in respect to other large metropolitan areas.

301

utilization of the potential options while discouraging agency isolation, inter-agency, and territorial hostilities, as well as gaps or duplications in service.

The closing of state hospitals is essentially a false issue. Buildings may be abandoned, sites changed, staff retained and redeployed, and services drastically altered—but services will continue to be provided to people by mental health workers on state payrolls. In this context, what are the recent developments that differentiate a state hospital located in a large metropolitan area from those in suburban or rural areas?

Catchment Responsibility and Unitization

Two of the most important recent developments affecting urban state facilities concern changes in their structure and organization. Assumption of the responsibility for manageable geographic areas (in the main, clusters of catchment areas conforming to federal Community Mental Health Center guidelines), has enabled state facilities to narrow their focus of concern from entire cities, boroughs, or mega-ghettos, to relatively small neighborhoods and health areas.[2] Catchmenting may complicate the efficient delivery of mental health services because such services tend to be concentrated in certain urban areas (e.g., center city), while certain high-risk population groups (e.g., alcoholics, homeless men, discharged patients, etc.) tend to live in other areas. However, these disadvantages are outweighed by the advantages of accountability and continuity of care that result from the staff serving a manageably sized population and dealing with a knowable number of agencies.

In addition, the attempt to unitize state hospitals serves to break up the monolithic institution into reasonably sized minihospitals of 100 to 200 inpatients and 500 to 1,000 outpatients.[3] In the big city the unitization of the state hospital allows it to begin to cope administratively with catchment responsibility, multiagency planning and service coordination, staff development, and the initiation of training programs so urgently needed for urban mental health workers.

The Team Approach

The adoption of the team approach in urban state hospitals has markedly altered the traditional patient-staff relationship for several reasons.[4] First, many of the paraprofessionals working in metropolitan state facilities have similar socioeconomic backgrounds to many of their patients, and come from urban minority groups and ghetto neighborhoods. Second, since the aide or attendant is expected to provide more than custodial care, his or her therapeutic input becomes even more valuable than previously. However, since many state hospital physicians are foreign-born and -educated, they lack the cultural familiarity necessary to deal optimally and optimistically with their ghetto patients. Likewise, while nurses, social workers, psychologists, and activity therapists are more likely to be American-born and English speaking, their predominately white, middle or working class backgrounds will perpetuate the cultural and socioeconomic gap between staff and patients.[5]

Optimal use of both the skills and knowledge of the professional as well as the know-how and reality orientation of the paraprofessional is dependent upon sophisticated team training programs. Such training should include a comprehensive exploration of the racial, cultural, subcultural, ethnic, religious, social, economic, and political differences that exist in all patients and staff groups. The essential goals of such training should be to provide a psychiatric frame of reference for the paraprofessionals or nonprofessionals and a cultural frame of reference for the professional staff members.

Full utilization of the team's resources, including using the aide's familiarity with the community, permits the treatment team to diagnose and treat the patient's illness more effectively, to utilize alternative services and programs, to discover helpful individuals in the community, and to pretest many ideas, plans, and proposals.

Unified Services

The passage of unified services legislation in New York State[b] has markedly altered the role of the state hospital, as well as the roles of most other providers of mental health care. Formerly, the state hospitals were primarily providers of mental health care, with little opportunity to plan or set policy. Now, even before the formal unified services programs are funded or implemented, there is an urgent need to undergo an extensive planning and coordination effort. In fact, in New York City, while unified services funding may never come to pass, the impact of unified services planning has already been felt.

The planning necessitated by the possibility of unified services funding requires that *all* providers of mental health services combine their efforts. Heretofore, the inpatient providers, whether city, state, or voluntary, provided the leadership and coordination, if there was any. Now, three other groups take part: the consumers of mental health services; the private, voluntary, or contract agencies; and the program analysts, from city and state governmental agencies. Consumers ask questions and provide input not otherwise heard. While sometimes peripheral, their concerns are often closer to reality in the community than that of the experts and facilitate program design and program acceptance in the area.

[b]Discussed in the previous chapter.

Voluntary agencies, some small, some highly specialized (along diagnostic, ethnic or age lines), and some bearing citywide rather than catchment responsibility, have also been added to the mix. While sometimes perceived as self-interested and elitist, they too have added a new perspective on the subpopulations in need of care in the urban community. And lastly, the governmental staff members have been introduced into the planning process at an operational rather than a purely policy level. While they too often serve only to add another layer of bureaucracy, they have the potential for providing an effective cohesive force and leadership, and for consultation to the provider/consumer group.

Periodic meetings involving city, state, and voluntary mental health care providers have already produced some remarkable benefits. The we/they attitude among agencies and institutions often gives way to the mutual problem-solving approach needed to resolve shared patient care responsibilities. In addition, discussion of existing services inevitably leads to the possibility of filling gaps in service networks. Identification of priorities, needs, and service inter-digitations is essential if planning is to move forward. In times of plenty, filling the gaps in service provides the catchment group with an opportunity to design new and more coordinated services. However, as in the recent past, characterized by economic restrictions, there has been a need to justify existing programs as well as to examine critically the allocation of resources. At best, this planning process can lead to creative solutions, such as staff-sharing, building flexibility, and interagency consultation. But there is the chance that the process may resemble dogs fighting for the same small bone, resulting in the development of suspicion concerning the motives for self-examination and self-appraisal. Frequently, at such times, the state's programs, often perceived as wasteful, inadequate, incompetent, and concerned with lower priorities (e.g., the chronically mentally ill), may become the target for criticism and fiscal raiding.

The impact of unified services planning on state facilities is already apparent. Plans for services are no longer arrived at unilaterally; staff members view their counterparts in the community with ambivalence, fearing their criticism and implied superiority, but welcoming their competence and expertise; and the morale of some members of the state facility goes up at the prospect of others helping to share the burden and frustration of caring for the chronic and severely mentally disabled population.

When unified services funding becomes a reality, it will enable the cooperating agencies to implement more creative program patterns, such as deploying staff according to community needs not institutional constraints, altering the utilization of space in and out of the hospital, and maximizing their deficiencies. For the state facility, this potential for flexibility in program and service delivery offers a great deal of hope in solving some of the more difficult problems.

For instance, joint staffing of a day care center gives unskilled workers from the state hospital the opportunity to gain community experience and to learn from the highly skilled staff of the community agency. In another situation, a general or voluntary hospital unable to generate new funding for personnel may contribute program space if the state facility contributes staffing.

Specialized Services

While the urban state hospital probably never became as much of an end-of-the-line custodial warehouse as its country cousin did, its role was all too often that of the passive receptacle for the ghetto's misfits and the city's homeless. With the hospital's assumption of more responsibility for more active intervention came the need for developing specialized services. These include services for diagnostic categories over-represented in urban areas, for example, alcoholics and drug addicts; for vulnerable age groups, for example, adolescents and the elderly; and for delivering specialized treatment modalities, for example, behavior modification, and social and vocational rehabilitation.[6]

Specialized services, while augmenting catchment services, must be thoroughly coordinated with and integrated into them. Staff must be retrained and deployed, and while considerable resistance is incurred in moving into unfamiliar areas, such retraining frequently motivates people previously regarded as rigid, noncontributory, and recalcitrant. The urban state facility, because of its responsibility for so many problem groups, must continue to see its future as shifting to serve these groups, utilizing these shifts in service delivery as opportunities to constantly retrain, rechannel and reenergize administrative and clinical staff members.

Inpatient Services

The conception of inpatient services has changed markedly in recent years, from that of caring for hopeless seniles and schizophrenics living out the rest of their lives in hospital settings, to providing active treatment and rehabilitation, enabling most patients to return to productive living and working.[7] Unitization and more active treatment have brought about different patterns in the utilization of inpatient services, with more patients spending fewer days as inpatients. Optimally, this results in a focus on active treatment and rehabilitation, rather than hoteling and custodial services. At its worst, however, it sets up the "revolving door," where patients are locked, not in inertia, but in constant shuffling and perpetual motion.[8]

In the urban state hospital, efforts are being made to reduce the difference in the quality and type of care provided by municipal county receiving hospitals and by the state units. In some instances, one or the other takes over total responsibility for all inpatient services. In other cases, the responsibility is

shared vis-à-vis the acute v. chronic differential, and in other situations the
responsibility is divided along geographical lines. Another recent development
is the provision of inpatient services in city or voluntary hospitals with shared
or co-equal staff from the hospital and state facility.

Movement of patients between service components in the mental health
network is sometimes facilitated by the placement of screening or admitting
teams in the receiving hospital, outpatient facility or mobile unit. Transfer
of patients from one facility to another then becomes a technical procedure
and minimizes the fighting, ping-ponging of patients and "rejection" by one
facility of another's referral. The multitude of facilities in an urban area makes
liaison relationships of critical importance.

Alternatives to Hospitalization

Because of the population density, obvious need and the availability of
public transportation, alternatives to inpatient hospitalization have been more
readily developed in urban areas by state hospitals. Day hospitals, day centers,
crisis teams, home care programs, night hospitals, and outpatient services have
sprung up both in state facilities and satellite locations. Whether funded and
staffed by unitary or multiple auspices, such services have provided an essential
link in the network of urban mental health services and will continue to serve
as alternatives to hospitalization.

Primary Prevention Services

Traditionally, state facilities have concentrated their services on secondary
and tertiary prevention. Now, in many instances, they develop active programs
of consultation and community education. Often such operations are focused
on the community network surrounding the chronically and severely mentally
disabled rather than the general population. For instance, broad programs of
consultation to the courts, schools, and seminars are less likely to be conducted
by state facilities than are case-oriented seminars with police, teachers, and
ministers around specific problems or patients. Programs of education in mental health are found more frequently in nonurban state hospitals, possibly
because in urban areas the private and municipally funded programs have traditionally performed this function, whereas in rural areas, the state hospital may
be the primary or only psychiatric facility. In addition, there continues to be
a great deal of resistance to the dilution of urban state hospital resources from
the primary mission of caring for the severely mentally disabled.[9]

Housing Problems

In the big cities, already plagued by a shortage of adequate housing, one frequently finds groups of discharged mental patients, who no longer require psychiatric inpatient care, living in deteriorated areas. In some cities, one can identify distinct neighborhoods to which specific groups gravitate. In other cities, representatives of these groups (alcoholics, homeless men, ex-convicts, the elderly, hardcore unemployables, and mental patients) all gather in the same area. In such areas, the strong all too often prey upon the weak and present a formidable problem.[10]

Urban state hospitals have attempted to cope with this seemingly overwhelming problem by building new facilities, developing scattered apartments for patients, and providing high quality services to existing hotels, flophouses, or hostels. In the past, society and its agents in municipal and voluntary hospitals have been accused of "dumping" into state hospitals, but lately this accusation has been directed at the state facilities themselves. Obviously, there should be no "dumping grounds," and the development of creative solutions to housing problems in areas of urban blight will continue to occupy all providers in metropolitan areas for many years.

Training

Recognizing that their changing role depends on the changing roles of their staff, state facilities have initiated substantial education and training programs. Urban state hospitals, with large numbers of poorly educated aides, are especially in need of such efforts. General educational strategies include high school equivalency programs, release time for study, and educational leave to pursue college or graduate work. The improvement of existing skills and acquisition of new ones is attained by in- and out-of-house programs that extend from floor buffing to family therapy, from supervisory techniques to long range mental health planning, and from cultural metaphors to foreign languages. Unique needs in urban areas include the understanding of symptoms in their cultural context, slang, and subcultural language use, cultural anthropology, and sociology. Team training, already mentioned, must incorporate understanding of all the ethnic, racial and social variables that exist in the population being served. In addition, managerial and administrative skills need to be taught to this new generation of generic mental health workers.[11]

Some urban state hospitals have developed their own training programs, others take advantage of community educational institutions, while others contract out such services or utilize regional state training or educational services. Most hospitals appreciate the advantage of utilizing community facilities, not only because of the economic advantage, but because of the interchange that develops between students and both institutions. Involvement of patients and consumers in such efforts further enhances their relevance and richness.

Relationships with Community Agencies

Because of the large number of agencies and institutions in large urban areas, relationships with them constitute a large portion of the state hospital staff's time and energy. Aside from the previously mentioned planning and training efforts, smooth functioning of the mental health network requires coordination, cooperation, and a great deal of continuous information-sharing. As a result, the number of community liaison meetings has created a subindustry in psychiatry. Negotiating skills, clear communication, and understanding mutual needs and offerings (e.g., trade-offs) become essential.

Techniques such as staff-sharing, joint educational programs, constant back and forth visiting, and staff interchanges help improve interagency relationships. Likewise, because distances are less formidable than areas around suburban or rural state facilities, tasks can be performed by cooperating staffs in the communities they serve with relatively little loss of time.

The Future

The fact that state hospitals in urban areas are so accessible to their communities leads some to hope that they can be phased out quickly and replaced by CMHCs, local hospitals, or community agencies. However, the state hospital's long-standing commitment to the severely mentally ill, coupled with the widespread lack of interest by others in dealing with such impoverished people, militates against an early demise. To the contrary, in spite of the state hospitals' chronic problems—civil service, budgetary restrictions, bureaucratic inflexibility, and incompetent or untrained staff—their potential to adjust and adapt to changing needs and priorities insures their continuing role in serving the severely mentally disabled in the urban community.

Notes

1. Foley, A.R.; Arce, A.; Greenberg, I.; and Gorham, P., "Collaboration Between Public and Private Agencies in Developing a Community Mental Health Service," *Hosp. and Comm. Psychiat.* 22:337-40, 1971; Wilder, J.F., Leven, G., and Zwerling, I., "Planning and Developing the Focus of Care," in *Practice of Community Mental Health*, H. Gruenbaum (ed.), Boston: Little, Brown & Co., 1970, pp. 383-409; Mesnikoff, A.M., "Unified Services: Promising Successor to the Mental Health Center," *NYSDB Bulletin* 15:8-9, 1973; Talbott, J.A., Restructuring of State Hospital Services To Bring About Comprehensive, Collaborative, Coordinated, Continuous, Community Mental Health Service: Fat Chance in Lean Times, unpublished manuscript.

2. Zusman, Jack, "Design of Catchment Areas for Community Mental Health," *Arch. Gen. Psychiat.* 21: 568-73, 1969.
3. Abrams, A.L., "Geographic Unitization in Large State Hospitals," *Hosp. and Comm. Psychiat.* 21:285-86, 1969; Ellsworth, R.B., Dickman, H.R., and Maroney, R.S., "Characteristics of Productive and Unproductive Unit Systems in VA Psychiatric Hospitals," *Hosp. and Comm. Psychiat.* 23: 261-68, 1972.
4. Shapiro, E.R. and Gudemen, J.E., "Using the Team Concept to Change a Psychoanalytically Oriented Therapeutic Community," *Hosp. and Comm. Psychiat.* 25: 166-69, 1974.
5. Talbott, J.A.; Ross, A.M.; Skerrett, A.F.; Curry, M.D.; Marcus, S.I.; Theodorou, H.; and Smith, B.J., "The Paraprofessional Teaches the Professional." *Amer. J. Psychiat.* 130: 805-808, 1973.
6. Klett, W.G. and Watson, C.G., "The Unit System: Current Staff Attitudes and Future Directions," *Hosp. and Comm. Psychiat.* 24: 539-42, 1973.
7. Paul, G., "Chronic Mental Patient: Current Status—Future Directions," *Psychol. Bull.* 71: 81-94, 1969.
8. Talbott, J.A., "Stopping the Revolving Door: A Study of Readmissions to a State Hospital," *Psych. Quart.* 48: 159-68, 1974.
9. Mazade, N.A., "Consultation and Education Practice and Organizational Structure in Ten Community Mental Health Centers," *Hosp. and Comm. Psychiat.* 25: 673-75, 1974.
10. Shapiro, J., *Communities of the Alone*, New York: Association Press, 1971.
11. Talbott, J.A. et al., "The Paraprofessional Teaches the Professional."

19

Operating Rural Community Programs Through a State Hospital

Roger Mesmer

Warren State Hospital's community psychiatry program is a comprehensive system of primary and tertiary prevention services that has been developed in the home county of a rural state hospital. Warren, Pennsylvania, is a county of 45,000 people about 100 miles south of Buffalo. The economy is fairly stable, with a base of diversified light industry. Warren county is hilly. Its population is made up mostly of Germans, Swedes, and Italians who have interbred. The percentage of elderly population is the highest in Pennsylvania. Unemployment is 4 percent, which is the lowest for northwestern Pennsylvania.

Not being near a city, Warren "does for itself" with active art, music, and intellectual groups, and active service clubs. Many of its young people migrate to cities. Industry attracts middle management and skilled personnel into the area. However, in-and-out migration is not common.

Warren State Hospital serves the thirteen counties of northwestern Pennsylvania, with a population of about 1,000,000 people in its catchment area, which amounts to about one-fourth of the state's area (seven MH/MR areas). In 1966 it started planning for two community programs, a community center for the elderly and a job placement service for long-term patients, based on European models described by Walter Barton and colleagues[1] and on the author's own observations.[2] With the cooperation of the Warren Council of Social Agencies, a committee was established that became the Board of the Warren Senior Center. The center opened as a community center for the elderly in 1968, helped by a three-year grant under the Older Americans Act. Gradually a day care program developed with a nurse in charge and a few geriatric patients from Warren State Hospital and the county home as its first clients, based on the simple program of daily living offered by Nuffield House in Nottingham, England. Day care patients arrived in the center's minibus with its friendly driver, read the paper, did some craft project, and then had lunch together. The afternoon was time when they could stop for their own needs and return home. They made friends quickly and began to improve in appearance and zest for living.

Also in 1968 a multidisciplinary team doing community job placement developed. It undertook the rehabilitation of patients who were good workers, but had no one to receive them back into the community. About thirty placements were made in Warren. The Community Job Placement Committee found these people jobs, housing, and a social club where they could meet together with volunteers from the Warren County Mental Health Association.

From 1969-71 the author was assigned to community work on a full-time

311

basis, until the exodus of the hospital's psychiatric staff to community mental health center positions necessitated resuming inpatient responsibilities. In those three years, consultations with the Bradford and Warren County Schools, and with Head Start and the Visiting Nurses Association were established.

After-care, previously the responsibility of family doctors, was provided by an after-care clinic for discharged Warren County patients. A mother's club at the YWCA proved to be a spawning ground for a number of lasting programs: a Lamaze class for expecting parents, two Montessori nurseries, and a nursing mothers' group. Widow-to-widow counseling[3] was added to the Warren Senior Center's services. A group of widows who had resolved their own grief were trained to listen to and support other recent widows. The group calls new widows one month after their husband's names appear in the obituary notices. They give them opportunity to express their grief, anger, and anxiety, and offer companionship at a time when the widow's family have left and she is alone.

Pastoral Counseling Seminars, case-centered seminars for groups of ten clergymen, were given regularly, in conjunction with the hospital's chaplains. The seminar's thesis was that counseling is part of a minister's function, that he should not be a minipsychologist, but should present an ethical position after listening to the problems. Cases of mental illness in the parish, sexual problems, aging, and alcoholism, were dealt with. Text for the seminar was Howard Clinebell's *Basic Types in Pastoral Counseling.*[4]

On the postseminar questionnaire, most of the ministers said they could refer more easily to mental health professionals. Several said they were more free to deal with certain problems; others felt they could better define the cases they should counsel and those they should refer. They also enjoyed the fellowship of the meetings, where the loneliness of bearing the burdens of parish life was relieved.

As soon as these programs were well established, interested residents participated in them as part of their training. One resident trained the widows and set up preretirement sessions at the Warren Senior Center. Three helped with the Warren County Schools. Another worked with the Day Care Program, and another with the Visiting Nurses. Weekly seminars, discussing what was taking place, and making future plans were held, relying heavily on the methodology of Gerald Caplan[5] for consultation technique.

The year 1971 was one of retrenchment for the community program, as the hospital became unitized. Time was spent working with Central Unit, which served the counties in which these consultation services were being given. Only the Warren County Schools and Visiting Nurses consultation could be offered that year. By now the Warren Senior Center was a strong community institution and carried on its own programs, adding a low-cost Meals-on-Wheels service.

Two group living arrangements were developed to help patients back into the community. A motel which was invariably underoccupied was utilized as a home for twenty-four patients who would be supported by the day care Program. Solid relationships with the churches through the Pastoral Counseling Seminar were helpful in the organization of "Community Concerns," a corporation consisting of the social action committees of six churches. Community Concerns bought a house in Warren for eight former patients who were capable of working. The mental health administrator, who by this time was funding Warren Senior Center's Day Care Program, hired the central unit caseworker to supervise these group homes.

Mutual interests created excellent cooperation between Central Unit's team and the local community Mental Health Center. By now, the after-care clinic and the eighty-year-old outpatient psychotherapy services had closed and the residents were transferred to the Mental Health Center for outpatient experience. The school consultation also sent many referrals to the Mental Health Center. Monthly meetings discussed these interfaces between hospital and community services.

By 1972 Central Unit was running smoothly and there was time for renewal of the community programs that had been lying fallow. The school consultation was integrated into the permanent structure of pupil personnel services by the school district's hiring a psychiatric nurse, an additional elementary guidance counselor, and a social worker to work with the hospital team.

The custom has been to see the referring teacher, the child, and the parents and to mobilize cooperative efforts. One-to-one tutoring by trained volunteers was often recommended. These had proven their usefulness in some schools that were now doing their own recruiting. Behavior modification with contingency contracting techniques was often useful. Many hyperkinetic children were treated with gross motor movements or Ritalin, depending on the ability of the consultee. Guidance groups have developed in some schools.

To the school consultation program was added a kindergarten-first grade preventive program. Title I funds were obtained by the school district. Three schools with high poverty incidence were chosen as test schools and matched with three similar schools. Aides were trained in gross and fine motor movements and assigned one-half day to each class in the test schools. Our basic theory was that many children who mature slowly or are unprepared culturally are defeated in their earliest school days. Teachers and principals of the test schools, therefore, were helped to de-emphasize the academic and allow the aides to work one-to-one and in small groups, giving the children tasks in which they could succeed until mature enough to learn to read. Ralph Ojemann's[6] Causal Approach materials were used in the first grade classes. Some group work was done by elementary guidance counselors with parents of troubled children. Test children were screened for perceptual problems. The test and control children are tested by the California Test of Personality and the Stanford Early School Achievement Test before beginning the project and after their third grades.

The Pastoral Counseling Seminar Took on a new format. Presentations

were given by members of the hospital team, describing the special needs of
people of different age groups in the parish congregations, for example,
expectant parents, preschool children and their families, aging and grieving,
etc. Next year the usefulness of this material in pastoral ministry, sermons,
and community action will be assessed in meetings with the clergymen concerned. Out of these meetings a Pastoral Counseling Service, a weekend
seminar of marriage enrichment for couples in the first year of marriage, and
a joint meeting of the Warren County Medical Society and the clergymen
have resulted to date.

A new consultation was begun with Warren County Children's Services.
Many cases needing that agency's help were seen at the school consultation.
A vigorous new director made the consultation highly feasible. Behavior
modification techniques were introduced to help families deal with their
children. One suggestion resulted in development of group counseling for
unwed mothers. The director presented many adminsitrative problems, and
good mutual exchanges occurred on the advisability of foster v. natural homes.

The Warren Senior Center is maintaining its social and clinical programs,
with a growing membership, and serves over 10,000 meals each year. A new
program has been added for the recruitment of elderly volunteers. This has
secured teacher-aides for the school program, one-to-one helpers for Head
Start, and workers in other programs, all of which give the volunteer significant work to do.

Advantages to Community and Hospital

The advantages in having this type of program emanate from a rural
state hospital are as follows:

1. In a rural area, concentration on psychological problems is facilitated.
There is less social unrest, less mobility, less violence, less drug usage, less
racial strife. There also is a paucity of established services, so stepping into
someone else's territory is no great risk. Long-term follow-up is possible
because of the community's relative stability.

2. The hospital has a residency training program. This provides man-
hours and meets the residents' needs for community experience. As the
program is considered part of training, consultative services are provided
to agencies that could not otherwise afford them.

3. The community program has sanctuary. As its participants are
already salaried to perform services, fluctuation in government funding
patterns and expiration of grants will be unlikely to destroy it.

4. Because the program is led by psychiatrists, it is economical. Services deemed necessary can be performed by the man responsible for the
decision, without having to wait for funds to bring in an outside expert.

The psychiatrist has community sanction at the start. His broad education gives him background to begin needed services and avoids a lot of dead endings.

The hospital itself has gained from its giving these community services with a better picture of community agencies and community care, very low readmission rate has resulted because of the insights afforded. The availability of community services is also an attraction for its residency program.

The psychiatric residency program has been enriched by the community program. Extramural work in the fields of early childhood, retirement, death, and dying are added. Experience is available in prevention of mental illness, as well as in consultation and outpatient management. An image of the psychiatrist as part of the care-giving network of society, and as a potential leader in this system is presented.

Experience in working with other agencies has fostered a successful team approach in Central Unit. Much more freedom and responsibility were offered the unit's staff through work with other agencies whose staffs were not under its direct control.

The Warren Senior Center and the Community Job Placement programs proved to be rich resources for rehabilitation when Central Unit became an entity. Many elderly patients left the hospital supported by Warren Senior Center's Day Care Program. Generally, the community's image of the hospital has become more favorable, giving better chances for staff and patients.

Plans for the Future

Many of the programs started are now healthy enough to be carried on under outside auspices. The Community Mental Health Center took over the Outpatient Department. Warren Senior Center is going into the county commissioner's hands and becoming an increasingly permanent institution. A county coordinator of aging is being established. Steps are being taken to place the center's building in the hands of the county commissioners.

The school consultation is becoming better known to teachers, many of whom feel they have been helped by it. This program will be much strengthened with return of a talented child psychiatrist now finishing his training. The preventive kindergarten-first grade program, if data indicate significant differences between test and control schools, will become a model used throughout the county schools. Increasing interest in the recruitment of one-to-one volunteers is developing, with the schools seriously looking to older school children as a most promising source for academic helpers. Mothers and retired persons will be utilized where relationship is especially important. The fact that the school district has hired additional pupil personnel is a most encouraging indication that the hospital work has been a lasting part of the school.

The Mothers' Club lasted a year at the YWCA and had to be curtailed when time for work outside the hospital became limited. It had three offspring: the Nursing Mothers' Club, two Montessori Nursery Schools, and the Prenatal Parents' Group (Lamaze). The Nursing Mothers' group existed for only a year while the interested mothers were nursing but several of its members still advise new mothers on methodology. The two Montessori schools are each completing their first year of service and looking to expand and to grant scholarships. The Lamaze group will undoubtedly lose its reason-to-be when a new obstetrician interested in Lamaze begins his practice in Warren this summer.

The Pastoral Counseling Seminar will continue last year's theme in greater depth, continuing to consider life stress periods, with emphasis upon how to listen, how to counsel, and when to refer during these same life stages. The Pastoral Counseling Service will give inexperienced clergymen an opportunity to be helped during their early days of counseling.

Summary

Warren State Hospital has given outpatient services for eighty years throughout its thirteen county catchment area. Its school consultation services began fifty years ago. It was the only mental health service agency in northwestern Pennsylvania. With this background of experience in community service, it was natural that the hospital would be the leader in the community mental health movement in its area.

Now there are eleven full- or part-time mental health clinics, and seven general hospital psychiatric inpatient units in the hospital's catchment area. The hospital's role in the care continuum varies depending on the capacity of the community service complementing the Hospital Unit. Appropriate patients are being defined as people with subacute or chronic psychoses. Its present population of chronic patients consists of those requiring long-term hospital care. Prehospital and posthospital care are provided by the basic service units. Aftercare placements are still mostly the responsibility of the Hospital.

The clinics are generally well enough staffed to give secondary preventive services. However, the hospital is still the chief provider of primary preventive services. These programs result from extra work by people salaried to perform late secondary and tertiary preventive services. Many of these programs are standing on their own as part of the fabric of the community care-giving system. It is hoped that these primary and tertiary programs will be supported by the state and encouraged to continue.

Notes

1.   Barton, W.E., et al., *Impressions of European Psychiatry*. Washington, D.C., American Psychiatric Assn., 1961.

2.   Mesmer, R.E.G., "European Psychiatry," *Pennsylvania Psychiatric Quarterly,* 1967, 7:47-63.
3.   Silverman, P.R., "The Widow-to-Widow Program," *Mental Hygiene,* 1969, 53:333-37.
4.   Clinebell, H.J., *Basic Types of Pastoral Counseling.* N.Y., Abingdon Press, 1966.
5.   Caplan, G., *Theory and Practice of Mental Health Consultation.* N.Y., Basic Books, 1970.
6.   Ojemann, R., *Education in Human Behavior.* Cleveland Educational Research Council of America, 1961.

20

Recent Trends in the Utilization of Mental Health Facilities

Carl A. Taube and *Richard W. Redick*

The number of patient care episodes in mental health facilities[a] in the United States[b] in 1971 totaled 4.2 million. This was almost one and one-half times greater than the estimated count of 2.6 million episodes in 1965 and two and one-half times greater than the approximate 1.7 million episodes in 1955. Moreover, the patient care episode rate per 100,000 population just about doubled between 1955 and 1971. Not only has there been this substantial increase in number and rate of episodes over the period 1955-71, but there has also been a significant shift in the locale in which these episodes have occurred. In 1955, 77 percent of all patient care episodes were in inpatient psychiatric services with the remaining 23 percent occurring in outpatient psychiatric services. By 1971 the outpatient care episodes accounted for almost three-fifths of all episodes while the proportion of episodes in inpatient services had decreased to 43 percent. Most of this decline can be attributed to the state and county mental hospitals where the proportion of inpatient care episodes had decreased from about half of all episodes in 1955 to slightly less than one-fifth in 1971.

The other notable change in inpatient care episodes has occurred with respect to general hospital inpatient psychiatric units where the number of patient care episodes has more than doubled since 1955. Most striking, however, has been the sixfold increase in number of outpatient care episodes over the time span 1955-71. In addition, the increasingly important role of the community mental

---

[a]The term mental health facilities as used here excludes those facilities organized primarily for the treatment of alcoholism and drug abuse, and also psychiatric care provided in other than organized mental health settings, for example, mental health professionals in private practice, and medical facilities such as neighborhood health centers, nursing homes, and general hospitals without separate psychiatric services. Recent research has highlighted the potential role of the general practitioner in the detection, treatment and referral of persons with mental disorders.[1]

Accurate, reliable estimates of the numbers and types of persons receiving psychiatric care in other than organized mental health settings are generally not available for the country as a whole, nor are any trend data available for recent years. For this reason, these areas are touched on only in the discussion section. The role of private psychiatrists in the spectrum of mental health resources[2] and the characteristics of persons they serve[3] have been discussed in the literature and will not be dealt with here.

[b]Patient care episodes are defined as the number of residents in inpatient facilities at the beginning of the year (or the number of persons on the rolls of inpatient facilities) plus the total additions to these facilities during the year. For more detail concerning this definition see: Redick, Richard W., "Patient Care Episodes in Psychiatric Services, United States, 1971." *Statistical Note 92,* August 1973. Rockville Md: Biometry Branch, NIMH.

health centers as locales for psychiatric care is evidenced by the fact that the proportion of patient care episodes in the inpatient and outpatient services of these centers more than doubled between 1967 and 1969—from 4 to 10 percent—and almost doubled again between 1969 and 1971, constituting 19 percent of all episodes in the latter year, as Table 20-1 and Figure 20-1 show. When the data on trends in patient care episodes by age are examined in Table 20-2, it is seen that between 1966 (the earliest year for which an age breakdown of these episodes was available) and 1971, both the number of episodes and episode rates per 100,000 population increased in every age grouping except that of sixty-five and over, where a substantial decline occurred. The magnitude of the increase was greatest for the youngest age groups, for example, the number of episodes in the eighteen to twenty-four age group more than doubled and the rate per 100,000 population increased 67 percent. This was closely followed by the under eighteen age group in which substantial increases in numbers and rate were noted. Increases of somewhat lesser magnitude were observed in the twenty-five to forty-four and forty-five to sixty-four age groups in that order. A more detailed examination of the age-specific patterns of change in patient care episodes by type of psychiatric service over the period of 1966-71 shown in Table 20-2 reveals the following highlights:

1. The pattern of increase in patient care episodes for the two youngest age groups (under 18 and 18-24) observed for all psychiatric services combined, was seen to have been repeated for every type of psychiatric service except the private mental hospital where a small decrease for the under eighteen age group was observed.
2. The overall increase in patient care episodes observed for the two middle age groups (25-44 and 45-64) was largely accounted for by substantial increases in outpatient care episodes (a doubling or more in both numbers and rates), since the patient care episodes among the various types of inpatient services for these two age groups exhibited for the most part either decreases or only relatively small increases.
3. The overall decrease in patient care episodes for the sixty-five and over age group was totally accounted for by the decline in episodes among each of the various types of inpatient services (community mental health centers excepted), inasmuch as outpatient care episodes for this age group more than doubled in both number and rate between 1966 and 1971.
4. The percentage distributions of patient care episodes by type of psychiatric service for each age group at the two time periods—1966 and 1971—indicate that the previously noted shift in locale of service taking place over time has been most predominant in the age group twenty-five years and over.

Figure 20-1. Percent Distribution of Patient Care Episodes by Type of Psychiatric Facility, United States, 1955 and 1971

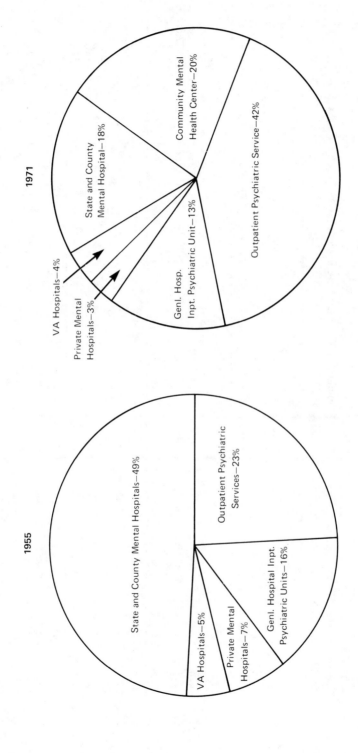

1971

Community Mental
Health Center—20%

State and County
Mental Hospital—18%

Outpatient Psychiatric Service—42%

VA Hospitals—4%

Private Mental
Hospitals—3%

Genl. Hosp.
Inpt. Psychiatric Unit—13%

1955

State and County Mental Hospitals—49%

Outpatient Psychiatric
Services—23%

VA Hospitals—5%

Private Mental
Hospitals—7%

Genl. Hospital Inpt.
Psychiatric Units—16%

Table 20-1
Number, Percent Distribution and Rate Per 100,000 Population of Patient Care Episodes in Psychiatric Facilities by Type of Facility, United States, 1955, 1967, 1969, and 1971

Year	Total All Facilities	Inpatient Services of:						Outpatient Psychiatric Services of:		
		All Inpatient Services	State and County Mental Hospital	Private Mental Hospitals[a]	General Hospital/Psychiatric Service	VA Hospitals	Comm. Mental Health Centers	All Outpatient Services	Comm. Mental Health Centers	Other
					Number of Patient-Care Episodes					
1971	4,038,143	1,721,389	745,259	126,600	542,642	176,800	130,088	2,316,754	622,906	1,693,848
1969	3,572,822	1,678,371	767,115	123,850	535,493	186,913	65,000	1,894,451	291,148	1,603,303
1967	3,139,742	1,659,391	801,354	124,258	578,513	128,196	27,070	1,480,351	97,351	1,383,000
1965	2,636,525	1,565,525	804,926	125,428	519,328	115,843	—	1,071,000	—	1,071,000
1955	1,675,352	1,296,352	818,832	123,231	265,934	88,355	—	379,000	—	379,000
					Percent Distribution					
1971	100.0%	42.6	18.5	3.1	13.4	4.4	3.2	57.4	15.4	42.0
1969	100.0%	47.0	21.5	3.5	15.0	5.2	1.8	53.0	8.1	44.9
1967	100.0%	52.9	25.5	4.0	18.4	4.1	0.9	47.1	3.1	44.0
1965	100.0%	59.4	30.5	4.8	19.7	4.4	—	40.6	—	40.6
1955	100.0%	77.4	48.9	7.3	15.9	5.3	—	22.6	—	22.6
					Rate per 100,000 Population					
1971	1967.8	838.8	363.2	61.7	264.4	86.2	63.4	1129.0	303.5	825.4
1969	1797.7	849.6	384.2	62.0	268.2	93.6	41.7	948.1	145.2	802.9
1967	1604.3	847.9	409.5	63.5	295.6	65.5	13.8	756.4	49.7	706.7
1965	1374.0	815.9	419.5	65.4	270.6	60.4	—	558.1	—	558.1
1955	1032.2	798.6	504.5	75.9	163.8	54.4	—	233.5	—	233.5

[a]Includes estimates of episodes of care in residential treatment centers for emotionally disturbed children.

Table 20-2

Number, Percent Distribution, Rate Per 100,000 Population, and Percent Change in Rate of Patient Care Episodes in Psychiatric Services, Type of Psychiatric Service, by Age, United States, 1966 and 1971

	Total All Ages		Under 18		18-24		25-44		45-64		65 and Over	
	1971	1966	1971	1966	1971	1966	1971	1966	1971	1966	1971	1966
Number												
Total all psych. services	4,038,143	2,772,089	771,874	485,729	681,641	334,422	1,433,133	959,959	888,231	678,965	263,264	313,014
All inpatient services	1,721,389	1,586,089	139,658	86,729	245,106	134,084	614,901	560,825	512,379	515,900	209,345	288,551
State & County Men. Hosps.	745,259	802,216	39,196	36,902	97,285	53,748	236,337	239,060	238,710	283,985	133,731	188,521
Private mental hosps.	97,963	103,973	7,668	7,794	14,095	11,154	34,253	41,361	29,525	30,486	12,422	13,178
Res. tx. ctrs/children	28,637	8,000	28,637	8,000	—	—	—	—	—	—	—	—
Genl. hosp. psych. serv.	542,642	548,921	46,065	34,033	94,569	66,968	231,376	216,824	132,863	166,872	37,769	64,224
VA hospitals	176,800	122,979	—	N.A.	20,967	2,214	59,738	63,580	79,885	34,557	16,210	22,628
CMHCs	130,088	N.A.	18,092*	N.A.	18,190*	N.A.	53,197	N.A.	31,396	N.A.	9,213	N.A.
All outpatient services	2,316,754	1,186,000	632,216	399,000	426,535	200,338	818,232	399,134	375,852	163,065	53,919	24,463
CMHCs	622,906	N.A.	194,877**	N.A.	92,609**	N.A.	221,796	N.A.	95,412	N.A.	18,212	N.A.
All other services	1,693,848	1,186,000	437,339	399,000	343,926	200,338	596,436	399,134	280,440	163,065	35,707	24,463
Percent Distribution												
Total all psych. services	100.0%	100.0%	100.0%	100.0%	100.0%	100.0%	100.0%	100.0%	100.0%	100.0%	100.0%	100.0%
All inpatient services	42.6	57.2	18.1	17.9	36.0	40.1	42.9	58.4	57.7	76.0	79.5	92.2
State & cnty men. hosps.	18.5	28.9	5.1	7.7	14.3	16.1	16.5	24.9	26.9	41.8	50.8	60.3
Private mental hosps.	2.4	3.8	1.0	1.6	2.1	3.3	2.4	4.3	3.3	4.5	4.7	4.2
Res. tx. ctrs/children	0.7	0.3	3.7	1.6	—	—	—	—	—	—	—	—
Genl. hosp. psych. serv.	13.4	19.8	6.0	7.0	13.9	20.0	16.1	22.6	15.0	24.6	14.3	20.5
VA hospitals	4.4	4.4	—	—	3.0	0.7	4.2	6.6	9.0	5.1	6.2	7.2
CMHCs	3.2	N.A.	2.3	—	2.7	—	3.7	—	3.5	—	3.5	—
All outpatient services	57.4	42.8	81.9	82.1	64.0	59.9	57.1	41.6	42.3	24.0	20.5	7.8
CMHCs	15.4	N.A.	25.2	N.A.	13.6	—	15.5	—	10.7	—	6.9	—
All other services	42.0	42.8	56.7	82.1	50.4	59.9	41.6	41.6	31.6	24.0	13.6	7.8
Rate per 100,000 Population												
Total all psych. services	1967.8	1433.2	1090.6	695.7	2862.8	1709.2	2964.7	2095.6	2105.0	1718.8	1310.2	1671.8
All inpatient services	838.8	820.0	197.3	124.2	1029.4	653.3	1272.0	1224.2	1214.3	1306.0	1041.9	1541.2
State & cnty men. hosps.	363.2	414.8	55.4	52.9	408.6	274.7	488.9	521.9	565.7	718.9	665.6	1006.9
Private mental hosps.	47.7	53.8	10.8	11.2	59.2	57.0	70.9	90.3	70.0	77.2	61.8	70.4
Res. tx. ctrs/children	14.0	4.1	40.5	11.5	—	—	—	—	—	—	—	—
Genl. hosp. psych. serv.	264.4	283.8	65.1	48.7	397.2	342.3	478.6	473.3	314.9	422.4	188.0	343.0
VA hospitals	86.2	63.6	—	—	88.1	11.3	123.6	138.8	189.3	89.5	80.7	120.9
CMHCs	63.4	—	25.6	—	76.4	—	110.0	—	74.4	—	45.9	—
All outpatient services	1129.0	613.2	893.3	571.5	1833.4	1023.9	1692.7	871.3	809.7	412.8	268.3	130.7
CMHCs	303.5	—	275.3	—	389.0	—	458.8	—	226.1	—	90.6	—
All other services	825.4	613.2	618.0	571.5	1444.4	1023.9	1233.8	871.3	664.6	412.8	177.7	130.7

N.A.—not applicable—only a few centers had begun functioning in this year and reporting was not requested.

* Under 20 years.

** 20-24 years.

**Number and Types of Psychiatric
Facilities 1972**

The distribution of mental health resources may be described either in terms of types of facilities (e.g., psychiatric hospitals, outpatient clinics, etc.) or in terms of the types of treatment modalities (inpatient, outpatient, and day treatment services) or both. Table 20-3 shows the number and types of facilities and the treatment modalities provided by these facilities as of January 1972.

In terms of types of facilities, 1,123, or 35 percent of the 3,200 mental health facilities, were free-standing outpatient clinics; 770, or 24 percent, were general hospitals providing separate psychiatric services; 482, or 15 percent, were psychiatric hospitals; 344, or 11 percent, were residential treatment centers for emotionally disturbed children; 295, or 9 percent, were federally funded community mental health centers. Overall, 46 percent of the facilities were operated under public auspices, and 54 percent under nonpublic auspices.

In terms of treatment modalities, there were 1,917 inpatient services, 2,279 outpatient services, and 989 day treatment services. About 46 percent of the inpatient services, 58 percent of the outpatient services, and 64 percent of the day treatment services were under public auspices.

Over a third of the inpatient services are located in general hospitals, a quarter in psychiatric hospitals (public and private), almost a fifth in residential treatment centers for emotionally disturbed children, and almost a sixth in community mental health centers.

About half of the outpatient services are located in free-standing outpatient psychiatric clinics; the other half are outpatient services of mental health facilities. Of those outpatient services affiliated with mental health facilities, about 28 percent are located in general hospitals, 29 percent in psychiatric hospitals, and 26 percent in federally funded community mental health centers (CMHCs).

Day treatment services, unlike outpatient services, are provided primarily within the program of a mental health facility offering also inpatient and/or outpatient care. Only 3.4 percent of the 989 day treatment services are free-standing. Day treatment services in CMHCs account for 30 percent of the total such services: psychiatric hospitals—21 percent; general hospitals—18 percent; and outpatient clinics—15 percent.

Inpatient Psychiatric Services 1966-72

Between 1966 and the beginning of 1972 the rate per 100,000 population of inpatient care episodes increased only about 2 percent, compared with an increase of 84 percent in the rate per 100,000 of outpatient care episodes over the same interval. The overall inpatient figure, however, masks wide variation in changes that occurred within different age groups and within different facility

Table 20-3
Distribution of Mental Health Facilities and Services and Admissions to These Facilities and Services by Type of Facility, United States, January 1972

Type of Facility	Number of Facilities	Number with:			Number of Annual Admissions to:		
		Inpatient Services	Outpatient Services	Day Tx. Services	Inpatient Services	Outpatient Services	Day Treatment Services
Total, all facilities	3,200	1,917	2,279	989	1,269,029	1,378,822	75,545
Psychiatric hospital	482	482	338	206	494,640	147,383	18,448
State and county	324	324	238	134	407,640	129,133	16,554
Proprietary	158	158	100	72	87,000	18,250	1,894
Veterans Administration hospitals	119	110	102	49	134,065	51,645	4,023
General hospital psychiatric services	770	653	322	174	519,926*	282,677	11,563
Public	158	141	86	47	215,158*	139,077	4,291
Nonpublic	612	512	236	127	304,768*	143,600	7,272
Residential treatment center for emotionally disturbed children	344	344	66	60	11,148	10,156	994
Federally funded CMHC	295	295	295	295	75,900	335,648	21,092
Day hospitals—free-standing	34	—	—	34	—	—	1,514
Outpatient clinics—free-standing	1,123	—	1,123	146	—	484,677	10,642
Public	588	—	588	79	—	273,358	7,737
Nonpublic	535	—	535	67	—	211,319	2,905
Other multiservice facilities	33	33	33	25	33,350	66,636	7,269

* Data shown for general hospital inpatient services are discharges, not admissions. Due to the short stay of admissions, discharges and admissions are approximately equal.

types. By age, the under eighteen and eighteen to twenty-four groups experienced almost a 60 percent increase in the inpatient episode rate between 1966-
71; the twenty-five to forty-four group had only a 4 percent increase; whereas
the forty-five to sixty-four and sixty-five and over groups showed decreases of
7 percent and 32 percent, respectively. These differential rates of change by
age are, of course, related to changes in the utilization of different types of
facilities. These changes are examined separately for each type of facility below.

State and County Mental Hospitals

Of the different types of inpatient psychiatric facilities, state and county
mental hospitals probably experienced the most change over the interval 1966-
72. A summary of these changes follows:

1. The resident population decreased from 452,089 in 1966 to 275,995 in
    1972, a decrease of almost 40 percent[c]
2. Total admissions increased from 330,399 to 390,000 over the interval,
    an increase of 18 percent. However, beginning with 1972, admissions
    began to decrease in number, reversing the trend of increasing admissions
    noted in previous years
3. The median stay of admissions during 1971 was forty-one days, with 75
    percent of the admissions released within three months of admission.
    This represents a dramatic change over the longer stays of earlier years.
4. The number of first admissions (no prior inpatient psychiatric care)
    decreased between 1969-72, reversing the trend of earlier years; while
    the number of readmissions increased,[d] accounting for 64 percent of
    the total admissions in 1972.
5. Average expenditures per patient day increased 168 percent, from $8 in
    1966 to $21 in 1972. Overall maintenance expenditures increased from
    $1.3 billion in 1966 to $2.1 billion in 1972.
6. Since the resident patient population decreased at a much faster rate
    than the number of full-time equivalent (FTE) staff between 1968-72,
    the ratio of FTE staff per 100 average resident patients has increased
    dramatically. Overall there was a 33 percent increase in this ratio, from
    57.7 in 1968 to 76.7 in 1972. Professional FTE staff per 100 average

---

[c]Changes in the age, sex, diagnostic characteristics of the resident population, and
admissions over this internal have been discussed in detail in a previous chapter and
therefore will be omitted here.

[d]The increase in readmissions is partially an artifact, resulting from a decreased use of
the long term or convalescent leave status in many states. Persons who previously would
have been placed on long term leave are now being discharged. Those who are readmitted
are therefore counted as readmissions rather than as returns from leave.

resident patients increased 36 percent, nonprofessional FTE staff per 100 average resident patients increased 19 percent, and the administrative and maintenance staff ratio increased 53 percent. While there was a decrease of 11.6 percent in the number of FTE psychiatrists, the ratio of FTE psychiatrists per average resident patients increased 25 percent, due to the faster rate of decrease in residents relative to the rate of decrease in FTE psychiatrists.

7. The number of state mental hospitals has increased from 312 in 1968 to 324 in 1972. This change reflects the net result of hospital closings, conversion of state mental hospitals to other uses, subdivision of large hospitals into separate administrative units or hospitals, and opening of new state mental hospitals.

350 CMHCs in operation as of that month included 540 inpatient services.[e] Two hundred and nineteen served CMHC patients exclusively, that is, all patients using the service were considered CMHC patients; while 321 served both CMHC patients and other patients. Of the 540 inpatient services affiliated with CMHCs, 20 percent were those of state and county mental hospitals, and 60 percent were those of general hospital psychiatric services.

While reliable trend data are not available on the age, sex, and diagnostic distribution of admissions to federally funded CMHCs, data are available on persons first admitted to the inpatient services during 1971, as shown in Table 20-13 below. Over half of such admissions were accounted for by two diagnoses—depressive disorders (27%) and schizophrenia (24%). Alcohol disorders constituted the third largest group, accounting for 13 percent of the total. By age, 28 percent of the first admissions were under twenty-five, 41 percent were twenty-five to forty-four years old, 24 percent—forty-five to sixty-four years old, and 7 percent—sixty-five and over.

Private Mental Hospitals

During 1971-72 the number of private mental hospitals increased, after remaining relatively stable over the three preceding years. In the interval 1968-70 there were about 150 such hospitals averaging around 90,000 admissions per year and about 10,500 resident patients. During 1971-72, the number of hospitals increased by twenty-seven, with consequent increases of 10,000 annual admissions, and about 1,000 resident patients as seen in Table 20-4.

The growth in number of hospitals has been due largely to new for-profit corporation hospitals that opened during this interval. The number of such

[e]CMHCs may affiliate with two or more inpatient facilities to provide inpatient care.

Table 20-4
**Trends in the Number of For-Profit and Not-For-Profit Psychiatric
Hospitals, Admissions and Residents, 1968-72**

		Number of:	
Year	Hospitals	Admissions	Residents
1968	150	89,138	10,454
1969	149	92,056	10,963
1970	150	87,106	10,677
1971	156	91,151	10,207
1972	177	101,198	11,193

hospitals increased 55 percent between 1968-72, while for-profit individually
owned or partnership hospitals decreased 30 percent in number, and the number of church not-for-profit hospitals also decreased by a significant amount
(24 percent) as seen in Table 20-5. Table 20-5 reflects the net change as a
result of both hospital openings and closings over this interval, whereas Table
20-6 shows the distribution of hospitals opening over the interval 1968-72.
Of the forty-eight hospitals opening, forty-one (21 single hospital corporations
and 20 multiple hospital corporations), or 86 percent were for-profit corporations.

Trend data on the age-sex-diagnostic composition of additions and resident
patients in private mental hospitals are available for the interval 1968-71.[4] The
data seem to indicate decreasing numbers and rates of admission in the twenty-
five to forty-four and forty-five to sixty-four year age group, and increasing
numbers and rates in the under eighteen and eighteen to twenty-four year age
groups, while the number and rates of additions for the sixty-five and over
group has remained relatively stable. These trends have resulted in changes in
the age composition of additions. For example, the proportion of additions
under twenty-five years of age increased from 17.6 percent in 1968 to 23.7
percent in 1971, while the percent for the twenty-five to sixty-four age group
decreased from 70.3 to 64.6 percent in the same interval.

The diagnostic distribution of additions to private mental hospitals also
appears to have changed only slightly during the period 1968-71. Approximately 40 percent of the additions were diagnosed with depressive disorders
and about 20 percent with schizophrenia. Among male additions the highest
proportion were diagnosed with depressive disorders, with schizophrenia and
alcoholism disorders alternately ranking either second or third over the four
year time period. For females the depressive disorders were the leading

Table 20-5
Trends in the Number of For-Profit and Not-For-Profit Hospitals by Hospital Control, 1968-72

Hospital Control	1968		1972		% Change 1968-72
	Number	Percent	Number	Percent	
Total hospitals	151	100.0%	177	100.0%	+ 17%
Not-for-profit, total	69	45.7	67	37.9	− 3
Church	17	11.3	13	7.3	− 24
Other	52	34.4	54	30.5	+ 4
For-profit total	82	54.3	110	62.1	+ 34
Individual/partnership	20	13.2	14	7.9	− 30
Corporation	62	41.1	96	54.2	+ 55

Table 20-6
Distribution of For-Profit and Not-For-Profit Hospitals Opening Over the Interval 1968-72 by Hospital Control

Hospital Control	Number	Percent
Total	48	100.0%
Not-for-profit	6	12.5
Church	—	0.0
Other	6	12.5
For-profit	42	87.5
Individual/partnership	1	2.0
Corporation	41	85.5
Single hospital	21	43.9
Multiple hospital	20	41.7

diagnoses during the period 1968-71 followed by schizophrenia, with "other neuroses" rather than alcoholism being the third ranking diagnosis.

In each of the four years, female additions outnumbered male additions in every diagnostic category except alcoholism (where the males exceeded the females by slightly more than 2.5 to 1), and drug abuse disorders. For drug abuse disorders, males relative to females increased gradually over the interval, and in 1972 there were 156 male additions for every 100 female additions in this diagnostic group.

The age distribution of resident patients at end of year in private mental hospitals exhibited some change during the period 1968-71. For both males and females, the number and proportion of residents under eighteen years of age and eighteen to twenty-four years of age increased during this time interval while the number and proportion of residents forty-five to sixty-four and sixty-five years of age and older decreased. The proportion of residents twenty-five to forty-four years of age fluctuated only slightly from year to year.

Changes in the diagnostic distribution of resident patients in private mental hospitals over the period of 1968-71 were for the most part relatively minimal. Organic brain syndromes showed a decrease, depressive disorders a slight increase. The sex ratios for resident patients by diagnosis are seen to be similar to those already noted for the additions to the private mental hospitals, that is, females outnumbered males in every diagnostic category except alcoholism and drug abuse disorders.

Veterans Administration Psychiatric Services

Total admissions to VA psychiatric inpatient services have almost doubled over the interval from 1968-73, increasing from 80,408 admissions in 1968 to 141,294 in 1973. This increase has been largely due to tripling of admissions to psychiatric inpatient services of VA general medical and surgical hospitals, increasing from 34,192 in 1968 to 90,612 in 1973. Admissions to the VA neuropsychiatric hospitals have fluctuated between 46,000 and 54,000 over the interval. The resident population in the VA neuropsychiatric hospitals has decreased dramatically since 1968, when the year end population was about 40,000. In 1973 the year-end population was just under 15,000 a reduction of over 60 percent in the six-year period. While the resident population has been decreasing, the year end resident population in the psychiatric services of the GM&S hospitals has more than doubled, increasing from 5,591 in 1968 to 11,976 in 1973.

While some of the decline in the resident population of the VA psychiatric hospitals can be attributed to the reclassification of psychiatric hospitals to general hospital psychiatric services, this administrative redefinition of hospital type certainly does not account for the major part of the drop in the resident population of the VA psychiatric hospitals. As shown in Table 20-7 below, there has been a decrease of 29,077 in the average operating beds in psychiatric hospitals between 1968-73, while over the same interval, the average operating beds in the psychiatric services of VA general hospitals increased by 8,117 beds.

Trend data on the age and diagnostic characteristics of admissions to VA psychiatric services are not available. Similar data on the resident population in VA psychiatric services, while not available for the most recent years, are available for the interval 1959-70. The discussion that follows examines these trends.

The largest proportion of mentally ill male residents under sixty-five years of age in VA hospitals in 1970 were diagnosed as psychotic, primarily with schizophrenia. The proportion that were psychotic ranged from 45 percent in

Table 20-7
Trends in the Number of Hospitals and Average Operating Beds, VA Psychiatric Hospitals and General Hospital Psychiatric Units, United States, 1968-73

	VA Psychiatric Hospitals		VA General Hospital Psychiatric Units	
	Number of:		Number of:	
Year	Hospitals	Average Operating Beds	Hospitals	Average Operating Beds
1973	28	17,896	92	14,892
1972	28	22,218	89	14,919
1971	33	31,770	80	12,087
1970	37	37,506	77	9,576
1969	38	46,176	79	8,670
1968	41	46,973	77	6,775

Source: VA Field Station Summary for each year.

the age group fifty-five to sixty-four to a high of 71 percent in the age group twenty-five to thirty-four. In the age groups sixty-five years and over, the majority of the residents were diagnosed with brain syndromes, the proportions ranging from 50 percent in the age group sixty-five to seventy-four to 83 percent for those eighty-five and over.

The most significant changes in the diagnostic distribution of residents under sixty-five years of age in VA hospitals over the period 1959-70 were the increase in the proportion of residents diagnosed with alcoholism, from 3 percent in 1959 to 14 percent in 1970, and the substantial decrease in the proportion of residents diagnosed with schizophrenia, from 75 percent in 1959 to 57 percent in 1970. The proportion of residents under sixty-five years with psychoneurosis showed some increase between 1959 and 1966 (from 5 to 11%) but no significant change since 1966, while those with brain syndromes and personality disorders showed almost no proportionate changes over the entire period.

For residents sixty-five years and over the only changes of note in their diagnostic distribution between 1959 and 1970 were a decrease in the proportion of schizophrenics from 45 to 35 percent and an increase in the proportion of those with brain syndromes from 41 to 52 percent.

In 1959 almost half (47%) of the resident population were under forty-five years of age whereas in 1970 only a third were in these age groups. Since residents under twenty-five years of age have shown some increase over the period, all of this decrease has occurred in the twenty-five to thirty-four and thirty-five to forty-four age groups. The increase in residents forty-five years of age and over has occurred for the most part in the age groups forty-five to fifty-four and seventy-five and over, especially the former group, which increased from 13 percent of the total in 1959 to one-third of the total in 1970.

Such changes, in general, are largely a function of the changing age distribution of the veteran population. For example, the number of veterans in the forty-five to fifty-four age group in the general population has increased over the period 1959-70 with a resultant general increase in the number of veterans hospitalized in this age group. However, owing to the fact that the resident patient population in this age group experienced a smaller rate of increase than the total veteran population forty-five to fifty-four years, the resident patient rate per 100,000 veteran population decreased from 270 to 150 per 100,000 population between 1959 and 1970. The resident patient rates decreased in every age group during this period except in the age group under twenty-five. This parallels the trend noted for resident patients in state and county mental hospitals and is more than likely a reflection of the increased availability and utilization of other types of care facilities such as outpatient psychiatric services, partial hospitalization programs, community mental health centers, and the like.

The median time on books of male veterans with mental disorders resident in VA hospitals has decreased from 6.8 years in 1959 to 10.5 months in 1970. This change was largely accounted for by decreases in the proportions of resident patients on the books twenty or more years (from 17% in 1959 to 12% in 1970) and ten to twenty years (from 24% in 1959 to 9% in 1970) as of each census date, and an increase in the proportion on the books less than three months as of each census date (from 10% in 1959 to 37% in 1970).

General Hospital Psychiatric Services

Of the 29.5 million inpatient discharges from nonfederal short-stay general hospitals in 1971, one million were discharged with a primary diagnosis of a mental disorder, which is almost 250,000 more than the 753,000 such discharges from these hospitals in 1967. Thus the number of psychiatric discharges increased 39 percent over the period 1967-71, which is more than three times the percentage increase in all discharges from short term general hospitals during the same interval (12%). While some of this increase may be an artifact, resulting from decreased reluctance to assign a psychiatric disorder due to increased insurance coverage for mental disorders, it is also a result of a greater utilization

Table 20-8
Discharges with a Primary Diagnosis of Mental Disorder, Nonfederal Short-Stay General Hospitals, United States, 1967 and 1971

	1967		*1971*		*% Change in number*
	Number	*Percent*	*Number*	*Percent*	*1967-71*
Total discharges with a primary diagnosis of mental disorder from all general hospitals	753,000	100.0%	1,050,000	100.0%	+ 39%
Discharges from separate psychiatric inpatient units	454,000	60.3%	649,000	61.8%	+ 43%
Discharges from general hospitals accepting psychiatric patients for diagnosis and treatment but with no separate psychiatric unit	125,000	16.6%	401,000	38.2%	+ 34%
Discharges from general hospitals admitting persons with known or suspected psychiatric illness on an emergency basis only or those who do not normally admit such patients	174,000	23.1%			

of general hospitals for psychiatric care. Of the one million discharges with a psychiatric diagnosis from nonfederal short-stay general hospitals in 1971 about 649,000 or 62 percent were from separate psychiatric inpatient units, while the remainder were from general medical wards of the hospitals (Table 20-8). There has been a 43 percent increase during the period 1967-71 in the number of discharges from separate psychiatric units, which is somewhat higher than the corresponding increase (34%) in psychiatric discharges from general medical services of general hospitals. This latter group may be conceptualized as two subgroups: (1) those treated and discharged from hospitals that accept psychiatric patients for diagnosis and treatment but that have no separate psychiatric service, and (2) those discharged from hospitals that admit psychiatric patients on an emergency basis only. For this last group, the hospital serves only a holding and referral function, and generally little treatment is carried out. Unfortunately, while the breakdown of discharges into these two groups is known for 1967, it is not available for 1971. As illustrated in Table 20-9 below, in addition to the 1,049,448 discharges from general hospitals with a primary diagnosis of mental disorder, there were an additional 682,474 discharges with a psychiatric diagnosis listed as the 2-5th diagnosis but with a nonpsychiatric primary diagnosis.

Table 20-9
Distribution of Discharges from Nonfederal Short-stay General
Hospitals by First Versus Second to Fifth Listed Diagnosis, Mental
Versus Nonmental Disorder, United States, 1971

Second to Fifth Listed Diagnosis	Primary Diagnosis		
	Mental	Nonmental	Total
Mental	251,921	682,474	934,405
Nonmental	797,517	27,573,206	28,370,723
Total	1,049,448	28,255,680	29,305,128

Table 20-10
Number of Nonfederal General Hospitals with Psychiatric
Inpatient Units

	Total	CMHC Inpatient Units	Other
March 1964	467	—	467
October 1967	617	—	617
January 1970	690	103	587
January 1972	815	162	653

Trend data on the number of separate psychiatric units in general hospitals presented in Table 20-10 show that between 1964 and 1972 the number of such units had almost doubled, from 467 in 1964 to 815 in 1972. Of the 815 such units in 1972, 162 were functioning as inpatient affiliates of federally funded community mental health centers and all of the patients served in such units were considered CMHC patients.

Residential Treatment Centers for Emotionally
Disturbed Children and Psychiatric Hospitals
for Children—1972

Since these facilities, prior to 1972, had never been surveyed comprehensively on a national basis, trend data are not available. Data are available for 1972, however, which provide a detailed description of these facilities.[5] As seen in Table 20-11 below, residential treatment centers accounted for about

Table 20-11
Distribution of Inpatient Psychiatric Episodes Under Eighteen Years of Age by Type of Facility, United States, 1971

Type of Facility	Inpatient-Care Episodes Under Eighteen Years of Age	
	Number	% Distribution
Inpatient psychiatric services, total	139,658	100.0%
Psychiatric hospitals, total	46,864	33.5
Children's psychiatric hospital	4,124	3.0
Child/adolescent units of psych. hosp.	19,167	13.7
Mixed age wards of psychiatric hosp.	23,573	16.9
General hospital inpatient psych. units	46,065	33.0
Residential treatment centers for emotionally disturbed children	28,637	20.5
Community mental health centers	18,092	13.0

21 percent of the inpatient episodes for the under eighteen age group in 1971; psychiatric hospitals for children accounted for only 3 percent; community mental health centers—13 percent; general hospital psychiatric services—33 percent; child/adolescent units in psychiatric hospitals—14 percent; and mixed age wards of psychiatric hospitals—17 percent. Table 20-12 below indicates that psychiatric hospitals for children serve a somewhat younger population than either RTCs or child/adolescent units in psychiatric hospitals. In addition, if the age distribution of children under eighteen served by general hospital inpatient psychiatric units is compared to that for the above three types of facilities, it is seen that an older group is served, with 65 percent of the general hospital discharges under eighteen years of age being in the age group fifteen to seventeen.

Federally Funded Community Mental Health Centers

The number of inpatient episodes in federally funded CMHCs has increased from 27,070 in 1967 to 130,088 in 1971, a reflection largely of the growth in the number of CMHCs becoming operational over this interval. CMHCs accounted for almost 8 percent of the total inpatient episodes in all types of psychiatric inpatient facilities in 1971.

CMHCs, for the most part, provide inpatient services through affiliation with preexisting psychiatric inpatient services. For example, in January 1973 the 350 CHMCs in operation as of that month included 540 inpatient services.[f] Two

---

[f]See footnote e.

Table 20-12
Age and Sex Distribution of Admissions to Selected Inpatient Facilities for Children, United States, 1971

Age and Sex	Residential Treatment Centers	Psychiatric Hospitals for Children	Inpatient Treatment Units–Psychiatric Hospitals
Total	11,148	2,089	11,268
All ages	100.0%	100.0%	100.0%
Less than 6	0.7	2.2	1.2
6-12 years	34.0	47.4	16.2
13-15 years	43.8	43.1	43.6
16-18 years	20.8	6.0	36.1
19 and over	0.7	1.3	2.9
Median age	14	13	15
Sex ratio	220	164	139

hundred and nineteen served CMHC patients exclusively, that is, all patients using the service were considered CMHC patients; while 321 served both CMHC patients and other patients. Of the 540 inpatient services affiliated with CMHCs, 20 percent were state and county mental hospitals, and 60 percent were general hospital services.

While reliable trend data are not available on the age, sex, and diagnostic distribution of admission to federally funded CMHCs, data are available on persons first admitted to the inpatient services during 1971, as shown in Table 20-13. Over half of such admissions were accounted for by two diagnoses— depressive disorders (27 percent) and schizophrenia (24 percent). Alcohol disorders constituted the third largest group, accounting for 13 percent of the total. By age, 28 percent of the first admissions were under twenty-five, 41 percent were twenty-five to forty-four, 24 percent were twenty-five to sixty-four, and 7 percent were in the sixty-five and over age group.

Outpatient Psychiatric Services

Outpatient psychiatric services may be categorized in terms of their organizational location as follows: (1) free-standing outpatient clinics, that is, those that are not administratively part of or affiliated with an inpatient psychiatric facilities; (2) outpatient services affiliated with psychiatric hospitals, public and private; (3) outpatient psychiatric services of general hospitals; and (4) outpatient psychiatric services of other mental health facilities such as residential treatment centers for emotionally disturbed children, outpatient services of

Table 20-13

Primary Diagnoses of Additions First Admitted to Inpatient Services of Federally Funded Community Mental Health Centers by Age, United States, 1971

Primary Diagnosis	All Ages	Under 15	15-19	20-24	25-44	45-64	65 and Over
				Age			
All diagnoses	75,900	2,137	8,276	11,068	31,286	17,859	5,274
All diagnoses	100.0%	100.0%	100.0%	100.0%	100.0%	100.0%	100.0%
Mental retardation	2.1	8.4	3.5	1.9	1.7	1.7	1.1
Organic brain syndromes	4.3	3.4	2.0	1.7	1.6	4.6	28.2
Schizophrenia	24.3	9.4	20.7	31.8	29.0	19.1	10.4
Affective & depressive disorders	26.8	6.3	16.7	25.5	28.8	30.6	28.5
Psychotic disorders (not elsewhere classified)	4.2	0.6	2.0	3.6	4.1	5.7	6.3
Alcohol disorders	13.1	0.3	0.9	3.8	14.5	24.8	8.8
Drug disorders	4.4	1.8	9.3	10.5	3.3	1.5	1.8
Behavior disorders of childhood & adolescence	4.3	53.8	25.6	0.0	0.0	0.0	0.0
All other	16.5	16.1	19.3	21.2	16.9	12.0	15.0

federally funded community mental health centers, and clinics of the Veterans Administration.

Of the total 2,279 outpatient psychiatric services in the United States, approximately 19 percent are affiliated with psychiatric hospitals, 14 percent are affiliated with general hospitals, and 49 percent are free-standing psychiatric services. These three types of clinics account for 15, 21, and 35 percent respectively, of the total caseload of outpatient services. Table 20-14 below gives the number of outpatient services and the distribution of admissions to these clinics by clinic affiliation.

As shown in Table 20-15, both the number of terminations from outpatient psychiatric services and the termination rate per 100,000 population increased steadily from 1963 through 1971. While the age composition did not change appreciably during these years, the number of terminations increased from an estimated 447,000 in 1963 to an estimated 1,271,000 in 1971, an increase of 185 percent. The corresponding termination rate per 100,000 population increased 157 percent from 241 in 1963 to 620 in 1971 (Table 12-15). For each age group shown, both the number of terminations and the termination

Table 20-14

Distribution of Outpatient Psychiatric Services and Admissions to These Services During 1971, by Clinic Affiliation, United States, 1972

Type of Facility Affiliation	Outpatient Services		Admissions to Outpatient Services	
	Number	Percent	Number	Percent
Total, all outpatient services	2,279	100.0%	1,378,822	100.0%
Psychiatric hospital	338	14.8	147,383	10.7
State and county	238	10.4	129,133	9.4
Proprietary	100	4.4	18,250	1.3
Veterans Admin. hospitals	102	4.3	51,645	3.7
General hospital psychiatric services	322	14.2	282,677	20.6
Public	86	3.8	139,077	10.2
Nonpublic	236	10.4	143,600	10.4
Residential treatment center for emotionally disturbed children	66	2.9	10,156	0.7
Federally funded CMHC	295	12.9	335,648	24.3
Outpatient clinics–free-standing	1,123	49.3	484,677	35.2
Public	588	25.8	273,358	19.9
Nonpublic	535	23.5	211,319	15.3
Other multiservice facilities	33	1.4	66,636	4.8

Table 20-15
Estimated Number, Rate per 100,000 Population, and Percent Distribution of Terminations from Outpatient Psychiatric Services[a], by Age, United States, 1963-71

Year	All Ages	Age at Admission						
		Under 18	18-24	25-34	35-44	45-54	55-64	65 and Over
				Number of Terminations[b]				
1963	446,601	159,648	56,166	82,441	77,863	42,191	17,896	10,396
1965	536,845	205,374	72,537	92,817	84,389	48,785	21,607	11,336
1967	703,054	255,452	101,532	125,339	107,789	67,194	30,771	14,977
1969	1,023,106	337,450	170,044	193,195	148,804	97,602	47,493	28,518
1971	1,271,225	436,202	205,951	240,545	179,415	118,538	59,543	31,031
				Rate per 100,000 Population[c]				
1963	241.1	234.4	342.5	381.6	322.0	198.6	110.1	59.6
1965	281.6	292.1	403.5	430.0	349.7	223.7	128.5	63.0
1967	361.0	361.4	512.9	567.2	453.1	300.9	176.6	80.4
1969	515.1	477.0	811.8	821.2	644.3	425.1	263.1	147.7
1971	619.5	616.3	865.0	941.6	787.1	504.4	318.5	154.4
				Percent Distribution				
1963	100.0%	35.8	12.6	18.5	17.4	9.4	4.0	2.3
1965	100.0%	38.3	13.5	17.3	15.7	9.1	4.0	2.1
1967	100.0%	36.3	14.5	17.8	15.3	9.6	4.4	2.1
1969	100.0%	33.1	16.6	18.9	14.5	9.5	4.6	2.8
1971	100.0%	34.4	16.2	18.9	14.1	9.3	4.7	2.4

[a]Includes outpatient services of the Veterans Administration and outpatient services of federally funded community mental health centers (CMHC's).

[b]For the years 1963, 1965, and 1967, data are for terminations from all outpatient psychiatric services. For the years 1969 and 1971 data on additions to CMHC's are combined with data on terminations from other outpatient psychiatric services. This merging of terminations and additions is based on the assumption that the number of terminations from outpatient services during a specific time period are considered to be a close approximation to the number of additions to such services during the same time period owing to the generally short length of time most patients remain on the rolls of these services.

[c]Base population used to compute rates is the estimated United States civilian resident population as of January 1, for the years shown.

rate per 100,000 population increased steadily throughout the period. In each year the termination rates were highest for persons aged twenty-five to thirty-four and lowest among persons aged sixty-five and over. However, the percent increase in the rates over the time interval 1963-71 varied according to age and ranged from a percent increase of 144 for persons aged thirty-five to forty-four to 199 for persons aged fifty-five to sixty-four. In general the largest increases in the rates occurred between 1967 and 1971, a time when the utilization of outpatient psychiatric services of community mental health centers was rapidly expanding.

Another indication of the growth of outpatient psychiatric services is in the proportion of total patient care episodes (patients on rolls at the beginning of the year plus additions during the year) in all psychiatric services that are outpatient. In 1971 outpatient care episodes accounted for 57 percent of the total as compared with 23 percent in 1955. The number of patient care episodes in outpatient psychiatric services has increased sixfold since 1955 (Table 20-1).

Day Care Services

In spite of dramatic increases in the number of day care programs and admissions to these programs, this modality still remains relatively unused in the total spectrum of mental health resources. Of the 4.2 million patient care episodes in mental health facilities during 1971, 3 percent or 118,343 episodes were in day treatment services, 55 percent or 2.3 million were in outpatient services, and 1.8 million or 42 percent were in inpatient services. In 1963 there were an estimated 114 day treatment programs that treated 7,689 persons during 1962.[6] As of January 1972 there were 989 day care programs that treated an estimated 118,343 persons during 1971. This represents an increase of over 700 percent in the number of such programs and a fourteenfold increase in the number of persons served. Table 20-16 documents the change in the number of programs over the interval from 1963 to 1967 and from 1967 to 1972. Between 1963 and 1967 the number of day care programs and admissions to these programs increased over 300 percent. Over the interval from 1967 to 1972 the number of day care programs increased about 100 percent and the number of admissions almost 200 percent (Table 20-17). In the earlier period the growth in day care programs was primarily accounted for by increases in the number of day care programs provided by psychiatric hospitals and general hospital psychiatric services. These two types of facilities accounted for 264 or 69 percent of the new day care programs that began operation between 1963 and 1967. Federally funded CMHCs accounted for an additional eighty new programs or 21 percent of the increase in this period. Between 1967 and 1972 the number of day care programs in general hospital and psychiatric hospitals increased by fifty-two, accounting for only 11 percent of the increase of 489

Table 20-16
Change in the Number of Day Care Services by Type of Affiliation, United States, 1963-67 and 1967-72

Time Period	All Day Care Services	Mental Hospitals	General Hospitals	Affiliation Outpatient Psychiatric Clinics	CMHC	Other Mental Health Facilities
1963-67						
Number of services						
1963	114	48	16	7	4	39
1967	500	170	158	36	84	52
Change in number of services 1963-67						
Absolute change	+386	+122	+142	+ 29	+ 80	+ 13
Percent distribution	100%	32%	37%	8%	21%	3%
Relative change	+339%	+254%	+888%	+414%	+200%	+ 33%
1967-72						
Number of services						
1967	500	170	158	36	84	52
1972	989	206	174	146	295	168
Change in number of services 1967-72						
Absolute change	+489	+ 36	+ 16	+110	+211	+116
Percent distribution	100%	7%	3%	22%	43%	24%
Relative change	+ 98%	+ 21%	+ 11%	+ 10%	+251%	+306%

Table 20-17
Distribution of Admissions to Day Care Services by Type of Affiliation, United States, 1967 and 1972

	Number of Admissions				Percent Change 1967-72
	Number		Percent Distribution		
Affiliation	1967	1972	1967	1972	
All day care services	26,595	75,545	100.0%	100.0%	+ 184%
State & county mental hospitals	8,715	16,554	32.7	21.9	+ 90%
Private mental hospitals	1,430	1,894	5.4	2.5	+ 32%
General hospitals	6,478	11,563	24.4	15.3	+ 78%
Community mental health centers	4,956	21,092	18.6	27.9	+ 326%
Outpatient psychiatric clinics	1,322	10,642	5.0	14.1	+ 705%
Other mental health facilities	3,694	13,800	13.9	18.3	+ 274%

new day care services beginning operation between 1967 and 1972. Federally funded CMHCs accounted for 211 or 43 percent of the increase; free-standing outpatient psychiatric clinics accounted for 110 or 22 percent of the increase; and other mental health facilities accounted for 116 or 24 percent of the increase.

Discussion

In this section several issues raised by the foregoing discussion of trends are examined. First, major differences still exist between the public and private sector in both the number and types of facilities and the types of persons served. These differences are illustrated by reviewing the differential utilization of public v. private facilities by whites and nonwhites, and then examining in some detail the characteristics of discharges from public v. private general hospital psychiatric inpatient units.

Second, the issue of increase in quantity versus an increase in quality or effective treatment is examined, using as an example the substantial increase in utilization of outpatient services.

Third, the imbalance in the geographic distribution of mental health resources is examined. And finally the issue of the adequacy of care for the mentally ill aged is discussed.

Public Versus Nonpublic
Psychiatric Services

Outside of the private practice of psychiatry, mental health services are for the most part provided in public facilities. Of the 2.5 million inpatient and outpatient admission episodes in 1971, 1.7 million, or 69 percent, were to public facilities. While there are variations in the distribution of admissions to public v. nonpublic facilities by age, sex, color, and diagnosis, the majority of the admissions within each of these subgroups were to public facilities.

Within this context however, nonwhites compared with whites, were much more likely to be admitted to public than nonpublic facilities. The admission rate for nonwhites to public facilities was four times the rate to nonpublic facilities, whereas for whites it was only twice as high. This color differential is particularly dramatic for nonwhite males, for whom the admission rate to public facilities is eight times that to nonpublic facilities (Table 20-18).

In general, these patterns hold true when inpatient and outpatient admissions are examined separately. However, these patterns are usually more accentuated among the inpatient admissions, and less accentuated among the outpatient admissions. For example, it was pointed out that the admission rate to public facilities for nonwhite males was eight times that to nonpublic facilities. For nonwhite male inpatient admissions, the admission rate to public facilities was fourteen times the rate to nonpublic facilities, while the admission rate to public outpatient facilities was only five times the rate to private facilities.

Some striking differences in the probability of admissions to different types of inpatient facilities by sex and color are as follows:

1. Males, in comparison with females, have a higher percent of admissions to state and county mental hospitals, and public general hospital psychiatric inpatient services, but a lower percent of admissions to private mental hospitals, nonpublic general hospitals, and community mental health centers.
2. Nonwhites, in comparison with whites, have a higher percent of admissions to state and county mental hospitals and to public general hospitals.
3. Almost half (48%) of the nonwhite female admissions were to state and county mental hospitals. This was higher than the percent of nonwhite males (41%) admitted to these facilities and considerably higher than the percent for white females (28%). Of the white female admissions, 39 percent were to nonpublic general hospital psychiatric inpatient services.

Detailed data for 1971 on discharges from psychiatric inpatient units in general hospitals serve to illustrate the differences in the utilization of public nonfederal general hospital units and of for-profit and not-for-profit hospital units.

Table 20-18
Ratio of Public to Nonpublic Admission Rates by Sex and Color,
Inpatient and Outpatient Psychiatric Services, United States, 1971

Sex and Color	Inpatient & Outpatient Combined	Inpatient	Outpatient
White	2.0	1.8	2.2
Males	2.6	3.0	2.2
Females	1.5	1.0	2.2
Nonwhite	4.0	7.7	2.6
Males	7.8	13.7	5.0
Females	2.4	4.4	1.7

Striking differences in the distribution of white and nonwhite discharges by hospital control are evident. Over 75 percent of the nonwhite discharges are accounted for by public nonfederal hospital units. Nongovernment hospital units account for over half of the total discharges from psychiatric units, but only 25 percent of the nonwhite discharges. While there are variations in these patterns within different age and sex groups, the public nonfederal hospital unit is still the predominant type of general hospital utilized by nonwhites for psychiatric care.

Referral patterns to and from general hospitals differ considerably for the two subgroups of hospitals. Almost a quarter of the referrals to public hospitals are by police, court or correctional agencies, as opposed to 4 percent of the referrals from such sources to nonpublic hospitals. Referral from private psychiatrists and other physicians account for almost half of the referrals to nonpublic hospitals, but only 14 percent of the referrals to public hospitals. On discharge, in the public hospitals, 30 percent go to psychiatric hospitals and 20 percent to organized outpatient psychiatric services; while in nonpublic hospitals, 64 percent go to private psychiatrists or other physicians.

The leading diagnoses for each of the two subgroups of hospitals are shown below:

Public Nonfederal	Nongovernment
Schizophrenia (39%)	Depressive disorders (41%)
Depressive disorders (15%)	Schizophrenia (18%)
Alcohol disorders (12%)	Other neuroses (11%)

In public nonfederal hospitals, the three leading diagnoses were schizophrenia, depressive disorders, and alcohol disorders. In nongovernment hospitals, depressive disorders and schizophrenia led the diagnostic distribution, but alcohol disorders were replaced by other neuroses as the third ranking diagnosis. In addition, there were significant differences in the distribution of disorders between hospital subgroups. While public nonfederal hospitals accounted for 41 percent of the total discharges, they accounted for 60 percent of all discharges with alcohol disorders, 70 percent of the total discharges with drug disorders, and 61 percent of all discharges with schizophrenia. Nongovernment hospitals on the other hand, with 50 percent of the total discharges, accounted for 80 percent of all discharges with depressive disorders.

The median length of stay for all discharges was twice as long in nonpublic (14 days) as compared to public hospitals (7 days). The longer stay in nongovernment hospitals held true within each age, sex, color, and diagnostic group.

Differences in the population served by the two subgroups of general hospitals results in differences in the method of payment used by their patients. Among discharges from nonfederal public hospitals, Medicaid which accounted for 43 percent of all dollar payments, was the single highest payment source. Among discharges from nonpublic hospitals, however, Medicaid accounted for only 10 percent of payments. A parallel situation existed for primary payment source: Medicaid was the primary payment source for 37 percent of nonfederal public hospital discharges but only 8 percent of nonpublic hospital discharges.

In contrast, nonpublic hospital payments were more heavily weighted by Blue Cross and commercial insurance plans: each of these accounted for 29 percent of dollar payments to such hospitals. Parallel percentages for dollar payments to nonfederal public hospitals were 7 and 8 percent for Blue Cross and commercial insurance plans respectively. Again, there was a close relationship to primary payment source. In nonpublic hospitals, Blue Cross and commercial insurance plans each appeared as the primary payment source 30 percent of the time. But in nonfederal public hospitals, Blue Cross and commercial insurance plans were the primary payment sources for only 7 and 11 percent of discharges, respectively.

Outpatient Services–Admissions v.
Services Provided

While the evidence presented earlier of an increase in use of outpatient psychiatric services can be interpreted as an indication of a movement away from the long-stay institutionalization of patients and of progress towards a goal of community care, some questions might be raised about the kinds and quality of services patients are receiving in outpatient facilities.

First of all, a significant proportion of the outpatient admissions represent those receiving aftercare services subsequent to an inpatient episode.

For instance, 40 percent of the total schizophrenic admissions to outpatient services in 1969 were to outpatient services of psychiatric hospitals (primarily the state and county mental hospitals), and, more than likely, a large proportion of these services represented after-care programs subsequent to an inpatient care episode. However, the high readmission rate of schizophrenics to inpatient services of state and county mental hospitals, raises questions about the success of these after-care programs.

Second, a primary function of outpatient services is that of diagnosis and evaluation, and for a sizable proportion of the total admissions to outpatient services, this is the only service the patient receives from the clinic. In Connecticut, for example, almost 9 percent of the terminations from general hospital psychiatric clinics, 14 percent of the terminations from community clinics, and 15 percent of the terminations from state mental hospital clinics received diagnostic and evaluation services only.[7] In Louisiana 10 percent of the terminations from mental health clinics and centers represented evaluations for other agencies.[8] For federally funded community mental health centers in Texas, about 20 percent of the outpatient admissions received diagnostic and evaluation services only.[9]

Third, a significant proportion of the total admissions to outpatient services during a given year receive intake services only, or initiate treatment services and subsequently drop out. High dropout rates are indicated by data from Indiana, where 30 percent of the outpatient cases were terminated during 1973 on the basis of a refusal on the part of the patient or the patient's family to continue treatment, and an additional 16 percent of the cases were closed because of failure of the patient to keep an appointment within a ninety-day period. Also, in Indiana 66 percent of the outpatient terminations during 1973 were treated; 16 percent received intake services only; 3 percent received psychological testing only; and 16 percent received diagnostic service only.[10] In Louisiana outpatient clinics and centers, 11 percent of the terminations received intake services only; and in Connecticut 12 percent of the terminations from general hospital psychiatric clinics, 14 percent of the terminations from community clinics, and 3 percent of the terminations from state mental hospital clinics received intake services only. In federally funded CMHCs in Texas, almost 40 percent of the outpatient admissions received intake and screening services only.

Another way of trying to assess the extent and type of service received by the increasing number of outpatient admissions is to look at the distribution of admissions by the number of outpatient visits made. This method represents more clearly the volume of services actually provided. For outpatient admissions to federally funded community mental health centers in Texas when followed for a one year interval, we find the following:

1. Of the 52,854 admissions, 21,565 or about 40 percent received intake and screening services. Of this group, 94 percent had only one visit.

2. An additional 10,792 admissions about 20 percent of the total, received diagnosis and evaluation services only. About 70 percent of this group had only one visit, an additional 18 percent had two visits, and 11 percent had three to five visits.
3. The remainder of the admissions, 20,697 or 40 percent of the total received treatment services. Of these patients entering a treatment program however, 35 percent had one visit only, and an additional 15 percent had two visits. In other words, half of the patients receiving treatment services received less than three visits.

Urban-Rural Distribution of Resources

Table 20-19 illustrates the imbalance existing in the distribution of resources between urban and rural areas. In 1970, 42 percent of the United States population lived in areas classified as either outside urbanized areas or rural by the Census Bureau; yet, the number of psychiatric facilities serving these areas represent a considerably smaller percentage of the total facilities. Public facilities relative to private facilities, in general, are more likely to be located outside urbanized areas. For example, about 51 percent of the state mental hospitals, 21 percent of the public general hospitals, and 57 percent of the free-standing outpatient psychiatric clinics are located outside urbanized areas. For the federally funded community mental health centers, 37 percent are located outside urbanized areas. In contrast, only 15 percent of the new for-profit multiple-hospital corporation mental hospitals were started outside urbanized areas.

While federally funded community mental health centers have undoubtedly increased services to rural areas, most of the problems of providing mental health services in rural areas still exist. As described by L.L. Bachrach, these include geographic isolation—with the attendant conditions of low population density, limited tax base, sparseness, and inaccessibility of facilities, manpower shortages, and negative attraction for new manpower.

Staffing must be mentioned separately as a very special problem at rural community mental health centers—certain characteristics of rural living exert inhibiting influences on optimal staff. Harvey Gurian stresses the professional loneliness of mental health practitioners in rural areas as being at the root of many of the difficulties in rural mental health care delivery. It has been noted that not only is it difficult to recruit staff for isolated facilities, but, once recruited, problems sometimes arise in local acceptance of outsiders. What is more, attitudes held by staff members themselves have a strong effect upon utilization patterns. A special study of twenty-four selected poverty CMHCs during 1972, eight of which were rural, concluded that an important urban/ nonurban difference among center staff was that:

Table 20-19

Percent Distribution of Psychiatric Facilities by Geographic Location (Urban-Rural), United States, 1972

Type of Facility	United States Total	Urban Total	Inside Urbanized Areas Total	Central City	Urban Fringe	Outside Urbanized Areas	Rural
Psychiatric hospitals							
Private	100.0%	97.1	83.5	51.4	32.1	13.6	2.8
State & county	100.0%	87.3	48.6	32.3	16.3	38.7	12.6
VA	100.0%	96.6	75.4	60.2	15.2	21.2	3.4
General hospitals							
Public (nonfederal)	100.0%	98.7	79.0	62.4	16.6	19.7	1.3
Nonpublic	100.0%	99.2	81.9	65.3	16.6	17.3	0.8
Outpatient psychiatric clinics							
Public	100.0%	93.5	43.8	27.6	16.2	49.7	6.5
Nonpublic	100.0%	97.2	63.5	44.5	19.0	33.7	2.8
Residential treatment centers for emotionally disturbed children	100.0%	90.0	72.7	53.6	19.1	17.3	10.0
Federally funded community mental health centers	100.0%	97.9	62.7	50.9	11.8	35.3	2.1

. . . urban staff (particularly outreach workers) tended to reflect more sophistication in their views of the unique needs of the poor. In particular, they reflected more sensitivity to the barriers existing between the poor client and traditional mental health services. Also they tended to address themselves more to the need for community involvement in making outreach efforts effective.[11]

Care of the Mentally Ill Aged

Much attention has been directed in recent years to the decline in the number of persons sixty-five years of age and over under care or coming under care in mental hospitals. Recent data on patient care episodes in psychiatric facilities illustrate this trend. As seen in Table 20-2, the number of patient care episodes in all psychiatric services increased from 2.8 million in 1966 to slightly over 4 million in 1971. However, during the same time period the number of patient care episodes aged sixty-five and over decreased from 313,000 to 263,000 and the corresponding patient care episode rate decreased from 1,672 to 1,310 per 100,000 population, or a 22 percent decline. All of this decrease occurred in the inpatient psychiatric services. It is noted that the number of patient care episodes for the sixty-five and over age group in outpatient psychiatric services more than doubled between 1966 and 1971 and constituted one-fifth of the total episodes sixty-five years and over in 1971 compared with only 8 percent in the earlier time period.

In 1971 state and county mental hospitals still accounted for the largest proportion of all patient care episodes in the sixty-five and over age group—50 percent, but the number and rate of episodes decreased substantially between 1966 and 1971 for these hospitals as did those for general hospital inpatient psychiatric services and Veterans Administration hospitals. Accompanying this decline was the increase in patient care episodes sixty-five years and over for the outpatient psychiatric services between 1966 and 1971 and also the emergence of the community mental health center (CMHC) as an alternate place of psychiatric care for the elderly. However, the number of elderly under care in community mental health centers and the other outpatient psychiatric services as a proportion of all patient care episodes in these facilities in 1971 is quite small—7 percent for the CMHC inpatient services, 3 percent for CMHC outpatient services and 2 percent for the other outpatient psychiatric services—this latter proportion showing no change over what it was in 1966.

Data from a 1969 NIMH survey of patients discontinued from the inpatient services of state and county mental hospitals showed that for the 37,000 discontinuations sixty-five years of age and over, the proportions referred to other types of psychiatric services were relatively small (e.g., 15 percent to outpatient psychiatric services, and equal proportions of 4 percent each to community mental health centers, to transitional mental health facilities, and to other mental hospitals) compared with the almost two-fifths referred to nursing homes or homes for the aged.[12]

The NIMH survey data, cited above, seem to infer that community-based psychiatric facilities (community mental health centers, outpatient psychiatric services, and transitional mental health facilities) are playing a relatively minor role in the care of the aged mentally ill as their numbers decline in psychiatric hospitals, whereas nursing homes and homes for the aged appear to be assuming a greater part of the burden of caring for this population.

This latter influence is given further support by the published findings of the most recent surveys of nursing and personal care homes conducted during 1968-69 by the National Center for Health Statistics.[g] When the data for these surveys are compared with those from earlier 1963-64 surveys of these facilities conducted by the same organization, it is seen that the 815,130 residents in 18,391 nursing and personal care homes in the United States in 1969 represent a 47 percent increase over the 554,000 residents in 17,400 such homes in operation during the earlier time period. More significant though was the near doubling of the number of mentally ill patients resident in these homes over the same interval from about 222,000 in 1963 to almost 427,000 in 1969. All but 14 percent of the mentally ill patients in nursing and personal care homes in 1969 were sixty-five years of age and over, their number increasing from 188,000 to 368,000 or 96 percent during the 1963-69 period.

The large majority of persons sixty-five and over with mental disorders resident in long-term institutions both in 1963 and 1969 were either in state and county mental hospitals or nursing and personal care homes (Table 20-20). In the earlier period almost two-fifths of this age group were in state and county mental hospitals and slightly over half were in nursing and personal care homes. However, by 1969 these proportions had changed dramatically with only a little

---

[g]The National Center for Health Statistics has conducted a series of ad hoc surveys of institutional health facilities that are part of the National Health Survey program to provide current health statistics on the nation. The first of these surveys was conducted in April-June 1963 and collected sample data on nursing homes, chronic disease and geriatric hospitals, and nursing home units and chronic disease wards of general and mental hospitals. The Resident Places Survey-2, which was conducted in May-June 1964, is the second of these ad hoc; it concentrated mainly on a sample of nursing homes and geriatric hospitals. This second survey collected more detailed information about each institution, its residents, and its employees. The 1968 Nursing Home Survey, conducted during April-September 1968, was the third survey. It was a census of all nursing homes in the United States. It collected detailed information on the characteristics of the facilities. The fourth survey, conducted in cooperation with the U.S. Bureau of the Census during June-August 1969, was multipurpose, collecting information about the nursing home, its residents, and its employees.

Table 20-20
Number and Percent Distribution of Patients with Mental Disorders Resident in Selected Long-term Institutions by Age and Sex, 1963 and 1969

Age and Sex	1963					1969				
	Total	State & County Mental Hospitals	Private Mental Hospitals	VA Hospitals	Nursing Homes[a]	Total	State & County Mental Hospitals	Private Mental Hospitals	VA Hospitals	Nursing Homes[a]
					Number					
Total	792,827	504,604	9,998	56,504	221,721	851,029	369,969	10,963	43,385	426,712
Under 65	437,257	355,762	6,795	40,654	34,046	359,888	258,549	8,503	33,710	59,126
65 and Over	355,570	148,842	3,203	15,850	187,675	491,141	111,420	2,460	9,675	367,586
Male	378,176	248,364	3,507	51,006	75,299	362,392	185,584	4,254	42,435	130,119
Under 65	244,710	187,642	2,427	36,877	17,764	204,739	140,775	3,545	32,870	27,549
65 and Over	133,466	60,722	1,080	14,129	57,535	157,653	44,809	709	9,565	102,570
Female	414,651	256,240	6,491	5,498	146,422	488,637	184,385	6,709	950	296,593
Under 65	192,547	168,120	4,368	3,777	16,282	155,149	117,774	4,958	840	31,577
65 and Over	222,104	88,120	2,123	1,721	130,140	333,488	66,611	1,751	110	265,016
Total	100.0%	63.6%	1.3%	7.1%	28.0%	100.0%	43.5%	1.3%	5.1%	50.1%
Under 65	100.0	81.3	1.6	9.3	7.8	100.0	71.8	2.4	9.4	16.4
65 and Over	100.0	41.9	0.9	4.5	52.7	100.0	22.7	0.5	2.0	74.8
Male	100.0	65.7	0.9	13.5	19.9	100.0	51.2	1.2	11.7	35.9
Under 65	100.0	76.7	1.0	15.1	7.2	100.0	68.8	1.7	16.0	13.5
65 and Over	100.0	45.5	0.8	10.6	43.1	100.0	28.4	0.4	6.1	65.1
Female	100.0	61.8	1.6	1.3	35.3	100.0	37.7	1.4	0.2	60.7
Under 65	100.0	87.2	2.3	2.0	8.5	100.0	75.9	3.2	0.5	20.4
65 and Over	100.0	39.7	0.9	0.8	58.6	100.0	20.0	0.5	0.0*	79.5

* Less than 0.05 percent.

[a] Includes residents diagnosed with advanced senility and with other mental disorders. The number of residents in this table is less than that shown in Table 2-14 of the chapter, "Trends and Projections in State Hospital Use," in this volume, which included residents with a condition of senility without psychosis.

over one-fifth in the state and county mental hospitals and three-quarters in nursing and personal care homes.

The reductions in the numbers of elderly persons resident in and admitted to inpatient psychiatric services, particularly state mental hospitals, in recent years appear not to have shifted the locus of care of these persons to community-based facilities (community mental health centers and other outpatient psychiatric services) to any great degree and have been accompanied by substantial increases in the number of mentally ill and mentally disturbed residents in nursing and personal care homes.

Others observing or studying the recent trend from mental hospital care to nursing home care for the elderly mentally ill, have similarly noted that, in but too few instances, the quality of care has remained generally unchanged— that of custodial-type care—with little or no benefit to the patient's condition.[13]

These circumstances prevail not only because of a lack of adequate numbers of appropriate staff in many nursing homes and because, as Lipscomb points out, of "the attitudes of nursing home staff which are mainly a reflection of lack of experience and training in handling patients who at times exhibit slightly more disturbed behavior than that normally expected in a nursing home";[14] but also because mental hospitals, particularly the state mental hospitals that have released large numbers of elderly over the past ten or more years, have failed to play a significant role in follow-up support of these released patients. In this respect, Frankfather notes that "only a very few State hospitals are actively involved with the nursing homes to which they discharged their patients, the range of activities includes preplacement visits, some follow-up services after placement, treatment supervision, and educational programs for nursing home staff. Unfortunately, such mental hospital-nursing home interaction is all too infrequent."[15]

Community mental health centers, as noted earlier, have performed a somewhat minimal role in the care of the mentally ill aged. In a recent study of eight community mental health centers,[16] which examined programs of services to the elderly, it was indicated that the services provided are largely of a clinical nature to those who seek out the center for help, and that there was little emphasis on programs oriented to those elderly in the community who are either receiving care in other community-based facilities (e.g., nursing homes, homes for aged, etc.), or are reluctant or unable to come to the CMHC facility, or are unaware of the availability of the center.

Notes

1. Goldberg, I.D., Consideration of Nonpsychiatric Medical Settings in the Delivery of Mental Health Services, paper presented at the National Conference on Evaluation in Alcohol, Drug Abuse and Mental Health

Programs, April 1974, Washington D.C.; _____ , "Psychiatry and the General
Practitioner," *WHO Chronicle,* February 1974; Shepherd M., "General
Practice, Mental Illness and the British National Health Service,"
American Journal of Public Health, (1964) 64:3; WHO, Psychiatry and
Primary Medical Care. Report of a Working Group, April 1973, World Health
Organization.

2. Sharfstein, S.S. et al., "A Response to the APA Task Force Report on Private Practice," *American Journal of Psychiatry,* in press.

3. Scheidemandel, P.L., "Utilization of Psychiatric Services," *Psychiatric Annals,*
   (1974) 4:1.

4. Bethel H., "Trends in Total Additions and Resident Patients at End of Year
   in Private Mental Hospitals, 1968-1971," *Statistical Note 99,* Rockville, Md.,
   Biometry Branch, NIMH.

5. Witkin, M.J., *Residential Psychiatric Facilities for Children and Adolescents:
   United States 1971-72,* Mental Health Statistics, Series A, No. 14. Division
   of Biometry, NIMH, 1974.

6. Conwell, M. et al., "The First National Survey of Psychiatric Day Night
   Services," in Epps, Robert L., and Hanes, Lee D. (eds.), *Day Care of Psychiatric Patients,* Springfield, Illinois: Charles C. Thomas, 1964.

7. Connecticut State Department of Mental Health, Outpatient Psychiatric
   Clinics in Connecticut, Statistical Tables for year ending June 30, 1972.

8. Louisiana State Department of Hospitals, Statistical Summary, Fiscal Year
   1971.

9. Texas Department of Mental Health and Mental Retardation, unpublished
   data.

10. Indiana Department of Mental Health, Statistics Branch, Annual Statistical
    Report for Indiana Mental Health Clinics, Fiscal Year 1973.

11. Bachrach, L.L., "Characteristics of Federally Funded Rural Community
    Mental Health Centers in 1971," *Statistical Note 101* Division of Biometry,
    NIMH, March 1974.

12. Redick, Richard W., "Referral of Discontinuations from Inpatient Services
    of State and County Mental Hospitals, United States 1969." *Statistical
    Note 57,* Division of Biometry, NIMH, November 1971.

13. Collins, J.A., Stotsky, B.A., and Dominick, J.R., "Is the Nursing Home of
    the Mental Hospital's Back Ward in the Community?" *Journal of the
    American Geriatric Society,* (1969) 15:75-81; Hefferin, E.A. and Wilner,
    D.N., "Opinions About Geriatric Patients in Public Mental Hospitals,"
    HSMHA Health Reports, (1971) 86:5, 457-71; Epstein, L.J. and Simon,
    Alexander., "Alternatives to State Hospitalization for the Geriatric Men-
    tally Ill," *American Journal of Psychiatry,* (1968) 124:7, 955-61; Markson,
    E.; Kwoh, A.; Cumming, J.; and Cumming, E., "Alternatives to Hospitaliza-
    tion for Psychiatrically Ill Geriatric Patients," *American Journal of Psychia-
    try,* (1971) 127:8, 1055-62; Sharfstein, Steven S., Mentally Ill Aged and

Neighborhood Health Centers, paper presented at the 127th Annual Meeting of the American Psychiatric Association, May 1974.

14. Lipscomb, Colin F., "The Care of the Psychiatrically Disturbed Elderly Patient in the Community," *American Journal of Psychiatry,* (1971) 127:8, 1069.

15. Frankfather, Dwight, Background and Position Paper on Mental Health Care for the Elderly, unpublished final report for the Planning Branch, Office of Program Planning and Evaluation, NIMH, p. 78.

16. Socio-Technical Systems Associates, Inc., Evaluation of NIMH Aging Programs with Special Focus on Services, (report prepared under contract for NIMH), 1974.

21

The Hospital Director's Viewpoint
Jonathan O. Cole

Introduction

A prevalent contemporary view is that state hospitals are finished. Ideally they should magically vanish in a puff of smoke to be replaced by better treatment facilities, preferably spread throughout the community. These new facilities will, of course, provide instant high quality service to all in present need with one hand, while preventing all future mental illness with the other, embracing a wide range of other human services with a third hand, and saving tax dollars with a fourth hand, while listening to advice from citizens and consumers with one ear and state officials and expert consultants with the other ear.

Faced with these awesome and frenetic expectations, the role of the superintendent or director attempting to guide his hospital rationally from a sedentary, decaying, unresponsive, overcrowded, isolated past to the frantic future is stressful to the incumbent and often frustrating to the various factions struggling over the still palpitating corpse of his hospital. The director has two major general problems. First, he's afflicted with a toxic dose of reality that keeps fouling up his own bright ideas for change as well as fouling up ideas imposed from outside. Second, he finds it very hard to plan the total abolishment of his own hospital. He wants it not to die but to change skillfully into the ideal mental health or human services or research facility of *his* dreams, not of someone else's dreams.

For this reason, if a state hospital is to be completely abolished, the final firm decision should be made by someone other than the director and a new acting director be brought in with the clear and explicit job of closing the place. This plan worked very well at Grafton State Hospital in Massachusetts. Another revealing look at problems facing heads of state hospitals can be found in the following account of the author's past six years as director of Boston State Hospital.

Boston State Hospital: 1967-73

At the time of assuming the directorship, it was clear that the hospital was already in transition.[a] A combination of programs (but chiefly creative hard

---

[a]The subject has been competently dealt with in Greenblatt, M. and Sharaf, M. *Dynamics of Institutional Change; The Hospital in Transition,* University of Pittsburgh Press, 1971.

work by chronic services staff), plus an embryonic community mental health program and a good triage and rapid treatment system had succeeded in cutting the inpatient population from 3,000 or more to about 1,300 over a ten-year period. In the meantime staff had risen from about 1,000 to about 1,300.

Utilization of the hospital and the carving up of the state into catchment areas had just occurred. Boston, the hospital's long standing catchment area, was divided into five mental health center areas. The Massachusetts Mental Health Center took, gradually, the total responsibility for its own area of Brookline, Brighton, and Jamaica Plains. A new facility, the Lindemann Mental Health Center, opened in 1971 with beautiful architecture and limited staff and now covers the North End, Charlestown, East Boston, and other parts of Suffolk County. A building for the Boston University Mental Health Center is now rising. This will serve the old core city and much of the black area. Tufts Mental Health Center serving South Boston has been trying to move out of Boston State Hospital and into a state public health hospital for two years. If all these moves are successful, the old Boston State Hospital (BSH) will be left with large grounds, about twenty large habitable or semihabitable major buildings, services for a permanent catchment area of 210,000 individuals, and maybe 400 extra, residual, chronic inpatients.

The normal fate of Boston State Hospital might then be considered to be its conversion to a local "South West Boston Mental Health Center." For a variety of reasons, this did not seem a viable solution. Some of the problems that surfaced and the ways we attempted to deal with them follow.

Should Mental Health Centers All
Leave the State Hospital?

It was decided to run the 210,000 person catchment area as two mental health centers each providing a full range of services. The smaller (in staff and problems) of these, serving a relatively homogeneous, white, Catholic, lower middle to middle class area, was on a successful course that could ultimately lead to its being self-sufficient and fully community-based with even its inpatient beds outside Boston State Hospital. The other mental health center could conceivably accomplish the same objective in its mixed racial community. What would then happen to the chronic patients that neither center wanted? Would the hospital then die or turn into a nursing home?

Should Good Chronic Services be Encouraged?

Boston State Hospital has had aggressive community placement programs for chronic patients (family care, cooperative apartments, halfway houses, nursing homes) and has done a good job of monitoring these ex-patients, often bringing them back to the hospital for day or work or rehabilitation programs. But all these good programs evolved out of an old line chronic service base, not out of mental health centers. The acute mental health centers did well on new chronics—almost no patients were transferred to the chronic wards from acute wards during my six-year tenure (about 10 a year)—but the centers were unwilling to take on hard-core chronic patients. Only one of the four other mental health centers in Boston had any interest in taking responsibility for their old chronic BSH patients. It seemed to us that for these patients, most of whom were very attached to the hospital and had no other real roots, a hospital-run placement and supervision program was preferable to arbitrary return to their ancient home catchment area of origin.

This moral and clinical commitment to a residual chronic group of mainly brain damaged and mentally retarded chronic patients, plus a few hard-core schizophrenics, left me chronically in conflict trying to allocate staff to help *both* the chronic programs *and* the mental health centers.

Let's Abolish the Medical Surgical Service!

This internal conflict between BSH's own mental health center and its chronic service over staff and other resources had a third force, the Medical-Surgical Unit. A peculiarity of Massachusetts State regulations made it very difficult to pay to have mental patients treated at ordinary hospitals. BSH was stuck with an expensively staffed medical-surgical building giving mediocre to poor care in the midst of major centers of medical excellence. Good surgical residents were obtained from Beth Israel Hospital; they tried to provide special surgical services and ended up doing surgery for seven surrounding state mental hospitals and schools that had even worse local situations. Finally, when all surgery had been transferred to the Shattuck Hospital, a state public health hospital half a mile away, it was learned that *that* hospital's budget was being cut and that *its* future was in doubt.

Mental hospitals do not belong in the medical-surgical business. They can rarely do it well and should not do it poorly. Before the transfer, attempts were made to improve the medical-surgical service; for example, consultants were incorporated to enable them to function on third-party payments. This plan failed owing to constant delays in payment by Medicare and Medicaid. In retrospect it appears it should have been phased out earlier.

Should the New Centers Dismember the Old Hospital?

The other Boston mental health centers posed another stress and problem. For a while no one noticed that BSH had achieved a 2:1 staff-patient ratio, but gradually pressure from all sides increased as census dropped to about 650 inpatients. Painful contracts had earlier been worked out with Tufts, Boston University, and Lindemann, assigning them certain state hospital positions. A few of these were being legally transferred to the books of the other facilities. Demands were beginning to mount for a larger share of the hospital's personnel pie.

Rightly or wrongly, major disbursements of positions were resisted. The other mental health centers were even persuaded to absorb some chronic patients being repatriated to Boston from distant state hospitals (where they had lived for 10 to 20 years). But concern over the issue of fairness in the allocation of resources led finally to the establishment of a management data system obtained through a Hospital Improvement Grant to try to fit tasks and needs to resources in some rational way. This is now in its second year.

Plant and Nonclinical Staff

The Hospital Improvement grant also helped resolve another problem, the crumbling state of nonclinical services. Years of mediocre bureaucracy and very low pay scales for nonclinical middle management had left the hospital dirty, poorly maintained, and full of unworkable interdepartmental frictions. Housekeeping, garage and grounds, plumbing, security, and all aspects of the laundry system *except* the actual washing were particularly bad and all service systems were antiquated. This part of the hospital actually tied up over 330 of the 1,300 employees. Worse still, even if patient census dropped to 300, and hospital buildings were mostly used for community or human services programs, most of the 300 employees might still be needed to service the plant, buildings, and grounds. For this reason any arbitrary splitting of BSH's staff evenly among the five or six mental health centers in Boston could not be done without demolishing the hospital.

Research and Training

Along with the above problems, it was attempted, with some success, to expand clinical research and training programs at the hospital, by robbing Peter to pay Paul creatively. For studies needing a large homogeneous patient sample, community mental health has spoiled state hospitals as research facilities. However, studies were made of tardive dyskinesia, drug therapy in chronic patients in the community, and drugs in the elderly with some success. Eventually, with the help of Dr. Milton Greenblatt and an effective architect-lobbyist a new research building was achieved, though new toilets might have been preferred. But the question of what happens to research and training if the hospital disappears out from under it remains.

New Uses for Old Positions

The program experimented with using personnel in new ways. Old-line hospital personnel and licensed practical nurses were used as community agents with success. Interdisciplinary teams were used whenever possible, often utilizing untrained personnel because we could not afford to hire trained professionals. We had particular success in using occupational therapists in the community in home treatment, in geriatrics, and in work with emotionally disturbed children. In fact, we were left with inadequate ward activity programs in most areas as the O.T.'s moved into the community.

The Boston Land Rush

Given a shrinking state hospital in an urban setting, the superintendent finds that he has—for a time—control over a unique asset, space. The buildings may be delapidated, poorly lit, and with inferior toilet facilities, but they are empty, heated, and almost rent free. Some informal arrangements were simple and useful. A building was used for classes for subtrainable retarded children with the staff provided by the Boston Public Schools. Another building was a halfway house for alcoholics, partially funded by the Welfare Department. Another building housed an excellent program for forty predelinquent boys, funded by Welfare and the Youth Service Board through a nonprofit foundation of our creation. We started this because there were no good residential programs for such youngsters, whom we began to see in large numbers on consultations with the local court. This excellent program became controversial when the youths damaged the building badly, but we survived the crisis.

We lent a building to the overcrowded public elementary school and got involved in trying to force the city to build a better school so we could get our building back (after the city had refurbished it!). We lent a building to the local black community to use as a community center for a time and got picketed for not providing good furniture, play equipment, and free milk too! We housed a self-help, state-contract-supported day program and halfway house for drug abusers. The hospital housed a nonprofit sheltered workshop supported by state rehabilitation funds.

The most controversial move was use of one building as the first (and only) prerelease (preparole) center for prisoners being returned to the community in Massachusetts. One lesson learned, however, is that state hospitals have neighbors who have already endured much, and zoning changes are not needed to use old buildings for new programs.

Recently, long standing plans to place a forty-five-bed, 300-day-student school for the retarded on one side of the hospital grounds were completed. Just when the retarded citizens' group was happy with the plans, the state's

new commissioner of human services objected to it and a community group
got interested, under a state senator, in having a voice in the future use of all
BSH's buildings and land. So the days of relatively free creative use of buildings at BSH appear to be numbered.

Human Services, a Curse or an Opportunity

The Department of Human Services now controls mental health, welfare,
public health, corrections, and rehabilitation in Massachusetts and a plan is
before the legislature to homogenize all departments down to the catchment
area level and to create an area human services director who could reassign
people and reallocate funds. Prolonged chaos appears possible if it passes the
legislature. Nevertheless, the hospital has gradually moved in that direction.
As inpatients decrease and mental health services are increasingly provided off
the hospital grounds, perhaps other state and local agencies should move in.
Welfare offices would have been the natural choice. One was invited to move
in but objected to the buildings. If we could have merged the hospital as an
institution with the Shattuck Public Health Hospital and the Juvenile Detention Facility, all within a half mile radius, fiscal savings and improved service
delivery could have resulted and may yet occur. A range of facilities for the
elderly and handicapped (apartments, maybe partial care hotels, nursing
homes) built on some of the vacant land, plus a branch of a junior college,
would also have been viable alternatives.

Bureaucracy and Politics

If one tries hard to be a creative administrator, one has to learn to circumvent or abide by a certain amount of red tape. However, the prospect of
added advisory groups, extra bureaucratic levels (all of which can say no and
none can say yes), increasingly rigid personnel policies at the state level,
arbitrary categorical budget cuts (e.g., 50 percent of an already inadequate
maintenance supply budget), and a spiralling number of inspections and
documentary requirements (joint commission, affirmative action, medicare,
public safety, public health) give one the feeling that one must run, like the
Red Queen in *Alice in Wonderland,* just to stay where one is and that any new
program is going to take so long to clear and fund and will take so many arguments that even eventual success in the venture turns to ashes in one's mouth.

Discussion

The role of the superintendent or director of a public mental hospital
is getting progressively more complex and stressful, particularly if his hospital
is "in transition", that is, likely to be changed into some different kind of

mental health care facility. One of the chief stresses is the lingering suspicion
that one is participating in a vast social experiment that may prove to have
serious or tragic side effects. It is clearly "good" for a state hospital to reduce
its census of chronic and acute patients and to treat everyone in the community.
That way someone else—usually the Welfare Department—pays for the impaired
patient's room and board. Hospital staff are freed for new programs (or more
likely, to adequately staff old programs at long last), and the graph showing a
declining hospital census plummets further. The lingering suspicion persists
that chronic patients may be less happy and less well cared for in boarding
houses or nursing homes than they were in the comfortable old state hospital
and that acute patients, excluded from the hospital, may be wreaking psychosocial havoc in the community. These two evils can be avoided if crisis, ambulatory, and chronic after-care programs are well run. But if they are not, how
can the "quality of life" of a chronic patient in various settings be measured or
cost accounted?

Another problem involves the allocation of staff from, for example, chronic
ward A to primary prevention in the schools. Even if one had data on incidence
and prevalence of school problems, and the efficacy of various new and old
programs, the director still has to make a value judgement. While decision
making has always been critical, what is new is the diversity of needs and services
to be dealt with (e.g., preschool nurseries, day care for the elderly, methadone
maintenance, sheltered workshops, consultation, and education) and the need
to allow for the value judgements of an increasing welter of other interested
parties (e.g., community boards, block associations, powerful individual citizens,
other service agencies, consumer groups, and members of the legislature).

A further complication for state hospitals developing new community-
oriented programs is the rigidity problem. Will existing personnel be willing
to move out into new programs. Will state rules (or the union) allow hospital
employees to work full or part time off the grounds? What if you need a
sheltered workshop director or child psychologist to start a new program
and no category exists in civil service for such a person and you cannot bootleg
them into a job that is at the right pay grade, but has different duties? Can
you hire college graduates into ward attendant jobs but use them as social
work assistants or lay therapists? What if your community wants a day care
program for disturbed children and you have adequate space, but the Fire
Department suddenly demands major building alterations in an old building
that had been approved by the same department when it was an inpatient ward
building? Then you get a community group to agree to pay for the alterations
but the state authorities insist on it being done the most expensive way and
the community group cannot afford that much.

To achieve new community activities in an old state hospital requires drive,
ingenuity, risk-taking, conniving, and stretching of regulations. Support from
higher echelons is necessary and some help in circumventing bureaucratic

death-traps is necessary. If the director is to move the hospital he needs power and freedom, and both are being whittled away as state budgets get tighter and state hospitals are viewed with disfavor.

At some point, state hospitals may have to be killed because they have been mummified in red tape. Already in Massachusetts the state juvenile delinquency program has abandoned its institutions and is contracting with ad hoc foundations just so as to be able to circumvent over-rigid state rules and regulations.

Hospitals can also be killed by physical decay. Boston State Hospital was able to cut census rapidly enough to empty its worst buildings before they were condemned. But the remaining buildings are by and large poorly lit, badly heated, and have inferior toilets and bathing facilities. Over 95 percent of patient toilets lack seats and privacy. It is hard to justify new buildings with a declining census. Since it can take between four and ten years to get new buildings in Massachusetts, it is possible that the physical plant may collapse and settle the future of the hospital once and for all.

One solution, offered only partly in jest, is that the state should give the whole hospital to a private corporation and give the corporation the same annual budget now provided, but abolish all state rules and regulations. It is possible that a private corporation could do a better job with fewer, higher paid staff, and even make money in the process. Government management of programs no longer makes me optimistic; civil service seems to be a fiasco. Unions impress me with their incompetence and distorted values. Citizen participation often leads to painful, unproductive, and prolonged confusions.

The best part of being a hospital director is the entrepreneurial role. If state hospitals are to move toward new diversified and therapeutic roles, the rules and regulations need to be changed to provide adequate freedom and flexibility for the director and to reward innovation. Higher personal financial rewards may also be necessary to recruit and maintain good people in a job that shows signs of going the way of the dinosaur.

22

Recent Developments in French Public Mental Health

Martin Gittelman, Jacques Dubois, Michel Gillet

There is considerable ferment in mental health practice and administration in many countries today as various approaches to efficient and continuous care are tried within the framework of public health services. Almost everywhere emphasis is on community-based services and a move away from institutionalization. But the organizational and financial means by which different countries are attempting to deliver adequate and effective care vary from country to country, and each system may have valuable suggestions to offer to others—ideas that may be adapted but not adopted, since conditions are not the same in different settings.

Recent developments in French public mental health focus on the system known as "sectorization." While the state of flux apparent in French services since 1972, and further changes doubtless in the offing make this difficult to describe, the concept of sectorization and the team approach it employs seem likely to prevail. For this reason, the French "solution" certainly warrants study by other countries.

There are other elements in the French system, including private practice. Until 1972 patients could see private psychiatrists of their choice as much as twice a week and be reimbursed fully by social security for their physicians' charges. However, the psychiatrists could tack on a surcharge if they liked, and could collect it! Under new regulations, there is a fixed fee for both reimbursement and for the surcharge; but in order to claim the surcharge, the psychiatrist must have more than the usual qualifications—he must, for example, be a professor or a chief of services.

France, like the United States, has a relative shortage of mental health personnel. Roughly one-fourth the size in population, France has only 2,000 psychiatrists compared with the United States total of 20,000. As early as the end of World War II, France began to try to cope with this problem, moving in the direction of maximal utilization of the available manpower and, above all, toward the development of public mental health services. This move has led to emphasis on prevention, rehabilitation, and community-based programs for all strata of society, under the umbrella of "sectorization."

The authors wish to thank Dr. R. Amiel, for his review of this paper and his helpful suggestions, and Mrs. Betty Appelbaum, for her valuable editorial assistance.

363

Historical Background

Formal intervention by public authorities in the care of the mentally ill in France dates from the seventeenth century (1660), when some space was officially reserved for the "insane" in general hospitals. During the seventeenth and nineteenth centuries, a few laws evolved that specified that the involuntary confinement of the mentally ill could be ordered by the king *(lettre de cachet)* or by a justice *(interdiction)*. After the French Revolution, these powers were delegated to municipal authorities.

It was during this period that the reform movements of Pinel, Esquirol, and their students generated ideas that led to the first law concerning the rights of the mentally ill—the law of 30 June 1838, which is still in force. This law provided for the establishment, on a departmental or regional basis, of "asylums for the insane"; it fixed the conditions for confinement and guaranteed individual liberties, making provision for the legal needs of those confined and arranging for the protection of their material possessions. With this law the mentally ill became rejects of society—no longer beings touched by the Divine Spirit or creatures "possessed" but sick human beings who had to be cared for in asylums that protected society from their possibly dangerous acts. But the chief concern of this law was to prevent the arbitrary application of its provisions and to remove the temptation for anyone to profit from the situation of the mentally ill by squandering or misappropriating their wealth.

Since the beginning of the twentieth century, psychiatry has moved away from its historical preoccupation with asylums and has accepted new tasks, particularly with respect to rehabilitation and social adaptation. This development has come within the context of the Industrial Revolution, a tremendous growth in population, urbanization, and significant social changes.

Political and social factors have had decisive influences on mental health care in France. In 1936 the socialist government of Leon Blum (the Front Populaire) introduced social security. The term "psychiatric hospital" was substituted for "asylum," and the medical personnel of the psychiatric hospitals began to be "radicalized"—a trend that was to be reinforced during World War II and the Occupation.

A number of ideas that had been latent for many years began to be expressed following the Liberation (1945). Social security was greatly expanded, in terms of both population covered and benefits provided. Dr. Lucien Bonnafe, chief of services at the Hopital Psychiatrique de Perray-Vaucluse, denounced the confinement and primitive care of the mentally ill. Dr. Georges Daumezon, chief of service at the Hopital Henri-Rousselle, defined the concept of sectorization and proposed the use of hospital-based teams to work in the community and provide after-care services. Daumezon also emphasized the importance of prevention. He called for wide-scale teaching of mental hygiene, expressing the view that physicians, social workers, teachers, and others should first learn,

and then teach, mental hygiene, with the support of readily available psychiatrists. He wanted psychiatrists to divide their time between care of the
hospitalized ill and care of the ill outside the hospital.

In 1952 the discovery of chlorpromazine, which permitted patients to
be treated outside the hospital, contributed greatly to an already developing
movement away from institutionalization. Mental hospital care was expensive,
it was inhumane, and for many patients it was unnecessary. With the aid of
the new drug treatment, French psychiatry began to reflect the influence of
the open hospital and community approach to mental care, introduced some
years earlier in Britain by Maxwell Jones.

Although many French psychiatrists have had some training in psychoanalyti-
cal concepts, psychoanalysis has played only a small role in French public psychiatry. Two ideological currents have gradually appeared: somatic or biologically
oriented techniques, such as electroshock and insulin shock therapy, and "dynamic"
treatment methods based on the interaction of patients with their milieux and
with others in that milieu, particularly those in a therapeutic relationship with
them. Under this latter heading would come the therapeutic community, insight-
oriented individual and group therapy, work rehabilitation, and other approaches
to altering the patient's mental and social functioning.

Practical moves have preceded legislative action in French public mental
health. In 1953 Daumezon arranged for each psychiatric hospital in the Paris
region to receive patients from a definite geographic sector. His example was
followed in the provinces by Lambert, Loechlin, and Le Guiliant.

In 1957 Philippe Paumelle attempted to put the principles of sectorization
into practice.[1] A private association—l'Association de Sante Mentale et de Lutte
contre l'Alcoholisme—supported by the staff of the Psychoanalytic Institute of
Paris, contracted with the social security system to provide community and hospital
treatment in what was at that time one of the poorest sections of Paris—the thirteenth arrondisement. Paumelle became the first director of this sector.

In 1960 collaboration between the director general of health and his psychiatric
advisers resulted in the Memorandum of March 15, which laid the groundwork
for true "sector psychiatry." Lack of space precludes a detailed discussion of
this legislation; briefly, it follows the guidelines and recommendations of the
World Health Organization, which had been greatly influenced by the ideas of
Paul Sivadon, a hospital psychiatrist who had been involved in the movement
for a long time and who is now director of the sixteenth arrondissement sector
and of Les Verrieres, a very modern, open hospital.

Sectorization

Much has been written about the outstanding work of the thirteenth arrondissement of Paris in developing comprehensive public mental health services in
France.[2] The aim of the thirteenth's plan was to create an entire range of

outpatient facilities, with clearly defined and organized roles, all centered
around a community mental health center and each serviced by a psychiatric
team. This plan, outlined in the above-mentioned Memorandum of 15 March
1960, provided for all the facilities and services required for patient care within
a relatively small geographic area—for geriatric centers; child guidance clinics;
foster home placements; day, night, and weekend hospitalization; vocational
and rehabilitation centers; halfway houses; an inpatient hospital; emergency
and crisis intervention services; and others. Most important, it defined the role
of the team as being responsible for the population residing in a specified geographic area: the team was to provide all the necessary services—inpatient,
outpatient, and rehabilitative—required by the inhabitants of its sector.

The thirteenth arrondissement has come to serve as a model for many
other sectors throughout France. All of France has now been decentralized,
or sectorized, for mental health purposes. This means that every region in the
country has been divided according to geographic and population factors and
plans have been developed to maximize the usefulness of the existing mental
health facilities and personnel of each area. The development of new services
and the coordination of existing services have not been uniform throughout
the country. Some local authorities and professionals have been quick to
grasp the implications of their new positions and have experimented with new
types of community service, whereas others have moved more slowly. But
with increased funds and more substantial salaries serving as "carrots" and
their allotments based on progress in achieving the goals of sectorization
acting as the "stick," most sectors are steadily moving toward community
psychiatry.

Since early 1972 there has been a new incentive for professionals to
become part of community treatment schemes. Hospital-based psychiatrists
have been given the choice of remaining in the hospital or becoming sector
psychiatrists. If they remain in the hospital, they continue to draw their low
salaries but retain their special prerogatives as state functionaries—a car, a
house (usually on the hospital grounds), and, frequently, servants. However,
if they choose to become sector psychiatrists, they lose these fringe benefits,
but their salaries are more than doubled ($14,400 to start, $24,000 per annum
for 14 years of service). They must work full time, initially devoting a
minimum of three-tenths of their work week to community services. They
may spend two-tenths of their work treating private patients in their community
public facilities and even have several beds available to them for private patients
in partial-hospitalization facilities. The improved working conditions have
induced most of these doctors to become sector psychiatrists.

In the Paris area, all mental health sectors are the responsibility of the
Prefecture de la Seine. Generally, sectors correspond to preexisting administrative districts that contain a population of 100,000-200,000. Thus, Paris
is divided into twenty arrondissements or neighborhoods, each corresponding

to a sector. A sector, in turn, is usually further divided into smaller units, each with its own mental health team. The thirteenth arrondisement, for example, has six teams, each responsible for a "minisector." Each team has a pavilion in the inpatient hospital serving the area—the Eau Vive. Currently there are about a hundred mental health teams in the Greater Paris area. Each is responsible for no fewer than 50,000 and no more than 100,000 people.

Besides teams for adult care, there is a parallel sectorization system for child care, with one child sector for every two adult sectors. Generally speaking, however, the child psychiatric sectorization program is lagging behind that for adult care.

It is important from the standpoint of community participation to note that an arrondissement has its own mayor and elected representatives. The latter meet and work with representatives of the medicosocial teams in mental health associations to discuss the operation of existing services and to plan for future needs and construction.

Included in the network of mental health services are both private and public facilities. Patients may be treated at a state or municipal service without charge. Patients covered under the social security system—and since 1968 this means almost all of the French population—are reimbursed, generally in full, for other care, and pay directly only when dealing with a private physician or, in some sectors, with a "private" nonprofit organization.

The funds for the French social security system are derived from an insurance plan under which the employee contributes a percentage of his salary and the employer contributes the rest. It must be noted, however, that a considerable proportion of the population can still fall between the cracks of the system because of ignorance of the provisions of social security or inability to adapt to the system's requirements. For example, "drifters" and others outside the general society make up a sort of underclass, a subproletariat, that never reaches the level of consumers of medical services, not to mention psychiatric services. Another payment system, a municipal one, takes over in such cases and becomes responsible for these people.

Coordination of Services

In setting up the sectorization system, the French Ministry of Health has attempted to deal with a situation in which services were rarely coordinated and in which residential and outpatient facilities were often located at great distances from each other. Before the advent of psychotropic drugs, there was little need for coordination between outpatient and inpatient facilities; once a patient entered a mental hospital, he usually stayed there a long time. But when psychotropic drugs were introduced, it began to be evident that prolonged hospitalization was less a response to treatment needs that to the difficulty of coordinating social readaptation and maintaining family ties. Provided follow-up care could be assured; medication often made it possible for the patient to be kept in, or quickly returned to, his community, which greatly facilitated his rehabilitation.

Coordination among mental health services is now effected through the "mobile team" approach. Within each sector, when a patient initially seeks help, he becomes the responsibility of a particular mental health team. Members of this team—psychiatrists, nurses, psychotherapists, social workers, rehabilitation counselors, and a hostess or receptionists—then work together to learn as much as possible about the patient, under conditions that cause him a minimum of difficulty (e.g., an evening consultation may be arranged so that the patient has little conflict with work or home responsibilities).

Once the diagnosis has been made by the psychiatrist, in collaboration with other team members, the patient is referred for treatment to one of the resources of the sector. However, he remains the responsibility of the team that saw him originally; in effect, the team "moves" with the patient to the appropriate and available treatment facility. This presents no problem since individual team members work in all of the sector's facilities.

The thirteenth arrondissement furnishes an example of how the mobile team operates. To meet the needs of the sector, there is a 175-bed hospital some twenty miles outside Paris. When a patient who has been seen at an outpatient center within the sector requires hospitalization, every effort is made to have him treated and followed by the same therapist he saw at the outpatient center. This, of course, requires that members of the medical teams travel from one treatment facility to another from day to day in a routine fashion. For the patient, the advantages of the continuity the mobile team provides are practical as well as psychological: not only does he not have to adjust to new people but he receives more intensive and effective treatment because less time is spent on rediagnosis, repeated workups becoming unnecessary when the same staff cares for him wherever he is treated.

The continuity of care this arrangement makes possible has also resulted in significant savings in funds, which can then be allotted to the construction of additional outpatient or community facilities. Although the overall ratio of beds for the mentally ill in France is 2.5 beds per 1,000 inhabitants, sectorization in some areas has reduced this ratio to 1 bed per 1,000 inhabitants—a remarkably low figure. In the seventh arrondissement, under the direction of Dr. P. Bailly-Salin, successful community care is being achieved with only forty-five beds for a population of 90,000, a ratio of 1 bed per 2,000 persons. Obviously such figures represent considerable savings in mental care costs.

To accelerate the establishment of closer connections between inpatient and outpatient services, plans are being discussed for the construction of an increasing number of mental health services in general hospitals within the geographic confines of the sectors. This should permit even closer collaboration between the community and the hospital and lead to greater emphasis on partial hospitalization.

Hospitalization v. Ambulatory Care

On the whole, French mental health practice is committed to the view that hospitalization may have iatrogenic effects and should, therefore, be avoided if at all possible. If it cannot be avoided, then it should be as brief as possible.

In keeping with this view, emergency treatment and home care are being stressed. Home hospitalization is, in fact, the *dernier cri* of French community psychiatry. It is a type of crisis intervention in which a team actually treats the patient in his home and concurrently offers family therapy and instructs the family in the patient's care. Visiting nurses are used extensively to administer the prescribed medicines. If necessary, a homemaker may be provided for up to eight hours a day to ease the burdens of maintaining the patient in his own environment.

Many sectors have walk-in treatment centers in which individuals and families can be treated immediately, without an appointment. At some of these centers a team may treat several families simultaneously: the families discuss their problems among themselves, with the assistance of the mental health team.

Intensive individual psychotherapy is available for those who need it, but it is not generally recognized as the sole treatment of choice. When appropriate and available, group therapy, psychodrama, family therapy, and psychomotor and relocation therapies may all be used. Patients who drop out of treatment or who do not appear for treatment may be visited at home. Pharmacological treatment is widely used as an adjunct to psychotherapy, under the supervision of physicians and/or nurses.

The Changing Scene

According to one authority,[a] sectorization *officially* entered the scene in March 1972. This date marks the recognition by official text of what had been happening all along by administrative fiat. Up until that time, although an enormous amount of sectorization—or community-based treatment—was being practiced, it was being done without overt official sanction. Hospital staffs who had developed after-care and community treatment services often had done so

---

[a]Dr. R. Amiel, who works with Dr. Paul Sivadon and is quite knowledgeable in these matters.

on their own initiative, and their salaries often continued to reflect only their hospital employment.

Still, administrators were, in many instances, paying full-time hospital salaries to psychiatrists engaged in part-time sector work; allocating funds slated for physical therapy to group therapy; paying mental health salaries from construction funds; offering social security payments to a psychoanalytically oriented treatment center treating upper-class patients if it would accept sectorization by agreeing to treat patients from working-class areas; and resorting to other administrative dodges in order to practice "psychiatry by stealth"—and in such a way as not to be overwhelmed by patients and to permit those concerned with public mental health to set their own priorities, without pressure from the hierarchy above or the consumers below.

Official recognition has brought this glorious "underground" movement to an end. Yet, in many ways the changes have really changed little: even the new salaries are not so significant considering that they are now officially quite similar to what they often were unofficially before, thanks to administrative finagling. But much of the romance that used to be associated with sectorization when it had an aura of conspiracy about it is now gone. It remains to be seen whether the French *chef du secteur,* accustomed to flexibility in juggling accounts, commingling funds (particularly with the aid of matching funds), and otherwise doing what he considered in the best interests of the population of his sector, will be able to function as effectively within the framework of officialdom.

Sectorization has been a hotly debated subject in France, much like community control in the United States. Underlying much of the discussion has been the problem of funding. Prior to 1972 there were several types of arrangements under which a sector could be provided with mental health care. In some sectors a private organization (e.g., as in the 13th arrondissement, as previously noted) or the psychiatric service of a trade union might assume responsibility for an area. The latter was the case, for example, in the sixteenth arrondissement, where both inpatient and outpatient care became the responsibility of the Psychiatric Service of the Mutuelle Generale de l'Education Nationale, a teachers' trade union.

Funding before 1972 was on a fee-for-service basis, each "act" of service being paid for by the social service system. However, the fee-for-service arrangement was found to be unsatisfactory for many reasons, not the least of which was that the fee schedule tended to influence the type of treatment given. In other cases, services that were important to the patient's recovery but were time-consuming, such as home visits and phone calls, were not covered by the fee schedule.

Under the new regulations, any contact or service provided to a patient is reimbursed on a flat fee basis. It is unclear how this arrangement will work out, but even now there are demands that budgets be allocated on an annual basis rather than on a fee-for-service basis.

In the early days of sectorization, from 1960 until about 1966, there seemed to be a quality of "movement," almost a "brotherhood" feeling, about working in the sector program. Now that sectorization has become policy and the government is moving toward closing the hospitals in favor of community treatment, some of the fervor is gone. Also, in about 1966 the influence of the "antipsychiatry" movement (e.g., Laing, Szasz) began to be felt. Opposed to the mental hospital, the antipsychiatry professionals spurned sectorization as largely a reformist program designed to effect institutionalization and conformity in a more subtle but effective manner. These people now believe that, with the government's espousal of sectorization, their predictions have been confirmed; and some view sectorization much as mental health professionals in the United States view the Department of Welfare. Many newly graduated psychiatrists are electing to work in the private sector, which consequently, for the first time in many years, is now growing.

Yet in spite of its problems, past and present, sectorization seems to be working in France. The combination of a carefully delimited geographic area serviced by mobile teams, working out of hospitals and ancillary mental health facilities and supplying continuous care, offers a viable solution to the problem of delivery of mental health services. The responsibility for patient care is clearly defined, and the financial means for meeting that responsibility are assured by social security funds to which both workers and employers contribute. Sectorization may not be *the* answer, but it is certainly an answer.

Notes

1. Paumelle, P. and Lebovici, S., "An Experience with Sectorization in Paris," in *International Trends in Mental Health,* ed. Henry P. David, New York: McGraw-Hill, 1966.
2. Pichot, P., "Recent Developments in French Psychiatry." *Brit. J. Psychiat.* 113: 11-18, 1967; Pichot, P., "Recent Developments and Trends in French Psychiatry." *Compreh. Psychiat.* 14: 1, 1973.

23

"State" Hospitals in the USSR: A Model of Governmental Psychiatric Care

Jimmie Holland

To determine the direction in which American state psychiatric hospitals should proceed, a review of all contemporary models of psychiatric care, including those in other societies, is required. The first and largest experiment by a government to give equal and free health care (including psychiatric) to all citizens, was attempted by the USSR in 1917. The results of this noble experiment almost sixty years later provide useful data at a crossroads of planning for the best future models of psychiatric care in the United States.

American physicians' reports of Soviet psychiatry since the Revolution are somewhat analogous to a physician's attempt to describe the gross anatomy of the liver from looking at several biopsy specimens. For a long period, visits were often restricted to certain psychiatric facilities only, and the opportunity to obtain an overview of Soviet psychiatry was difficult. In the early years after the Revolution, the particular political bias of the visiting physician also contributed to either a strongly positive or a negative assessment of the Soviet medical accomplishments. Hopeful and idealistic accounts from the thirties[1] were followed by more objective reports from the Krushchev and post-Krushchev era. In the sixties, M.G. Field presented several particularly perceptive and comprehensive studies of Soviet medicine.[2] A flow of accounts during the sixties, beginning with a broad review of psychiatric services in the USSR by N.S. Kline[3] was followed by increasingly more frequent and extensive views of Soviet psychiatry.[4] Ziferstein's year of work at the Bekhterev Institute in Leningrad in 1966 gave a new perspective to our understanding of the variety of approaches to treatment in the USSR.[5] His descriptions suggested that there may be no typical "Soviet psychiatry," just as there is no typical "American psychiatry," but diverse approaches in different geographic areas in both countries. Differing major schools of psychiatric thought can be discerned in Moscow, Leningrad, Kiev, and Tbilisi. There is little question, however, that the Moscow School, headed by Snezhnevsky at the Psychiatric Institute of the Academy of Medical Sciences, has a dominant position in influencing major national trends in philosophy of approach and treatment.

The first official United States mission on mental health was led by Stanley F. Yolles.[6] Since then, accounts of specific aspects of psychiatric services, research, and treatment have emerged as scientific exchange has increased. A clearer picture of organization of psychiatric services,[7] forensic psychiatry,[8] group therapy,[9] emergency services,[10] work therapy and psychotherapeutic activities,[11] child psychiatry and psychology[12] and physician education[13]

has developed. The Health Agreement of 1972 between the United States and
the USSR included collaboration in biological research in schizophrenia, the
first official joint work approved by both governments in the psychiatric area.
Under the agreement, exchange of scientists and physicians has broadened
somewhat. An assessment can now be made that provides a more balanced
analysis of assets and liabilities of the Soviet system of psychiatric care, as
nearly as outsiders can ever appreciate the complexities of psychiatric care in
another culture.

A collaborative study of classification of schizophrenia provided opportunity for the author to work with Soviet psychiatrists in Moscow in the winter
of 1972-73 as consultant for the National Institute of Mental Health in the
Soviet Union.[14] Collaboration with the staffs of the Psychiatric Institute of
the Academy of Medical Sciences, the Psychiatric Training Faculty, and
Kaschenko Hospital provided opportunity for full participation as a staff member in the day-to-day operation of an acute admission ward in a psychiatric
hospital. The eight months of working with acutely psychotic patients in
Kaschenko Hospital provided basis for these observations on psychiatric
services.

Historical Development of Psychiatric Services

Psychiatry more than any other specialty of medicine uniquely reflects
the social customs, culture, values, and politics of the society in its theory
and practice. Many diverse cultural and ethnic groups make up contemporary
Soviet society. The evaluation of psychiatric theory and practice is briefly
traced in relation to the rest of medicine and critical events in Russian and
Soviet history.

A rich and remarkably varied cultural history exists for the area now
geographically known as the Soviet Union. Particularly important in early
history were the highly developed cultures in Central Asia and Armenia of
the first and second centuries in which there was church-supported care by
the monks for the poor and sick.[15] By the tenth century, physicians from
Syria and Armenia began medical work in Kiev. By the fifteenth century,
European physicians, particularly from Holland and Germany, came to Russia
to work. They principally cared for the nobility while the churches continued
to assume responsibility for care of the indigent ill.

Foreign doctors also came at the request of the Czars during the seventeenth and eighteenth centuries to serve as military physicians and surgeons
under a system organized and financed by the state. Peter the Great encouraged
foreign physicians to come to Russia in the eighteenth century and sent Russian
physicians to Europe to study. In 1707 a military hospital in Moscow became
the site of the first medical school and the Academy of Sciences was founded.

Later, schools for feldshers (the first model for physicians' assistants) and nurses developed. Medical care for serfs was still, however, virtually nonexistent and epidemics took a constant toll on the population. With the freeing of the serfs in 1864, local governments (Zemstvos) were given some authority in self-government, which included responsibility for public health. Each Zemstvo developed a system of medical care (though primitive) that provided services for the total population in the given geographic area. Each district was autonomous and developed their own network of dispensaries, medical stations and hospitals. Physicians, feldshers, and midwives were employed by the local government. The Zemstvos took over, in 1892, the psychiatric wards and insane asylums, which numbered thirty-four hospitals containing 9,055 beds and were staffed by ninety psychiatrists.[16] Though Zemstvo medicine was comprised of less than a third of all physicians, it nevertheless represented the first organized care for the poor and attracted many young dedicated physicians, including Chekhov.

During this period the founders of Russian psychiatry, Korsakov,[17] Kandinsky[18] and Bekhterev[19] made significant contributions to psychiatric knowledge through description and differentiation of discrete psychopathological states. Psychiatry followed closely along the Kraeplinian concepts of the Germanic school. The concepts of Pinel and Rush, which proposed more humanistic care of the mentally ill, were rapidly inculcated in Russian psychiatry. Their first appearance in Russian literature was by I.M. Balinsky[20] in 1858. These views have remained a cornerstone of psychiatric practice.

The significant work of Pavlov on conditional reflexes and higher cortical activity contributed strongly to the biological orientation of psychiatry.[21] Freudian psychology with its emphasis on "hidden forces" or "the darker side of man's nature" seemed to oppose the Marxist ideology of dialectical materialism and thus was never allowed significant development. Pavlovian principles of man's ultimate conscious control over his actions provided ideal support for socialist ideological views in the first half of the twentieth century, and for a time were utilized in furthering ideology. In spite of the emphasis on Pavlovian psychological principles in societal development, psychiatry has not, to an outside observer, received as much support as other medical specialities. Limited funds for health have been deployed more generously in areas concerned with physical rather than mental health.

The Bolsheviks, in 1917, moved to place medical care and public health in the expansive centralization of all services. The model of Zemstvo medicine was reshaped within a year into a centralized existing structure under a Commissariat of Health Protection.[22] Resistance of many physicians, epidemics, and starvation prevented total implementation. Early five-year plans were forced to deal largely with epidemics, particularly typhus, which at times threatened to destroy the beginning of the socialist society.

Medical schools were largely separated from universities as six-year

vocational schools (beginning after secondary education). A three-year specialized secondary education program trained feldshers, nurses, mid-wives, and
technicians. Similar models of medical education continue today.

Current Psychiatric Care System

The Soviet system of psychiatric care is a single pyramidal "state" system,
with decisions for planning and implementation made at the top. The Ministry
of Health in Moscow is responsible for actual care through the system of
psychiatric facilities. The Academy of Medical Sciences, through its Psychiatric
Institute and Central Training Faculty, monitors psychiatric research and training. While there is planning at all levels with input to higher levels, nevertheless, final decisions are made at the highest levels. In this type of organization,
a change in practice or treatment can be effected quickly in all facilities in the
system. However, because of its size and the import of a single change, they
are usually incorporated slowly and there is little opportunity for innovation
on a smaller scale. As in earlier state hospital systems in the United States, the.
tendency has been toward conservatism in viewing change, with maintenance
of the status quo being a major objective.

Psychiatric care, while part of the total highly organized medical care
system, actually exists as a parallel complex rather than an integral unit. Entry
for a patient to psychiatric care is initially through the medical system, but he
then is treated wholly within the range of psychiatric facilities and services
with consultation from other specialities only as considered necessary by the
psychiatrist. Psychiatric facilities are geographically separate; logistics alone
discourage close integration and frequent consultation with the rest of medicine. Soviet hospitals in general are highly specialized, as are the physicians
who staff them. This is in sharp contrast to the American traditional general
hospital staffed by physicians of various specialties available for consultation
in one setting. Soviet psychiatrists have proposed more psychiatric units in
general hospitals but current numbers are small and plans for more move
modestly.

Psychiatric care is administered primarily through neuropsychiatric dispensaries[23] and large psychiatric hospitals. The mental hospitals have more
prestige since they constitute the academic teaching centers where the chairs
of psychiatry are usually located; also, prestigious psychiatric research institutes
are often in close proximity. Adequate psychiatric hospital beds are still felt
to be in short supply due to the destruction of hospitals during World War II.
The emphasis on innovative outpatient care methods in the post World War
II period may have been more a matter of necessity due to a lack of adequate
psychiatric beds than a philosophical alternative choice away from the
hospitalization.

A single "state" system has certain advantages while presenting some liabilities (Table 23-1) in contrast to the multiple systems of care in the United States. As employees of the state, Soviet psychiatrists can be distributed more equitably geographically and deployed in such a way as to be responsible for segments of population that are similar in size to catchment area populations in the United States. No economic or social considerations determine the type of treatment recommended by the psychiatrists. The same care is given by similarly trained professionals who number about 25,000 psychiatrists in the USSR. They are located in large numbers at the neuropsychiatric dispensaries (where as many as 30 to 35 may be working at one large dispensary), and in the hospitals. The only other professional group involved in psychiatric care is nursing. There are no social workers, no clinical psychologists (no psychological testing), and no occupational therapists, although there are active work therapy programs for those able to participate. Use of the psychiatric ward milieu as a therapeutic social system is not as yet extensively recognized.

Detection of mental illness and follow-up become much more efficient under this system. Emergency services are particularly well developed in Moscow and Leningrad where they are coordinated with emergency medical services organized through a "911" telephone system. Psychiatrists are on twenty-four-hour duty to take emergency calls in ambulances.[24] Psychiatric examinations may be requested by an individual, his family or co-workers, but only the psychiatrist can admit a patient to a psychiatric hospital. Most admissions are voluntary since all cases are considered as such when the requesting family or co-worker agree to the admission, even though the patient himself does not consent.

There is, in practice, no legal review of ordinary psychiatric admissions nor is there any mechanism similar to a writ of habeas corpus by which the patient can request legal review of commitment. There is, in general, a much greater feeling of assurance that the psychiatrist makes a just and proper decision and thus legal safeguards are not necessary. Aside from the forensic psychiatric system that handles all criminal issues as they relate to psychiatrically ill individuals, there is little contact between the psychiatric-medical system and the law in handling ordinary psychiatric patients. The single psychiatric care system appears to emphasize a "we-know-what-is-best-for-you" approach to the patient, offering less protection of patients' legal rights. Historically, the United States state hospital in general had a similar philosophy.

Following discharge from the hospital, a patient receives after-care at the neuropsychiatric dispensary in his geographic area. If he does not keep an appointment for a follow-up visit, the psychiatrist and nurse go to his home to see him. They know patients well in their district and often have a long and close relationship with a patient over time. Continuity, defined as care by a single psychiatrist or a team at all levels of psychiatric service to a patient, seems a yet-to-be-attained goal in the USSR as in the United States. There is

Table 23-1
A Comparison of Psychiatric Practice Between the United States and the USSR

	USSR	*United States*
Psychiatric services	one system	many systems
Distribution of psychiatrists	XXXX	XX
Detection and follow-up	XXXX	XX
Emergency services	XXXX	XX
Continuity of care	XX	XX
Psychopharmacology	XXXX	XXXX
Psychotherapeutic approach/emphasis	XX	XXXX
Psychiatric professionals (other than psychiatrist)	Few	Many
Confidentiality	0	XXXX
Emphasis on doctor/patient relationship	X	XXXX

X = Rating unit on a scale 1-4.

little contact between psychiatric hospital and neuropsychiatric dispensary staffs beyond formal referral. Psychotherapy given with frequent visits in a psychodynamic therapeutic model is not used. A friendly social relationship exists between psychiatrist and patient coupled with heavy reliance on psychopharmacological drugs. Minimal emphasis is placed on relationship between doctor and patient as a therapeutic tool, though in Leningrad there seems to be more use of the relationship, utilizing the psychiatrist in a directive role as "teacher of life."[25]

Significantly in the USSR, psychiatrists, as indeed all physicians, are employees of the state and thus bear responsibility both to the state and to the patient. Concern that a psychiatrist may have conflict in serving both his institutional (state) obligation and his obligation to his patient is unusual since social structure in general is geared to place concerns (rights) of the group ahead of the individual. The psychiatrist as physician and member himself of the collective group, is responsible both to treat the patient's illness and to return him to a productive role in the group. The active role is assumed of model, teacher, and healer to the patient. The psychiatrist has considerable authority as a social agent to place a patient on temporary or permanent disability with pension, or to intervene in job situations. Character training of all young individuals in the USSR includes the concept of responsibility for others in his group.[26] The doctor's skills make his responsibility and thus his *right* to intervene, more clear. The teaching of "skills of life" is the highly developed concept of A.S. Makarenko,[27] an educator whose ideas have had profound effects on both child rearing and psychotherapeutic techniques.

In general, stress is placed on the biologic aspects of mental illness[28] as opposed to social aspects. Pharmacologic therapy, insulin, and ECT are often used for schizophrenia. Lithium is used for manic-depressive illness. The pyramidal structure tends to support greater uniformity in treatment methods. An example in point is the decision made in the1950s by an All-Union Conference that psychosurgery was inhumane. It is not performed today nor is it considered a potential area of experimental interest.

A single system assures the psychiatrist of full access to a patient's history since his medical record, often since birth, is on file in his dispensary. The release of psychiatric records does not require a patient's approval nor is there any way that information deemed confidential can be withheld by the psychiatrist. The stigma of mental illness has consequences similar to those in this country. Individuals with a history of mental illness are more closely scrutinized to assume responsibilities and prerogatives requiring emotional stability. While having fully available records is helpful in diagnosis, there is a curtailment of the right of privacy for the patient.

In the USSR there is less social tolerance for deviance from the norm in style of clothes, hair, or acceptable social behavior. This leads to a wider range of behaviors being called into question as possible mental illness or deviance, which might require psychiatric examination or hospitalization. Whereas in the United States, attempts are underway to increase tolerance of eccentric behavior by greater acceptance of the mentally ill in the community, quite the contrary appears to be true in the USSR. Historically, rural Russian villages tolerated the mentally ill very well. The change from a rural to an urban socialist society may have resulted in less flexibility in dealing with an unproductive collective member in their midst. It may now be easier to provide a special facility for those individuals than to maintain them in society. Psychiatric hospitalization by virtue of societal attitudes of society may occur early in the course of illness and be lengthy.

Longer hospitalizations may be encouraged by the absence of financial pressure; both the physician and patient are relieved of concern for cost, thus accepting hospitalization as an alternative more easily and for a longer time than in the United States.

New Directions

Many of the innovations in psychiatric care in the United States utilizing social clubs, transitional living facilities, and volunteers are not apparent in the USSR. There is, however, increasing emphasis on the "total rehabilitation of the psychiatric patient" in Leningrad,[29] which sets forth several concepts:

1. The principle of partnership involving the patient in his own rehabilitation. An atmosphere of trust and cooperation is indispensible; a set of relations between the physician and the patient (or more correctly, among the physician, intermediate medical and nonmedical personnel, the patient, his relatives, and close friends) must be created. To quite a few, such a statement sounds like a truism (as, however, does much else having to do with rehabilitation); but, unfortunately, very little has been done in psychiatric institutions to change the traditional patterns of working with patients; and most psychiatrists need little convincing of how shoddy this work is.
2. The principle of a variety of actions, restructuring patients' attitudes in all aspects of life.
3. The principle of unity of psychosocial and biological methods of intervention.
4. The principle of staging of efforts, and interventions into a systematic process.

The Leningrad group are progressively concerned with socially oriented techniques involving partial hospitalization,[30] prevention of "invalidism" in patients with severe and chronic psychoses,[31] use of active and passive participation in music, work, and occupational programs in institutions.[32] One senses in these concepts an emerging concern for change of the large state psychiatric hospitals in the USSR that are largely traditionally biologically oriented toward stronger emphasis on social therapeutic aspects. There is also a move to examine Western concepts of dynamic psychotherapy[33] and even a reexamination of psychological theory of an unconscious.[34]

Lessons for Planning

Historical precedent in Zemstvo medicine existed for a state system of psychiatric care in the USSR that was centralized in 1918 to a single system. Organized on a geographic basis, it gives free and equal psychiatric care to all citizens. The system allows a better distribution of psychiatrists, earlier detection, and better follow-up of the ill. It tends to diminish patients' legal rights at all levels of care through entry, hospitalization and follow-up, with considerable reliance on the objectivity of the psychiatrist's judgment. It does assure care for those patients who cannot assume responsibility for themselves and eliminates patients "falling through the cracks" of levels of care.

While in general psychiatric care is biologically oriented, there has been a long-standing use of work-therapy and maintenance of the patient in the community when psychiatric beds were unavailable after World War II. A movement exists towards increasing examination of all social factors and possible social intervention in total rehabilitation of the psychiatric patient, and a cautious reappraisal of Western concepts of dynamic psychotherapy in Leningrad.

The Soviet model of care approximates a complex of community mental health centers that geographically cover the country. There is, however, a wide gap between hospital and neuropsychiatric dispensary care so that continuity is met only on an administrative level. The value of a highly organized system is readily apparent in areas of professional allocation, detection, and follow-up. The most valuable quality attained by the Soviets is a total system of services, equally accessible and available to all. Willingness to innovate with a diversity of treatment methods, and philosophical concern for the individual and his rights are notably absent in the USSR service delivery model.

Parallels in historical development are readily apparent in the state-supported Soviet system of psychiatric care and the United States state hospital systems. Groups of American state hospitals, financed by each individual state, are close to the model of Zemstvo medicine supported by autonomous units of local government in prerevolutionary Russia. The organization of Zemstvo units into a single tightly organized government-supported system in 1918 has no American counterpart. Centralization did not occur; financing and control were maintained in the individual states.

Large state hospitals in which care was geared to long hospitalization, organic therapy, and little emphasis on social milieu was a similar pattern in both the USSR and the United States until about three years ago. Diversity of approach from one state to another with more flexibility may have supported easier change than in the USSR, though varying quality of care from state to state was a liability of the lack of centralization. With the drug revolution, which occurred in both countries in the fifties, there was a strong movement in the United States toward exploration of social aspects of psychiatric hospitals, and use of the ward as a therapeutic milieu. Psychiatric hospitals in the USSR have largely maintained the same philosophical approach without increasing consideration of social aspects, with the exception of the Leningrad School. Availability in the United States of multiple state hospital systems may have made innovation in treatment methods easier than in the Soviet single system.

Many have seen the United States movement toward total geographic coverage by federally supported community mental health centers as a positive move toward the Soviet model,[35] and indeed the gains of planned, equally available care for all citizens is an exciting goal, especially when our current patchwork systems are viewed. Equal care for all has been idealistically attempted by the Soviets, but there are lessons to be learned from their experience. A similar federal system in the United States would require safeguards against some of the problems that the Soviet system highlights: The right of the patient to participate in decisions about his care; the confidentiality of his records; and the legal review of psychiatric administrative and therapeutic procedures for his protection are critical. Most valued in American psychiatric philosophy is concern for the uniqueness of each patient in whom the therapeutic goal is to support and promote his individuality. A large system geared to equal care may tend also to equalize individuals. A federal psychiatric care model would require immediate attention to the critical balance between an individual's right to refuse treatment and the responsibility to require treatment or a person who is a clear danger to himself or others. A centralized system can curtail the right of self-determination in accepting treatment and may promote more concern for the society's protection than that of the individual.

The responsibility of the psychiatrist to the patient versus institution would need safeguards against abuse. Likewise, protection of medical care from political influence, in a single government system, would be critical to prevent possible abuse for political or nonmedical purposes.

The USSR has served the world with a model of psychiatric care for all which, as an ideal, is notable. The liabilities that can accrue from such a single governmental system are also real and movement toward a centralized system of community mental health centers in the United States must take careful account of both the gains and losses that are visible from the Soviet experience.

Notes

1. Sigerist, H., *Socialized Medicine in the Soviet Union,* New York: Norton Publishing Company, 1937.
2. Field, M.G., "Approaches to Mental Illness in Soviet Society: Some Comparisons and Conjectures," *Social Problems,* 7:277-97, 1960; Field, M.G. and Aronson, J., "The Institutional Framework of Soviet Psychiatry," *Journal of Nervous and Mental Disorders,* 138:305-22, 1964; Field, M.G., "Soviet Psychiatry and Social Structure, Culture, and Ideology: A Preliminary Assessment," *American Journal of Psychotherapy,* 21:230-43, 1967.
3. Kline, N.S., "The Organization of Psychiatric Care and Psychiatric Research in the Union of the Soviet Socialist Republics," *Annals of New York Academy of Science,* 84:147-224, 1960.
4. Kolb, L.C., "Soviet Psychiatric Organization and the Community Mental Health Center Concept," *American Journal of Psychiatry,* 123:439, 1966; Hein, G., "Social Psychiatric Treatment of Schizophrenia in the Soviet Union," *International Journal of Psychiatry,* 6:346-61, 1968; Gorman, M., "Soviet Psychiatry and the Russian Citizen," *International Journal of Psychiatry,* 8:841-54, 1969.
5. Ziferstein, I., *Soviet Psychiatry: Past, Present and Future in Social Thought in the Soviet Union,* Simurenko, A. (ed.), Chicago: Quadrangle Books,

1969; Ziferstein, I., "Group Psychotherapy in the Soviet Union," *American Journal of Psychiatry,* 129:595-600, 1972.

6. National Institute of Mental Health, *First Mission on Mental Health to the U.S.S.R.*, Yolles, Stanley F., chairman. Public Health Service Publication #1893, Washington, D.C.: U.S. Government Printing Office, 1969.

7. ibid.; Gorman, "Soviet Psychiatry"; Allen, M.G., "Psychiatry in the United States and the U.S.S.R.:" A Comparison, *American Journal of Psychiatry,* 130:1333-37, 1973.

8. Morozov, G.V. and Kalashnik, I.M. (eds.), *Forensic Psychiatry,* International Arts and Sciences Press, White Plains, New York, 1967 (translated from Russian); Bazelon, D.L., *Introduction to Forensic Psychiatry,* Morozov, G.V. and Kalashnik, I.M. (eds.), White Plains, NY: International Arts and Sciences Press, 1967.

9. Hein, "Social Psychiatric Treatment of Schizophrenia."

10. Torrey, E.F., "Emergency Psychiatric Ambulance Services in the U.S.S.R.," *American Journal of Psychiatry,* 128:153-57, 1971.

11. Ziferstein, "Group Psychotherapy."

12. Rollins, Nancy, "The New Soviet Approach to the Unconscious," *American Journal of Psychiatry,* 131:301-17, 1974; Bronfenbrenner, Urie, "Theory and Research in Soviet Character Education," Chapter VII in *Social Thought in the Soviet Union,* Simurenko, A. (ed.), Chicago: Quadrangle Books, 1969.

13. Daniels, R.E., "A Comparison of Physician Education in the U.S.S.R., and the United States," *American Journal of Psychiatry,* 131:316-17, 1974.

14. Holland, J., Shakmatova-Pavlova, I., and Nadjharov, R., "Concept and Classification of Schizophrenia in the Soviet Union," in press, *Schizophrenia Bulletin,* NIMH, 1974.

15. Field, M.G., *Soviet Socialized Medicine,* New York: The Free Press, 1967.

16. Sigerist, *Socialized Medicine.*

17. Korsakov, S.S., *Kource Psykiatrii,* T. 1-2, Moscow, 1901.

18. Kandinsky, V. Kh., *O pseudogallulsinatiejach,* Moscow: 1952.

19. Bekhterev, V.M., *Gipnoz, vnushenie, psikhsterapiya i ikh lechebhoe znachenie,* St. Petersburg, 1911.

20. Balinsky, I.M., *Lektsii po psikhiatrii,* Moscow: 1958.

21. Pavlov, I., *Conditional Reflexes and Psychiatry,* International Publishers, New York, 1941.

22. Field, *Soviet Socialized Medicine.*

23. Snezhnevsky, A.V., "Dispensary Method of Registering Psychiatric Morbidity and the Soviet System of Psychiatric Services," *Living Conditions and Health,* 1:236-41, 1959.

24. Torrey, "Emergency Psychiatric Ambulance Services."

25. Ziferstein, *Soviet Psychiatry.*

26. Bronfenbrenner, "Theory and Research."

27. Makarenko, A.S., *Pedagogicheskaia poema Leningrad: Leningradskoie*

gazetno-zhurndnoie i knizhnoie izdalelstvo, 1949, (in English, *The Road to Live.*), translated by Ivy and Tatiana, L., Litvinov, Foreign Publishing Press, Moscow, 1951; Makarenko, A.S., *The Road to Life,* Moscow: 1955.

28. Portnov, A.A. and Fedotov, D.D., *Psychiatry,* Moscow: Mir Publishers, 1969.

29. Kabanov, M.M., "Basic Principles in the Rehabilitation of Psychiatric Patients," *Soviet Neurology and Psychiatry,* 5:7-16, 1972.

30. Ibid.

31. Volovik, V.M., "Differentiation of Forms and Methods of Rehabilitation in Clinical Psychiatry," *Soviet Neurology and Psychiatry,* 5:17-30, 1972.

32. Brusilovsky, L.S., "A Two Year Experience with the Use of Music in the Rehabilitation Therapy of Mental Patients," *Soviet Neurology and Psychiatry,* 5:100-108, 1972; Levitin, L.V., "Characteristics of the Occupational Rehabilitation of Chronic Mental Patients," *Soviet Neurology and Psychiatry,* 5:17-30, 1972.

33. Ziferstein, "Group Psychotherapy."

34. Rollins, "New Soviet Approach to the Unconscious."

35. Holland, J., "A Comparison of Soviet and American Psychiatry," (Translated by V. Moshalenko), *Korsakov Journal of Psychiatry,* in press, 1974.

**Part V
Epilogue**

Introduction to Part V

We are particularly pleased to be able to present a comment on the current state of psychiatric treatment by Dr. Lawrence Kubie. Dr. Kubie, who passed away shortly after preparing this chapter, was a long-time critic of the community mental health movement by reason of his concern with the neglect of certain needs of seriously ill psychiatric patients. Much to the distress of the proponents of community mental health, he often appeared in print, questioning and criticizing their work. In the chapter that follows—undoubtedly one of the last things he wrote before his death—he continues to express his concerns with the essentials of patient care.

24

The Responsibility of the Medical Profession to Provide Hospital Treatment

Lawrence S. Kubie

Hospital psychiatry of all kinds is at present being subjected to vicious, destructive, and totally ignorant attacks. One group involved regards itself as the ultimate defenders of human freedom and human liberties. What they fail to recognize is the imprisoning and restrictive processes of psychological illness itself. They fail to realize that the very essence of psychological illness is the impairment of actual loss of psychological freedom; that is, of the freedom to change and to learn from experience. They do not realize that this is of far greater importance than the restriction of external liberty that may sometimes be necessary in the care of mental patients, not merely for the protection of the patient and his family and society, but just to make possible a study of his illness and its treatment. The mentally sick individual cannot avail himself of external liberty, even if unrestricted.

This group further betrays its ignorance of the fact that there are some patients who can be evaluated only if they are under the trained scrutiny and observation of many observers and not just one. (This is true in all fields of science where multiple observers are the best way of eliminating the sources of error in each observer.) They are further ignorant of the fact that some patients need to be studied around the clock, when they are asleep, when they are awake, in multiple relationships with many different kinds of people; that is, with other patients, attendants, physicians, etc., and also through an extensive follow-up period. All of this is possible only with a hospital population.

Because of their ignorance, these critics, by eliminating hospital care, would deprive psychiatry of any opportunity to learn about the more severe and chronic forms of illness.

There is another group of critics whose arguments are purely short-sighted and mercenary. They want to eliminate hospital psychiatry because they erroneously think that it would save the taxpayer's money.

They have failed to learn the lesson pointed out by the Swiss historian of psychiatry, Ackerknecht, that it was a fatal development when psychiatry in Germany split into two camps—the "Anhalts—Psychiater" and the "Staats-Psychiater." The effects of this split arrested the maturation of German psychiatry for many decades; it has not recovered fully to this day. (The late Adolf Meyer was an observer of this disaster and commented on it frequently.) One effect of this split was to make it impossible to study disorganization. This reenforced the illusion that there was no relationship between the two.

Still another group of critics focuses entirely on the state hospital, over-looking the fact that their critical attitudes increase the very failings that they deplore. They are making it more difficult for these hospitals to secure adequate financing from state or federal legislators. They criticize these hospitals for what they do not do, without realizing that it is the lack of adequate funding that makes it impossible for them to have adequate staffs and adequate facilities. That the lack of adequate staffs and facilities is deplorable is certainly true; but these attacks contribute to the starvation rations on which the hospitals are required to live and then are criticized for what they cannot supply.

Again these critics are scientifically blind in their failure to realize that we must study statistically adequate, random, cross-section samples of the total population, if we are to understand the relative importance of social, economic, national, racial, and cultural differences in the genesis of illness, in the evolution of the process of illness, in the psychopathological process and in its therapy. Therefore, we need both public and private facilities, both public and private psychiatric hospitals, public and private outpatient facilities, public and private community facilities, public and private practice, if we are to make scientific progress.

Although it might present difficulties, the staffing of public and private facilities, inpatient and outpatient, ideally ought to rotate. A rotation of staff every ten years would result in an enormous growth in the maturity of the staff itself. Though difficult to plan and implement, this is a worth-while goal for the future. Finally, the value of foundation funding to private institutions is illustrated in this opinion often expressed by the late Alan Gregg, who was for many years medical director of the Rockefeller Founda-tion and later vice-president of that foundation. Whenever his conscience hurt him about putting so much Rockefeller money into private hospitals and medical schools, the heads of our great public and state institutions came to him and pleaded with him to continue to fund these private institu-tions generously. They would say, "The example they set with the facilities you create and the kind of work which this makes it possible for them to do, is the only effective weapon we have in dealing with stupid, restrictive and 'penny-wise-pound-foolish' legislators."

Index

Academy of Medical Sciences, USSR, 373, 374, 376
Accessibility, of programs, 11
Accountability, of mental hygiene structure, 139, 292, 295, 304
Ackerknecht, 389
Action for Mental Health, 286
Activity therapists, 303
ADA (average daily attendance), 249 251
Adams, A.S., 136
Adjudication, 104. *See also* Courts
Adjustment, of community, 225, 226. *See also* Change
Administration, at Camarillo State Hospital, 181*f*
  law and, 61
  Orange County, 272, 278-279
  reform of, 72
  and token economy program, 169, 174
Administrators, 127, 132, 137, 360
  and behavior modification, 186
  French, 370
  public mental health, 25
Admissions, 16, 91-109, 214-215
  admitting teams for, 306
  for alcoholism, 54
  in California, 265
  costs and, 250*t*
  to day care services, 342*t*
  distribution, 325*t*
  first, 38-39, 326
    age distribution of, 47*t*
    projected numbers of, 43
  Fort Logan Mental Health Center, 239-240, 243, 245, 246, 249, 250*t*
  geriatric, 191
  halfway house, 207-208, 210-211
  involuntary, 54, 114-115 (*see also* Commitment)
  and length of stay of, 326
  numbers of, 32
  nursing home, 193

outpatient, 345
  procedure for, 289
  of resident patients, 33*f*, 34*t*
  for schizophrenia, 346
  standards of, 112
  to state hospitals, 326
  voluntary, 97, 98, 99, 113, 114
Adolescent Division, at Ft. Logan Mental Health Center, 241
Adolescents, 305
  planning for, 24
  residential centers for, 277
  treatment programs for, 273. *See also* Children
Adult Psychiatry Division, At Fort Logan Center, 243
Adults, mentally ill, 21-22
  psychiatric offenders, 23-24
Advisory boards, 123
Advocacy, for mentally ill, 71. *See also* Rights
Advocates, 100
After-care, 11, 267, 279, 312, 345, 346,
  in USSR, 377
Age, care episodes and, 320
  and first admissions, 40*t*, 43, 47
  of halfway house residents, 218
  and inpatient psychiatric episodes, 335*t*
  and outpatient services, 339*t*
  and patient distribution, 43, 44*t*, 45*t*, 46*t*, 50, 52
  and private mental hospitals, 329-330
  of resident populations, 32-37
  and type of psychiatric services, 323*t*
  of VA hospital patients, 330-331
Aged, homes for, 350
  mentally ill, 52, 349-352. *See also* Elderly
Agencies, community, 308
  family, 11
  voluntary, 304. *See also* Centers
Aggression, of patients, 166

391

About the Editors
and Contributors

Thomas S. Ball is associate research psychologist at the UCLA School of Medicine and the Neuropsychiatric Institute-Pacific State Hospital Research Group, Pomona, California.

William B. Beach, Jr., is deputy secretary for mental health and medical services of the Commonwealth of Pennsylvania and associate clinical professor at the University of Pennsylvania School of Medicine.

Elmer F. Bertsch is clinical instructor in psychiatry and assistant to the director of the Department of Psychiatry at the E.J. Meyer Memorial Hospital in Buffalo, New York.

Irving Blumberg is executive secretary of the New York Citizens Against Mental Illness and executive vice-president of the International Committee Against Mental Illness, New York City.

Ethel Bonn is director of the Fort Logan Mental Health Center in Denver, Colorado.

Paul Binner is chief of program information and analysis at the Fort Logan Mental Health Center in Denver, Colorado.

Mildren Cannon is a staff member in the Biometry Branch of the National Institute of Mental Health in Rockville, Maryland.

William A. Carnahan is a practicing mental health attorney; a clinical associate professor of forensic psychiatry in the Department of Psychiatry of the State University of New York at Buffalo; and a lecturer in law and psychiatry on the Faculty of Law and Jurisprudence at the State University of New York at Buffalo.

Jonathan O. Cole is professor and chairman, Department of Psychiatry, Temple University, and a former superintendent of Boston State Hospital.

John Cumming is clinical professor of psychiatry at the University of British Columbia School of Medicine.

Harold W. Demone, Jr., is executive vice-president of United Community Planning Corporation, Boston, and clinical professor, Laboratory of Community Psychiatry, Department of Psychiatry, Harvard Medical School.

William J. DiScipio is director of psychology at the Bronx Children's Psychiatric Center, and assistant clinical professor of psychiatry at the Albert Einstein College of Medicine, Bronx, New York.

Jacques Dubois is associated with l'Hôpital Vinatier in Lyons, France.

Bruce J. Ennis is staff counsel of the New York Civil Liberties Union, New York City.

The Hon. Franklin N. Flaschner is chief justice of the District Court of Massachusetts, West Newton, Massachusetts.

Hyman M. Forstenzer is special consultant to the commissioner of mental hygiene for the state of New York.

Michel Gillet is associated with the l'Hôpital Vinatier in Lyons, France.

Martin Gittelman is chief of the Children's Services, Queens-Nassau Mental Health Service of the Health Insurance Plan of Greater New York, and associate professor, New York School of Psychiatry, Ward's Island, New York.

Leonard E. Gottesman is senior research psychologist of the Philadelphia Geriatric Center.

Irvin P.R. Guyett is psychology consultant to the Pennsylvania Department of Public Welfare and assistant clinical professor of psychiatry at the Western Psychiatric Institute, University of Pittsburgh.

Jimmie Holland is associate clinical professor, Department of Psychiatry, Albert Einstein College of Medicine, Montefiore Hospital and Medical Center, Bronx, New York.

Helen M. Huber is director of nursing services at the Fort Logan Mental Health Center in Denver, Colorado.

Ernest W. Klatte is director of the Orange County (California) Department of Mental Health and associate professor of psychiatry at the University of California at Irvine.

Lawrence S. Kubie was clinical professor of psychiatry, University of Maryland School of Medicine, and senior associate in research and training, Sheppard and Enoch Pratt Hospital, Towson, Maryland.

Robert Paul Liberman is associate research psychiatrist at the UCLA School of Medicine and director of the program in clinical research and the Clinical Research Unit at the Camarillo-Neuropsychiatric Institute Research Center, Camarillo State Hospital, California. He is also deputy program leader in the Ventura County Community Mental Health Department in charge of the Oxnard (California) Community Mental Health Center.

Peter A. Magaro is associate professor of psychology at the University of Maine.

Noel A. Mazade is assistant professor of mental health program administration, Community Psychiatry Division, Department of Psychiatry, School of Medicine, University of North Carolina.

Roger Mesmer is director of community psychiatry at the Warren State Hospital, Warren, Pennsylvania.

Alan D. Miller is commissioner of mental hygiene of the state of New York.

Charles R. Orndoff is director of Transitional Services, Inc. of Buffalo, New York.

Michael Alfred Peszke is associate professor in the Department of Psychiatry at the University of Connecticut.

Earl S. Pollack is deputy director of the Division of Biometry at the National Institute of Mental Health.

Richard W. Redick is assistant chief, Survey and Reports Branch, Division of Biometry, National Institute of Mental Health.

William R. Roy is a member of Congress from the Second District of Kansas and a member of the House Subcommittee on Public Health and Environment.

Herbert C. Schulberg is vice-president of United Community Planning Corporation, Boston, and associate clinical professor, Laboratory of Community Psychiatry, Department of Psychiatry, Harvard Medical School.

John L. Sheets is a medical fellow in the Community Psychiatry Division, Department of Psychiatry, School of Medicine, University of North Carolina at Chapel Hill.

Lois Sibbach has been the charge nurse for the token economy at Pacific State Hospital since 1967.

John A. Talbott is director of the Dunlap-Manhattan Psychiatric Hospital, Ward's Island, New York City.

Carl A. Taube is chief of the Survey and Reports Branch, Division of Biometry, National Institute of Mental Health.

Charles Wallace is supervisor, Clinical Research Unit, Program in Clinical Research at the Camarillo-Neuropsychiatric Institute Research Center, Camarillo State Hospital, California.

Jack Zusman is professor, Department of Psychiatry, School of Medicine, State University of New York at Buffalo; formerly director of the Division of Community Psychiatry.